MOSBY'S
TEXTBOOK FOR THE
HOME CARE AIDE

MOSBY'S TEXTBOOK FOR THE HOME CARE AIDE

THIRD EDITION

Joan Birchenall, RN, MEd
Trenton, New Jersey

Eileen Streight, RN, BSN
Hamilton, New Jersey

ELSEVIER

3251 Riverport Lane
St. Louis, Missouri 63043

MOSBY'S TEXTBOOK FOR THE HOME CARE AIDE   ISBN: 978-0-323-08433-8

Notices

Knowledge and best practice in this field are constantly changing. As new research and experience broaden our understanding, changes in research methods, professional practices, or medical treatment may become necessary.

Practitioners and researchers must always rely on their own experience and knowledge in evaluating and using any information, methods, compounds, or experiments described herein. In using such information or methods they should be mindful of their own safety and the safety of others, including parties for whom they have a professional responsibility.

With respect to any drug or pharmaceutical products identified, readers are advised to check the most current information provided (i) on procedures featured or (ii) by the manufacturer of each product to be administered, to verify the recommended dose or formula, the method and duration of administration, and contraindications. It is the responsibility of practitioners, relying on their own experience and knowledge of their patients, to make diagnoses, to determine dosages and the best treatment for each individual patient, and to take all appropriate safety precautions.

To the fullest extent of the law, neither the Publisher nor the authors, contributors, or editors, assume any liability for any injury and/or damage to persons or property as a matter of products liability, negligence or otherwise, or from any use or operation of any methods, products, instructions, or ideas contained in the material herein.

Previous editions copyrighted 2003 and 1997

Library of Congress Cataloging-in-Publication Data

Birchenall, Joan M.
  Mosby's textbook for the home care aide / Joan Birchenall, Eileen Streight.—3rd ed.
    p. ; cm.
  Textbook for the home care aide
  Includes index.
  ISBN 978-0-323-08433-8 (pbk. : alk. paper)
  I. Streight, Mary Eileen.   II. Title.   III. Title: Textbook for the home care aide.
  [DNLM: 1. Home Care Services—United States.   2. Home Health Aides—United States. WY 115 AA1]
  610.73—dc23

                                      2012030042

Content Strategist: Nancy O'Brien
Senior Content Development Specialist: Maria Broeker
Publishing Services Manager: Deborah L. Vogel
Project Manager: Pat Costigan
Designer: Paula Catalano

Printed in The United States of America.

Last digit is the print number: 9   8   7   6   5   4   3   2   1

In memory of
Horace M. Streight,
Anne Ryan,
and
Margaret B. Birchenall,
who taught us the meaning and essence of caring.

To the members of our families and friends for their patience,
sacrifices, understanding, and support.

To home care aides who provide selfless care for their clients.

Reviewers

Leah Erickson, RN, BSN, PHN
Nursing Assistant Educator
Hennepin Technical College
Eden Prairie, Minnesota

Patricia Graham, MSN, RN, CNE
Nurse Aide Program Director
Front Range Community College
BSN Instructor
Regis University
Boulder, Colorado

Tiffany Jakubowski, RN
Nurse Aide Instructor
Front Range Community College
Longmont, Colorado

Marianna D. Krivda, RN, BS Ed.
Nursing Instructor
South Tech Academy
Boynton Beach, Florida

Debra Mackey, MS, RN
Central Florida Institute Coordinator for
    Health Programs
College of Central Florida
Ocala, Florida

Nancy J. Moore, RN, BS, MSN Ed.
Medical Academy Coordinator
South Tech Academy
Boynton Beach, Florida

Acknowledgments

For their invaluable assistance during the preparation of this third edition, we gratefully acknowledge the following:

Tara Ryan Schill, BSN, RN, and Todd Schmitt, MEd, for their suggestions and support.

Marianne Sims, for her assistance in the preparation of Chapter 25.

Sandra Robbins, Ambest Surgical Supply Co., Ewing, New Jersey, for her expertise concerning home care equipment and supplies.

Casey M. Golazeski, Ewing, New Jersey, for providing the technical assistance in preparing the manuscript.

Mike DeFilippo, photographer, St. Louis, Missouri, for sharing his skills and artistry.

The reviewers of the manuscript provided many helpful suggestions that were incorporated into the material. We appreciated their careful and conscientious reviews.

Special thanks to Maria Broeker, Senior Content Development Specialist, whose enthusiasm and technical expertise were gratefully appreciated during the entire process of preparing this third edition. Her attention to detail and helpful suggestions made our work an enjoyable venture. We could not have asked for a more competent staff member.

Pat Costigan, Project Manager, assisted us through the production process. Many thanks for his patience and skills.

Finally, our thanks to Nancy O'Brien, Content Strategist, Nursing Division, for her advice and recommendations as decisions were made concerning the details of preparing the third edition.

Instructor Preface

Mosby's Textbook for the Home Care Aide, third edition, is designed to prepare the student with the necessary knowledge, skills, and abilities for employment in a community home care agency. It has been written solely to reflect care given in the home. Careful attention was given to making the text "user friendly" in both the presentation of content and format.

The text incorporates the national HomeCaring Council's curriculum for home care aides. The role of the home care aide is emphasized. Reporting to the supervisor and functioning as an important part of the home care team are stressed.

A continuing feature is the use of scenarios depicting real life situations that the home care aide may encounter in the care of the client. Four home care aides and one supervisor are introduced in Chapter 1. Then, situations are presented throughout the text that include one or more of the characters. These scenarios are meant to enhance the student's understanding of key principles discussed in the chapter and to help bring real life situations into the classroom. The scenarios show how the characters use critical thinking skills to handle typical situations.

The home care aide works in the home alone with the client and family. The supervisor is not "down the hall," but, rather, a phone call away. Therefore, it is critical that the home care aide understands his or her legal responsibilities, limitations, and scope of practice. The text emphasizes the aide's role and responsibilities in typical situations.

Expanded content and emphasis are placed on the following:

Special Notes—Have been expanded and updated to emphasize important information.

ORR—This designed format appears when the text discusses the aide's responsibility to Observe, Record, and Report. Appropriate chapters include these important points.

Pain—The right of the client to have relief of pain is discussed. This information incorporates the requirements of JCAHO (Joint Commission on Accreditation of Health Care Organizations).

Client Care Situations—Have been expanded and updated to reinforce principles of client care.

Cultural Diversity—Is emphasized throughout the text and is reflected in scenarios and other home care situations in the text and workbook.

Infection Control Reminders—The latest information on standard (universal) precautions and bloodborne pathogens is included. Chapter objectives emphasize the importance of infection control in the home.

Updated Content—Major changes include:
- Chapter 10—Reflects the latest information from the U.S. Department of Agriculture about the 2010 Dietary Guidelines for Americans. The MyPlate Food Guide is discussed in detail and the chapter discusses ways in which the home care aide can plan and prepare meals utilizing the Food Guide and Dietary Guidelines.
- Chapter 23—Reflects research and newest information on end-of-life experiences for both client and family.
- Chapter 25—Includes use of computers, websites, and electronic resumes as part of job-seeking skills.
- Definition of the term "scope of practice" and an explanation of the role of the home care aide is included. Confidentiality is stressed, especially in the areas of electronic communication and social networking.

Study Questions and Workbook Exercises—These features are designed to help the student meet the objectives of each chapter. Also, they are structured to develop the student's critical thinking skills.

Throughout the text, careful attention has been given to emphasizing the responsibility of the home care aide to follow the care plan, respect the dignity of the client, act as a guest in the client's home, and keep confidential all information about the client and family.

Part 1 provides the foundation of the program. For the remaining chapters, it is the instructor's choice to present the information in whatever sequence seems appropriate.

Mosby's Workbook for the Home Care Aide, third edition, was developed as an additional resource to both instructor and student. It is designed to reinforce student learning through a variety of activities. With guidance from the instructor, it offers the student an opportunity to apply newly acquired knowledge and skills to "real life" situations presented in the workbook. The workbook also contains a Skills Competency Checklist for every procedure in the textbook. These checklists may be used to assist in teaching these skills and/or to evaluate the student's performance of these procedures.

Finally, the Instructor's Guide, which accompanies both student text and workbook, recommends a wealth of teaching strategies and student learning opportunities. It has been updated and expanded to reflect the new content in the textbook. In addition to being available in print, this important resource is now available on the companion EVOLVE website, http://evolve.elsevier.com/Mosby/homecare/.

Student Preface

This book was designed to help you learn the skills and information needed for employment as a home care aide.

As you learn to be a home care aide, you will join an important group of people in the community—the home care team. You will also work closely with sick people and their families. You may also work with well mothers and their infants. While in the home, you are the eyes and ears of the home care team. Team members rely on your accurate observations and reports. Also, you are a guest in your client's home and have a chance to make a difference in his or her life.

In Chapter 1 you will be introduced to four home care aides and one supervisor who are employed in a home care agency. You will learn more about them in later chapters as they give care to their clients. We hope you enjoy learning about them and their experiences.

Chapter 1 also gives details about how to use the textbook, how to study, and tips for taking tests. This is a very important chapter because it gives the basics needed to get the best out of this book.

On the next few pages, you will see the special features that were designed to help you learn.

- *Objectives* tell you what you will learn in the chapter.

- *Key Terms*, with definitions, are listed at the beginning of the chapter and in blue print when they first appear in the chapter content.

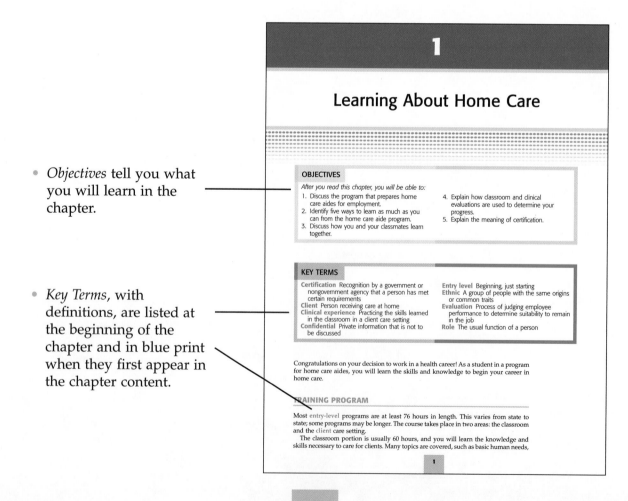

1

Learning About Home Care

OBJECTIVES

After you read this chapter, you will be able to:
1. Discuss the program that prepares home care aides for employment.
2. Identify five ways to learn as much as you can from the home care aide program.
3. Discuss how you and your classmates learn together.
4. Explain how classroom and clinical evaluations are used to determine your progress.
5. Explain the meaning of certification.

KEY TERMS

Certification Recognition by a government or nongovernment agency that a person has met certain requirements
Client Person receiving care at home
Clinical experience Practicing the skills learned in the classroom in a client care setting
Confidential Private information that is not to be discussed

Entry level Beginning, just starting
Ethnic A group of people with the same origins or common traits
Evaluation Process of judging employee performance to determine suitability to remain in the job
Role The usual function of a person

Congratulations on your decision to work in a health career! As a student in a program for home care aides, you will learn the skills and knowledge to begin your career in home care.

TRAINING PROGRAM

Most entry-level programs are at least 76 hours in length. This varies from state to state; some programs may be longer. The course takes place in two areas: the classroom and the client care setting.

The classroom portion is usually 60 hours, and you will learn the knowledge and skills necessary to care for clients. Many topics are covered, such as basic human needs,

1

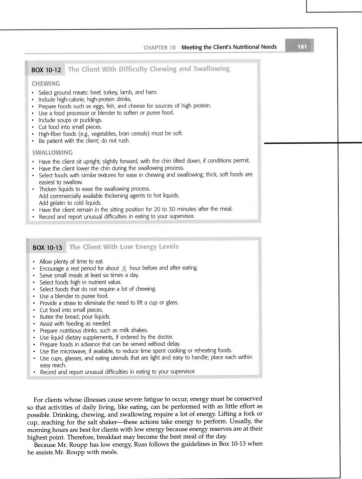

- *ORR highlights* reinforce the importance of Observing, Recording, and Reporting.

- *Special notes* throughout the book appear in magenta print and point out important topics and reminders.

- *Scenarios* are examples of "real life" situations that you may experience while caring for a client at home.

- *Boxes* and *Tables* list rules and guidelines. They stress important information.

- Document the client's response to care.
- Record what the client tells you; use direct quotes; do not record what you think he or she told you.
- Be concise.
- Use correct spelling and proper English.
- Do not leave blank lines or empty spaces that someone else could fill in; print N/A (not applicable) in the space that is not used.
- Sign your initials or full name and title according to agency policy.

REPORTING TO THE AGENCY

The agency should be notified when you observe changes in the client's physical or mental condition. Also, report any client complaints about his or her physical condition or care. Report anything that seems unusual or out of the ordinary. Before you call, have a pen and paper ready so that you can write the instructions you receive.

When you call your supervisor to report information about your client, give the following information:
1. Your name
2. Client's name, address, and telephone number
3. Your observations, such as
   - What you saw: The client is crying.
   - What you heard the client say: "I feel sick to my stomach. I don't want to get up; let me sleep."
   - What you felt (to the touch): The client's skin is hot and dry.
   - What you smelled (if anything): A fruity odor to the breath.
4. How long the client has had the problem
5. How you handled the situation; if you were unable to follow the care plan, give the reason

IT IS YOUR RESPONSIBILITY TO FOLLOW THE CARE PLAN, RECORD THE CARE GIVEN, AND REPORT ANY CHANGES IN THE CLIENT'S CONDITION. IF YOU BELIEVE THAT THE CARE PLAN NEEDS TO BE CHANGED, NOTIFY YOUR SUPERVISOR AND RECORD YOUR FINDINGS ON THE CLIENT'S CARE RECORD. YOUR SUPERVISOR, CASE MANAGER, OR ANOTHER HEALTH PROFESSIONAL ARE THE ONLY PEOPLE WHO CAN CHANGE THE CARE PLAN.

INCIDENT REPORTS

As Anna Petrova was walking up the stairs to Mr. Smirnoff's apartment, she tripped and fell. She scraped her hands and knees on the concrete steps. They hurt, but she tried to ignore the discomfort while she cared for Mr. Smirnoff.

During the visit, Anna's hands and knees became stiff and swollen. The pain became worse. Before leaving Mr. Smirnoff's apartment, she decided to call Mrs. Quick, her supervisor, on her cell phone to explain the situation. Mrs. Quick told Anna to go to the emergency department at the local hospital to be checked. "You'll have to fill out an incident report when you return to the office, Anna. In the meantime, I'll notify your next client, Mr. Abrams, that you will not be coming this afternoon. I hope you'll be feeling better—talk to you later."

BOX 10-12 The Client With Difficulty Chewing and Swallowing

CHEWING
- Select ground meats: beef, turkey, lamb, and ham.
- Include high-calorie, high-protein drinks.
- Prepare foods such as eggs, fish, and cheese for sources of high protein.
- Use a food processor or blender to soften or puree food.
- Include soups or puddings.
- Cut food into small pieces.
- High-fiber foods (e.g., vegetables, bran cereals) must be soft.
- Be patient with the client; do not rush.

SWALLOWING
- Have the client sit upright, slightly forward, with the chin tilted down, if conditions permit.
- Have the client lower the chin during the swallowing process.
- Select foods with similar textures for ease in chewing and swallowing; thick, soft foods are easiest to swallow.
- Thicken liquids to ease the swallowing process.
  Add commercially available thickening agents to hot liquids.
  Add gelatin to cold liquids.
- Have the client remain in the sitting position for 20 to 30 minutes after the meal.
- Record and report unusual difficulties in eating to your supervisor.

BOX 10-13 The Client With Low Energy Levels

- Allow plenty of time to eat.
- Encourage a rest period for about ½ hour before and after eating.
- Serve small meals at least six times a day.
- Select foods high in nutrient value.
- Select foods that do not require a lot of chewing.
- Use a blender to puree food.
- Provide a straw to eliminate the need to lift a cup or glass.
- Cut food into small pieces.
- Butter the bread; pour liquids.
- Assist with feeding as needed.
- Prepare nutritious drinks, such as milk shakes.
- Use liquid dietary supplements, if ordered by the doctor.
- Prepare foods in advance that can be served without delay.
- Use the microwave, if available, to reduce time spent cooking or reheating foods.
- Use cups, glasses, and eating utensils that are light and easy to handle; place each within easy reach.
- Record and report unusual difficulties in eating to your supervisor.

For clients whose illnesses cause severe fatigue to occur, energy must be conserved so that activities of daily living, like eating, can be performed with as little effort as possible. Drinking, chewing, and swallowing require a lot of energy. Lifting a fork or cup, reaching for the salt shaker—these actions take energy to perform. Usually, the morning hours are best for clients with low energy because energy reserves are at their highest point. Therefore, breakfast may become the best meal of the day.

Because Mr. Roupp has low energy, Russ follows the guidelines in Box 10-13 when he assists Mr. Roupp with meals.

- *Procedures* give step-by-step, easy-to-understand directions for those skills used to care for clients at home.

- Color *illustrations* and *photographs* show key ideas and procedure steps.

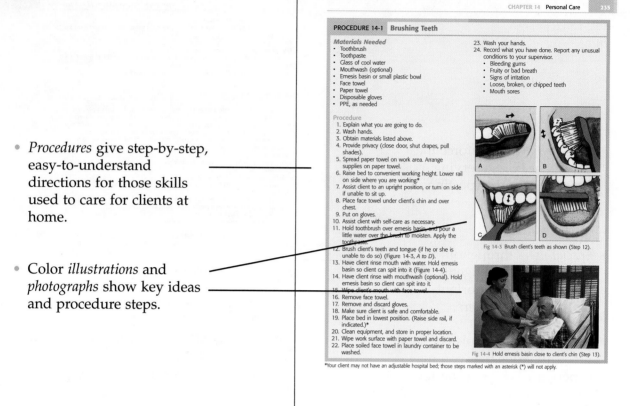

- *Chapter Summaries* review main points presented in the chapter.

- *Study Questions* help you learn by using the information presented in the chapter.

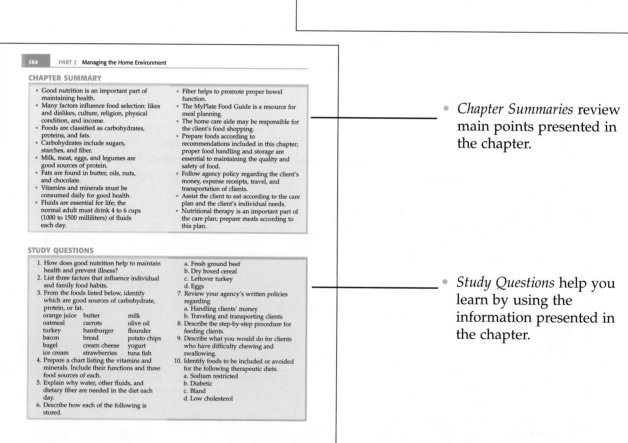

Contents

Procedures

Learning About Home Care

OBJECTIVES

After you read this chapter, you will be able to:

1. Discuss the program that prepares home care aides for employment.
2. Identify five ways to learn as much as you can from the home care aide program.
3. Discuss how you and your classmates learn together.
4. Explain how classroom and clinical evaluations are used to determine your progress.
5. Explain the meaning of certification.

KEY TERMS

Certification Recognition by a government or nongovernment agency that a person has met certain requirements

Client Person receiving care at home

Clinical experience Practicing the skills learned in the classroom in a client care setting

Confidential Private information that is not to be discussed

Entry level Beginning, just starting

Ethnic A group of people with the same origins or common traits

Evaluation Process of judging employee performance to determine suitability to remain in the job

Role The usual function of a person

Congratulations on your decision to work in a health career! As a student in a program for home care aides, you will learn the skills and knowledge to begin your career in home care.

TRAINING PROGRAM

Most entry-level programs are at least 76 hours in length. This varies from state to state; some programs may be longer. The course takes place in two areas: the classroom and the client care setting.

The classroom portion is usually 60 hours, and you will learn the knowledge and skills necessary to care for clients. Many topics are covered, such as basic human needs,

Fig 1-1 Students and instructor in a classroom setting.

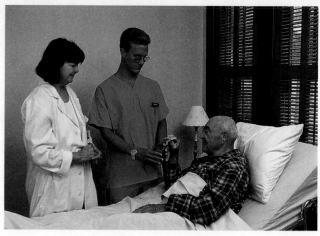

Fig 1-2 A student and instructor in a clinical setting (client's home).

communications, normal growth and development, the aging process, and working with ill persons. Nutrition, special diets, and home management are also discussed (Figure 1-1).

Classes are taught by a registered nurse instructor and other specialists in home care. They will demonstrate and explain the procedures you need to know to give personal care in a client's home. Your learning will be evaluated through written tests and return demonstrations.

You will spend 15 hours in a **clinical experience**. This is a supervised field practice in clients' homes where you use the skills learned in the classroom. You will be evaluated on how well you perform the skills learned in this program (Figure 1-2).

SUGGESTIONS FOR SUCCESS

There are some basic actions that will help you to be successful in this course:
- Attend every class.
- Arrive on time and ready to take part in class. If you bring a cell phone to class, turn it to "mute" or "off."
- Bring all necessary materials to class: books, notebook, pens, pencils, and eyeglasses, if you need them for reading.
- Pay attention to the instructors.
- Watch all demonstrations carefully.
- Read all of the assignments in the textbook and all handouts before and after class.

These are important ways to learn as much as you can in your home care aide program.

USING THE TEXTBOOK

When using this book, begin your reading with the chapter objectives and key terms. When you have finished the chapter, return to the objectives. Ask yourself, "Can I do what the objectives say I should be able to do?" If your answer is "yes," test yourself by answering the questions at the end of the chapter. If your answer is "no," read the chapter again and continue with the objectives and this "test yourself process."

Overview of the Textbook

This book is divided into five sections, as follows.

Part 1, Orientation to Home Care, introduces basic information about the home care industry, communication skills, human needs, body systems, and working with sick and/or disabled people.

Part 2, Managing the Home Environment, discusses home safety, healthy environment, and nutrition.

Part 3, Home Care Procedures, presents the basic skills needed to care for clients in their homes. You will also learn about infections and how to prevent their spread.

Part 4, Meeting the Client's Special Needs, covers the care given to infants, mothers, older adults, and those with a mental illness. You will also learn how to care for clients with specific disease conditions, with final illnesses, and in emergency situations.

Part 5, Professional Skills, helps you with the transition from student to employee and discusses ways to get a job and keep it.

The role of the home care aide is stressed in every section of the book, helping you to understand what is expected of you and what actions are appropriate.

Throughout the book, you will read about some home care aides and their supervisor as they care for their clients in the home. This will give you the chance to learn about the work of the home care aide and to meet some of their clients.

Meeting the Caregivers

Please meet the caregivers who appear in the book.

CHARLOTTE QUICK, Nurse Supervisor

"My mother was a military nurse during the Korean Conflict in the 50s. As I was growing up, I remember the stories she told me about caring for the sick and injured. When I was very young, I decided that I wanted to be a nurse, too. Right after high school, I enrolled and graduated from a college nursing program. I've always worked in home care because I like serving clients, where they are most comfortable" (Figure 1-3).

Fig 1-3 Charlotte Quick, nurse supervisor.

Fig 1-4 Anna Petrova, home care aide.

Fig 1-5 Betty Randolph, home care aide.

"I teach a program to prepare home care aides once a year, but I prefer to be working with them on the job. They are the eyes and ears of the home care team. We rely on them to give us information about the client's progress."

"My nursing career gave me the chance to work part time while caring for my two children. Now, they are adults and have their own children. Five grandchildren, and another on the way! I can't believe it! I've been working full time since my kids were in high school. I just received an award as 'Home Care Nurse of the Year.' What a nice surprise after 25 years of service! My husband would have been so proud. He died last year. I miss him. We were a great team."

ANNA PETROVA, Home Care Aide

"Seven years ago, we came to this country from Russia—Sergei, my husband; Katrina, my baby daughter; and me. It was difficult to find work because we couldn't speak or read English very well. Sergei got a job driving a taxi, and I cleaned houses. We lived with our cousins in the city" (Figure 1-4).

"After our son was born, I took a home care aide course and began to work part time. My relatives took care of the kids, and we worked hard to get our own home. Today, both children are in school and I can work full time. Sergei and I are studying to become citizens; we love our new country."

BETTY RANDOLPH, Home Care Aide

"I've worked with Mrs. Quick ever since I got this job—15 years ago. Believe me, I was really scared when I first got started, but she taught me what I needed to know, and every month, we have classes about new and changing things" (Figure 1-5).

"Sometimes, when I have a long day, I'm almost too tired to feed and play with my three dogs. But, they lift my spirits; they're really good company. I'm sure glad that I don't have anyone to take care of. Another thing that lifts my spirits is singing in the gospel choir at my church. After practice, my mother and two sisters get together for coffee and to catch up on what's happening."

"I really enjoy taking care of my clients. In fact, I volunteer to work with those who are very sick and near death. I am blessed to be able to do this kind of work."

Fig 1-6 Russ Larson, home care aide.

Fig 1-7 Rosina Chavez, home care aide.

RUSS LARSON, Home Care Aide

"I really didn't know what I wanted to do when I graduated from high school, so I worked in menswear in a large department store in the mall. I was there for a few years, but I didn't like it. My girlfriend decided to be a medical secretary. I thought, 'Why not try a new career?' I took some tests at the community college, and they suggested that nursing might be the career for me. I thought it over and thought, 'Why not?' So here I am, a first-year nursing student. I took the home care aide course to see if I like this type of work. And I do" (Figure 1-6).

"This gives me experience working with sick people of all ages and the chance to earn money while I'm going to school. With rent to pay and textbooks to buy, the money I make sure helps a lot. Shawn, Bill, and I are on a tight budget. We share a tiny apartment in town, and we love to eat. I keep telling them that we have to cut down on the snacks, but it's not working very well! They like to party, too. And sometimes, I have to take care of them afterwards!"

ROSINA CHAVEZ, Home Care Aide

"This is my last year. I have worked all my life. I've been married to the same man for 30 years and raised my four children. It hasn't been easy, but we've survived. It's been 20 years since I first became a home care aide. Now, I'm ready to retire and enjoy my seven grand-children. They all live near me and enjoy my good Mexican cooking. I love to have all of them in the kitchen. It's mass confusion, but it's great" (Figure 1-7).

"I will miss my clients—they're very special to me. Some tell me not to retire; they say they need me. The best part is that they tell me that they love me! But, it's time for me to go. So this will be my last year. How time flies!"

Using the Index

The Index, on p. 500, lists, in alphabetical order, all of the topics covered in this book, and it lists the page numbers on which the topic is discussed. The following are some examples:

- Absorbent undergarments, 268: This means that you will find information on absorbent undergarments if you turn to p. 268.

- Vitamins, 143-144, 143t, 144t: This means that you will find information about vitamins on pp. 143 and 144. Also, you will find information about this topic in tables found on pp. 143 and 144.

Rather than going through the book, page by page, looking for a certain topic, do the following:
- Go to the Index section of the book (p. 500).
- Find the topic for which you are looking, using the first letter of the topic (e.g., bath, hair care, temperature of bath water).
- Use paper and pencil to write the page number where the topic will be found (e.g., "bath, 240").

Turn to the pages where you will find the information on these topics.

Using the Glossary

The Glossary, on p. 496, lists, in alphabetical order, all of the key terms, with definitions, found in the book. Remember that each key term has been defined the first time it is used in a sentence. For example, the term *disability* is defined in Chapter 3. Suppose you are reading Chapter 5 and the word *disability* appears. You are not sure of its meaning and want to refresh your memory about the correct meaning. You should do the following:
- Go to the Glossary section of the book on p. 496.
- Find the term *disability* by using the first letter of the term *(d)*.
- Read the definition and/or use paper and pencil to write down the definition.
Use of the Index and the Glossary saves time and helps you to learn.

USING THE WORKBOOK

The workbook that accompanies this textbook is designed to help you gain the knowledge and skills you need to begin your career as a home care aide. Before using the workbook, you should first read the assigned chapter. Each set of activities in the workbook will help you to meet the chapter objectives. All of the answers for workbook activities can be found in the corresponding chapters of this textbook. Using the workbook gives you a chance to be involved in the learning process and to test yourself to see what you have learned—or still need to study.

STUDY "HELPS"

An excellent "help" and guide to studying is the PQRST method, which gives suggestions for studying.
- **Preview:** Flip through the chapter, paying attention to headings and words in bold print.
- **Question:** Read the objectives. Ask, "What am I supposed to learn?"
- **Read:** Sit in a comfortable, well-lit, and quiet place.
- **Study:** Review important points in the chapter.
- **Test:** Answer questions at the end of the chapter.

ASKING QUESTIONS

Have you heard the saying, "The only dumb question is the one that is not asked"? This is very true. YOUR INSTRUCTOR WANTS YOU TO ASK QUESTIONS IF YOU DO NOT UNDERSTAND. Do not be shy or afraid. Remember, there is usually at least one other classmate who did not understand either. Be sure to ask right away. Do not wait and ask classmates to explain it to you after class; they may not know what is correct. Your instructor wants you to succeed and to learn the right information the first time. ASKING QUESTIONS HELPS YOU AND YOUR CLASS-MATES TO LEARN.

COMPLETING ASSIGNMENTS

Your instructor will give assignments to be completed on your own time or during class. These assignments may require that you

- Read pages of your textbook.
- Complete workbook questions.
- Report to class on a special topic.
- Perform a task related to the topic.
- Answer questions given by your instructor.

An assignment is given to help you learn more about the topic you are studying. Or it may be given to help you prepare for a new topic to be covered next time. It is important that these assignments are completed with care. Your instructor may give a test to find out whether your assignment was completed properly. Your final grade for the program will include how well you completed your assignments. Set aside a period of time each day or evening when you will study and do your assignments for the next class.

TAKING TESTS

Tests are given to show how well you know the subject material or how well you perform a set of tasks or procedures. They are guideposts that show you and your instructor what you have learned and what areas need improvement. During the program, oral quizzes may be given. These are brief tests in which students answer the instructor's questions in class. Sometimes, your instructor will ask you to take the test at home. Directions for completing the test will be given. If the test is "on your honor," it means that your instructor is relying on your honesty to complete the test without any assistance.

During the program, you will have a lot of practice in taking tests. Your workbook has sample test questions to help you in the process of learning.

Here are some tips to help you take tests.

- Relax: Take a few deep breaths before you begin.
- Read each question carefully.
- Read the question again.
- Watch for the words *all, always, never,* and *none* in the statements you read. The statement is *usually* wrong.
- Do not read into the question something that is not there.
- If you do not know the answer, do not spend a lot of time on it. Go to the next question.
- Return to the unanswered question after you complete the test.
  For multiple-choice questions, the following suggestions are helpful.
- Read all of the answers carefully.
- Select the one *best answer*.
- There may be two or more answers that are partly correct, but choose the one that most closely fits the answer you would give.

WORKING WITH CLASSMATES

You and your classmates make up another "family"—a family of people who are preparing for a career in home care. You have chosen this career because you like people and want to give the best care to your clients. It is important that you show the same caring concern for your classmates. RESPECTING OTHER PERSONS' POINTS OF VIEW AND LISTENING TO WHAT THEY HAVE TO SAY ARE IMPORTANT QUALITIES OF A HOME CARE AIDE.

Often, your classmates will be from a background that is different from yours. This is an opportunity to learn about another person's heritage, customs, and beliefs. The respect you show your classmates in these areas will prepare you for your future work with clients of various ethnic backgrounds.

Perhaps your instructor will ask two or more of you to work together on an activity. The way you work with others shows your instructor how well you will cooperate with members of the home care team. Team work is very important in this profession. Classroom activities will help you improve your communication, listening, and cooperation skills.

EVALUATION

The process of judging how well you have learned the information and skills required to be a home care aide is called evaluation. There are two types of evaluation: classroom and clinical.

The person responsible for evaluating your performance in both areas is your instructor. Other people may have a role in this process, such as part-time classroom instructors. The client and family also may be asked to give information for the clinical evaluation, but the final evaluation is your instructor's job.

CLASSROOM EVALUATION

This type of evaluation is a way for your instructor to determine how much you have learned from classroom instruction and the areas in which you need improvement. Evaluation is helpful to both you and your instructor.

Your instructor will use a variety of ways to help you learn the information and skills necessary to be a home care aide. Each person has special ways they use to learn, so a variety of methods are used. Some of these ways have already been discussed. The instructor also uses a variety of ways to evaluate each student's learning.

At the beginning of the program, your instructor will discuss the specific ways that will be used to evaluate your performance. Many instructors use the ratings of *acceptable/ unacceptable* or *satisfactory/unsatisfactory*. The rating includes such areas as
- Completes assignments on time
- Contributes to classroom discussions
- Successfully passes tests
- Follows the rules and regulations of the school/agency and classroom

Evaluations of your classroom performance will occur at specific times during the program. BE SURE TO ASK YOUR INSTRUCTOR TO EXPLAIN ANY AREA OF THE CLASSROOM EVALUATION PROCESS THAT YOU DO NOT UNDERSTAND; IT IS BETTER TO ASK RIGHT AWAY THAN TO BE WORRIED ABOUT THIS IMPORTANT PART OF YOUR PROGRAM.

The following are some questions to ask yourself during the classroom part of the course: "How well am I
- participating in classroom discussions?"
- contributing my knowledge and experiences to the topics being discussed?"
- cooperating with classmates in activities assigned?"
- completing assignments in and out of class?"

- passing written and oral tests?"
- performing the skills needed to be a home care aide?"
- listening, cooperating with others, showing respect, and handling difficult classroom situations?"
- coming to class on time?"
- handling suggestions for improvement given by my instructor?"

CLINICAL EVALUATION

Clinical evaluation shows how well you perform your duties as a home care aide in the client's home. The questions listed below are answered by your instructor with help from the client and family:

"How well do you

- perform correctly the tasks assigned?"
- give safe, considerate care?"
- report back to your supervisor?"
- record your activities according to agency policy?"
- respect the culture of your client and family?"
- communicate with your client and family?"
- know the policies of your agency and act according to them?"

Your instructor will explain how often these evaluations will occur. The instructor will meet with you to review the results. This is the time for you to discuss the evaluation and to ask questions; you can then work on any areas needing improvement.

THE EVALUATION CONFERENCE

Your instructor will meet with you privately to review the written evaluation of your performance, both classroom and clinical. This is the time to discuss the evaluation and to ask questions. If there are areas in which you need improvement, ask your instructor for suggestions of ways to make progress.

You will be asked to sign and date the evaluation form at the end of the conference; this means that you have reviewed the written evaluation. If you believe that the evaluation is not correct, you may write comments about it in a place on the form. Each written evaluation is kept as a part of your permanent, confidential school record.

CERTIFICATION

STATE CERTIFICATION

When you successfully complete the program, your agency or school will send this information to the state agency responsible for the certification of home care aides. You will receive a certificate that permits you to practice as a home care aide.

NATIONAL CERTIFICATION

Some agencies require that you pass a national test to determine that you have the skills and knowledge needed for the job. Your instructor will give you information about applying to take the test. You must complete an approved program before taking this national examination.

Welcome to the home care training program!

CHAPTER SUMMARY

- Home care aides are prepared in the classroom and clinical settings.
- Ways to learn include the following:
  Read the textbook.
  Complete the workbook.
  Observe demonstrations carefully.
  Use the PQRST method of study.
  Work with your classmates.
  Ask questions.
  Complete assignments.
- Progress is measured by classroom and clinical evaluation.
- Certification is the means by which home care aides are recognized as meeting requirements for working in the home.

STUDY QUESTIONS

1. Describe your training program and include the following:
   a. Classroom hours
   b. Clinical areas
   c. Topics that will be presented
2. List five important things that will help you to be successful in this program.
3. Discuss how you and your classmates learn together.
4. What is classroom evaluation? What is clinical evaluation? List three ways in which the instructor may evaluate your learning.
5. Explain the meaning of certification.

2

The Home Care Industry

OBJECTIVES

After you read this chapter, you will be able to:

1. Explain the importance of home care.
2. Discuss the types of clients who require care.
3. Identify two types of home care agencies and two sources of payment.
4. Describe five members of the home care agency team and a function of each.
5. Identify resources in the community that assist the client at home.
6. Discuss the qualities necessary to be a member of the team.
7. Explain the role of the home care aide as a part of the team.

KEY TERMS

Acute illness Illness with a rapid onset and severe symptoms and of short length

Assess To determine the client's needs for home care services

Behavior Actions and interactions with clients

Chronic illness Disease with little change and slow progress and of long duration; not an acute illness

DRG (diagnosis-related group) Listing of diagnoses used to establish reimbursement by Medicare and Medicaid for hospitalization and medical care

Hospice Program of care that assists the dying client to maintain a satisfactory lifestyle during the end stage of an illness

Hospital discharge planner Person who arranges for the care of a patient on release from the hospital; may be a professional nurse or social worker

Medicaid State and federal insurance program that pays for hospitalization and health care for low-income persons of all ages

Medicare Federal program of hospitalization, prescription drugs, and health care insurance for persons older than 65 years and/or those with permanent disabilities; participation is voluntary

Policy, policies Set of rules and regulations

Reimbursement To make payment for an expense incurred

Scope of practice A term used by licensing agencies that describes what procedures and actions are permitted by law for a home care aide to perform

Standard Gauge that is used as a basis for judgment

Home care agencies have been in existence for many years. In the 1880s, visiting nurse societies were established to provide home health services to immigrants in cities, the rural poor, and others in need. Over the years, home care agencies have expanded staff and services to meet the growing needs of society.

GROWTH OF INDUSTRY

Several factors have influenced the growth of the home care industry. One major influence originated in 1965 when the U.S. Congress passed the Medicare laws that allowed funds for home health services for older adults. These new laws caused the number of home care agencies to increase rapidly. Today, it is estimated that the number of home care aides needed by these agencies will also increase. In fact, it will grow faster than average for all occupations through 2018.

Another influence on the industry's growth was the 1983 passage of federal legislation that created diagnosis-related groups (DRGs). A DRG is a list of specific diagnoses used to determine the typical length of stay and the cost of treatment allowed for patients with that particular group of illnesses. The hospital receives only the dollar amount specified in the DRG for Medicare and Medicaid patients. If the patient leaves the hospital after less time than specified in the DRG, the hospital gets to keep the excess funds. If the patient stays longer than the time allowed, the hospital loses money. This is one reason that patients are sent home from the hospital as quickly as possible. Other reasons for early hospital discharge include the following:

1. *Medical and surgical advances:* Modern treatment has reduced the length of time spent in the hospital.
2. *Lower costs:* Home care is less expensive. Many times, home care costs about half that of hospital care. Technical improvements in equipment and supplies make it possible to do many of the same things at home as in the hospital.
3. *Greater comfort:* Most people prefer to recuperate in the familiar surroundings of home. Children and older adults often feel more at ease—more comfortable—at home with their family and friends (Figure 2-1). They can follow their own schedules

Fig 2-1 Most people prefer home care.

for eating and sleeping. Many people say they recover more quickly at home than in the hospital.

4. *Lower risk:* The risk of hospital-acquired infection is reduced because patients' exposure to others who may carry infection—hospital staff, other patients, and visitors—is reduced.

When people come home sooner, they may also come home sicker. An estimated 10 million Americans will need ongoing specialized care each year. Home care agencies in the United States provide care on a short-term, long-term, or live-in basis to more than 7.2 million people. Home care is a large part of the nation's health care budget.

HOME CARE AGENCIES

Home care agencies are as varied as the clients who use them. Each is uniquely organized to best serve the needs of the clients in the community.

ORGANIZATION AND REGULATION

Home care agencies are organized and administered in many ways. They may be classified as follows:

1. *Governmental or official:* Sponsored by local or state government and supported by tax monies, usually a part of the department of health
2. *Voluntary, nonprofit:* Governed by a volunteer board of directors and financed through tax-deductible contributions and/or fees for service (e.g., visiting nurse associations and church-sponsored home care agencies)
3. *Private, for-profit:* Operated by individuals through a franchise or as part of a local or national company (e.g., Interim Health Care)

The agency director is responsible for the day-to-day operations of the entire organization. Office staff provide clerical and bookkeeping services. Other staff members who are responsible for client care are discussed later in this chapter.

The activities of home care agencies are regulated by state or local authorities. Licensure as a home care agency may be required. These regulations vary in each community. Agencies that participate in the care of Medicare clients must also meet specific governmental standards. The state department of health or other designated organization conducts regular inspections to make sure that the agency complies with Medicare regulations.

SOURCES OF CLIENTS

Home care agency clients come from many sources, which include the following.

1. *Hospitals:* When care needs to be continued at home but not at the level provided by the hospital, the hospital discharge planner arranges a transfer of information and doctor's orders to the home care agency
2. *Rehabilitation centers:* When a person has reached the highest level of ability after injury or accident but still needs assistance with routine care and therapy at home
3. *Hospice:* When a terminally ill person wishes to be cared for at home

4. *Personal referral:* When a family member finds that caring for an ill or disabled relative is too much to handle alone
5. *Doctor's office or clinic referral:* When a patient needs care at home

TYPES OF CLIENTS

Just as there are many sources of clients, there are many types of clients. A large number are older adults who have been recently discharged from the hospital after an **acute illness**. Other examples of clients include the following.
- New mothers and their babies
- People with **chronic illnesses**
- Sick children
- People who have had recent surgery
- People with fractures
- People with amputations
- **Hospice** clients
- Frail older adults
- People with disabilities
- People who need special treatments/medications

PAYMENT FOR SERVICES

Services provided by home care agencies cost about half that of similar care offered by hospitals. But who pays for it? Agencies can turn to several sources for **reimbursement**, or payment, for their services.
1. *Out of pocket:* The client or client's family may be responsible for paying a deductible and/or specific percentage of the cost of care, depending on the type of health insurance of the client. Sometimes a client must pay "out of pocket" for all care because he or she has no insurance or has exhausted the insurance coverage or because the client's insurance does not pay for home care.
2. *Health care insurance/health maintenance organizations:* An individual or group insurance plan may pay a part or all of the cost of medical care and services. The services and payment for them vary depending on the insurance company and the client's type of insurance.
3. *Medicare:* With this federal health insurance program for older adults and individuals with disabilities, the agency is reimbursed according to required types of assessment and record keeping.
4. *Medicaid:* This federal- and state-supported program provides health care for people with limited income and individuals with disabilities, including children and pregnant women.
5. *Other state and federal programs:* Services are available to eligible clients through special programs for older adults and individuals with disabilities.
6. *United Way and other charitable programs:* Grants are given to certain agencies for client services.

The type of care and service provided are limited by the provisions of the programs listed here. ACCURATE RECORD KEEPING IS ESSENTIAL TO SHOW EXACTLY WHAT CARE WAS GIVEN. IF CARE IS NOT PROPERLY RECORDED, THE AGENCY MAY NOT RECEIVE PROMPT REIMBURSEMENT. Most agencies expect you to submit a daily report that lists the exact services performed and the hours worked. This report is signed by the client and is used to complete your payroll record so you can be paid. The report is also necessary to bill the client and/or insurance company for reimbursement.

THE HOME CARE TEAM

A team is a group of people who work together to accomplish a common goal. Each team member has a specific responsibility. The home care team is made up of many members, and they must work together very well to meet the client's special goals (Figure 2-2).

TEAM MEMBERS

Listed here are the types of professionals, in addition to the doctor, who may be included on the home care team. Some typical functions for each member are also included.

Case Manager
- Assesses the client's physical, emotional, social, and environmental needs
- Develops a plan to meet these needs
- Recommends services of other professionals
- Reviews or reassesses the client's progress, and adjusts the plan as needed
- Coordinates the plan of care

Registered Nurse (RN)
- Assesses, plans, and implements the nursing care required
- Carries out the doctor's orders
- Teaches the client and family members about care techniques and procedures
- Supervises care given by the home care aide and licensed practical/vocational nurse

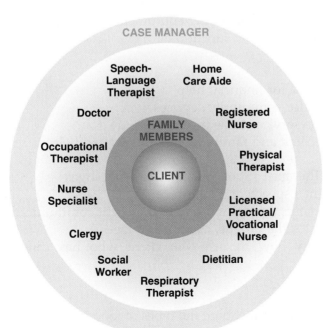

Fig 2-2 The circle of home care.

Nurse Specialist (RN)

- Provides complex nursing care to clients with special needs (e.g., children, infants, clients with cancer)
- Teaches other nursing staff about new procedures
- Acts as an advisor to other agency members about clients with special needs

Licensed Practical/Vocational Nurse (LPN/LVN)

- Gives nursing care under the supervision of an RN
- Cares for clients whose conditions are stable and do not require complex nursing care

Home Care Aide

- Provides personal care according to the client's care plan
- Performs required housekeeping services
- Works under the supervision of an RN and/or therapist
- Reports activities performed according to agency policy

Physical Therapist (RPT)

- Assesses the client's muscle strength, balance, and movement of joints
- Plans and implements the physical therapy program
- Teaches the client and family exercises to strengthen muscles and improve movement
- Supervises care given by the home care aide

Occupational Therapist (OTR)

- Assesses movement of the client's arms, hands, and fingers
- Determines how well the client is able to perform activities of daily living (ADL), such as eating, bathing, and dressing

Respiratory Therapist (RRT)

- Assesses the client's ability to breathe with ease
- Plans and implements the respiratory therapy program
- Explains the proper use of breathing equipment
- Checks equipment for proper functioning

Social Worker

- Determines the need for financial help
- Assesses the need for community services
- Arranges for these services to be provided
- Ensures that the client and family receive the needed help

Speech-Language Therapist (Speech-Language Pathologist)

- Assesses the client's speech and language
- Plans and implements a program to help the client communicate
- Teaches exercises for the tongue, mouth, and face
- Teaches the family how to help the client who has difficulty speaking and swallowing

Dietitian

- Teaches the client and family about the types of food needed to maintain or improve health
- Teaches proper menu selection and preparation according to the diet ordered by the doctor

Others
- Clergy
  - Provides spiritual support to the client and family
- Volunteer
  - Gives service to the agency or the client without being paid
  - Performs tasks that do not require complex skills, a license, or certification
  - Is supervised by the agency

FORMING THE TEAM

The types of team members who are selected will vary according to the needs of each client and family. First, the case manager meets with the client and family to assess the types of services needed. Information received from the hospital's discharge planner (mentioned earlier) is also considered. The case manager may be the registered nurse, the physical therapist, the occupational therapist, or the speech-language therapist if there is only one skilled service needed in the home. Next, the case manager determines the type and amount of services. The following information is used:
- Client's health and physical condition and abilities
- Treatments ordered by the doctor
- Family members or others able and willing to give care
- The family as a social group—strengths and problems
- Reactions of family members to the need for help
- Home environment needs—housekeeping required
- Other services needed, such as Meals On Wheels, special equipment, and transportation
- Financial resources of the client to obtain services needed
- Length of service needed and expected results

As an example, the client who must receive medications by injection and requires oxygen therapy to help breathe more easily may have a team that includes a registered nurse and a respiratory therapist.

THE CARE PLAN

ESTABLISHING THE GOAL

The case manager develops the goals to be met by the team according to the needs of the client and family. For the client who is disabled, the goal may be to help restore as much function as possible. The goal for a mother and her newborn baby may be to help her gain independence in caring for herself and the baby. For the client who is dying, the goal will be to give the physical care and emotional support needed so that death can occur with dignity. The plan may also include support for the family.

DEVELOPING THE PLAN

The plan of care to meet the goal is based on the information obtained by the case manager while assessing the types of services needed (Box 2-1). The plan includes the following:
- The activities to be performed, who will perform them, and how often
- Other agencies performing activities

Several health professionals may be required to give service to the client, such as a physical therapist, respiratory therapist, and registered nurse. Each will develop a plan of care, implement the plan, and evaluate the client's progress. However, the case manager coordinates the total plan of care (Figure 2-3).

> **BOX 2-1**   Plan of Care for Mrs. Stevens
>
> ### GOAL
> • Mrs. Stevens will gain ½ lb per week until she reaches normal weight (134 lb).
>
> ### ACTIVITIES
> • Weigh her once a week.
> • Rosina Chavez, home care aide, will visit on Fridays at 10:00 AM.
>
> ### OTHER AGENCIES PROVIDING SERVICES
> • Meals On Wheels will provide noon meals from Monday through Friday.
> • The local church will provide noon meals on Saturday and Sunday.

Fig 2-3 The case manager coordinates the services of team members.

Fig 2-4 A client receives a home-delivered meal.

USING COMMUNITY RESOURCES

The case manager may recommend that resources in the community be used to assist clients and their families with various tasks. Perhaps the client is not able to prepare meals or perform housekeeping duties. Other family members may be at work and unable to help. Community agencies and organizations offer services that may help the client to remain at home rather than to be placed in an institution (Figure 2-4).

TABLE 2-1   Examples of Community Programs

TYPE OF SERVICE	PROGRAM	SERVICE PROVIDED
Nutrition services	Home-delivered meals (Meals On Wheels) *Sponsor:* State, county, or local community agencies, civic organizations	Provides one or more meals a day, at least 5 days a week. Food is delivered by a volunteer. A hot meal arrives, ready to be eaten. A cold meal—usually a sandwich, fruit, and milk—may be eaten later.
Social services	Volunteer-friendly visitor program *Sponsor:* Local community agencies; senior citizens' clubs; civic organizations	Offers a chance for the homebound person to socialize with mature men and women on a regular basis. The volunteer makes weekly home visits. Activities include writing letters, reading aloud, playing cards, or just talking about topics of interest with the client.
	Telephone reassurance *Sponsor:* Civic organizations; senior citizens' clubs; police departments; nursing home residents	A volunteer calls the client at a prearranged time each day. The conversation with the volunteer may be the only contact with another human being for the entire day.
	Religious activities *Sponsor:* Church/temple/ mosque/synagogue	Religious groups provide a variety of services. Visits by clergy and members link the client to the life of the congregation.
Household services	Volunteer services *Sponsor:* Local community	Volunteers run errands, do routine home repairs, or perform light housekeeping tasks.
	Housecleaning services *Sponsor:* Local community businesses	For a fee, the service provides all types of housecleaning tasks according to the needs of the client.

Table 2-1 gives examples of community programs that provide valuable help to both the client and family.

YOU, AN ESSENTIAL PART OF THE TEAM

THE DUTIES YOU PERFORM AS A HOME CARE AIDE ARE A VITAL PART OF YOUR CLIENT'S CARE. IN SOME CASES, YOU WILL BE THE PERSON WHO HAS THE MOST CONTACT EACH WEEK WITH THE CLIENT AND FAMILY. INFORMATION YOU SHARE WITH OTHER MEMBERS OF THE TEAM IS VERY IMPORTANT. THE TEAM RELIES ON YOUR VALUABLE CONTRIBUTIONS SO THAT THE PROPER CARE AND TREATMENT CAN BE GIVEN.

You will be expected to
1. LOOK AND ACT PROFESSIONAL
2. PERFORM YOUR DUTIES PROPERLY
3. WORK AS PART OF THE TEAM

Fig 2-5 Good grooming is an important requirement for the home care aide. **A,** A properly groomed male home care aide. **B,** A properly groomed female home care aide.

LOOKING AND ACTING PROFESSIONAL

Looking Professional

Your appearance says a lot about the way you will perform your duties. A neat, clean, and properly dressed person conveys an image of one who is ready to perform tasks properly (Figure 2-5). Your appearance says, "I am proud to be a home care employee." Remember, first impressions are usually lasting ones. Clients and families will appreciate your professional look. Your employer has policies about proper dress and appearance that you will need to follow.

The tips given in the Appearance Checklist will help you present a professional appearance.

Appearance Checklist

Clothing

- Wear a clean uniform each day with undergarments that fit properly and do not show through the uniform.
- Iron and repair clothes as needed.
- Wear your name pin and agency badge above the waist at all times, unless it interferes with client care.
- Do not wear dark lens eyeglasses because clients cannot see your eyes. This may be frightening to your client.

Shoes, stockings, or socks

- Wear comfortable, low-heeled shoes with nonskid soles and heels to help prevent accidents.
- Polish your shoes daily, if appropriate.
- Keep shoelaces clean.
- Buy the best shoes you can afford that offer support for walking, standing, and squatting.
- Keep shoes in good repair.
- Wear clean, properly fitting stockings or socks each day.

Jewelry, cosmetics, hair, and nails

- Wear only wedding bands.
- Wear a watch with a sweep second hand.

- Do not wear dangle earrings, bracelets, or pendants.
- Do not wear a lot of makeup.
- Do not wear perfumes, colognes, or after-shave lotions.
- Maintain a neat hairstyle that is easy to manage and off the face and neck.
- Keep your hair clean and free of heavy hairspray.
- Keep your fingernails short.
- Wear nail polish according to your agency's policy.
- Do not wear artificial nails, nail extenders, and so on

  For men:
  - Keep your beard and/or mustache, if worn, trimmed and clean.
  - Shave daily.

Daily hygiene
- Bathe each day.
- Apply underarm deodorant or antiperspirant immediately after bathing.
- Brush your teeth before coming to work and, if possible, after each meal.
- Use mouthwash as directed by your dentist.
- Avoid foods that produce bad breath (e.g., garlic, onions).
- Keep your teeth in good repair; see your dentist regularly.
- Avoid smoking before client care (if you must smoke) because this produces an offensive odor.

Acting Professional

Healthy habits and a positive attitude are keys to acting in a professional manner. As a member of the home care team, you show that you have good personal habits and a positive attitude about yourself and others. The client and family will look to you as an example of the right kind of personal health care practices. You are a role model.

Maintaining Healthy Habits. The proper balance of food, exercise, and rest is an important factor in keeping healthy.

Food. Eating the right kinds of food in the right amounts provides the body the energy needed to function well. Without proper nutrition, you will not have the energy or stamina to correctly perform your duties. Information about daily food requirements is found in Chapter 10.

Exercise. Your job will require lifting and moving clients. It is important that your muscles and joints are in good working order. Your doctor is the best person to offer advice about a daily exercise program. Almost everyone can benefit from rapid walking three times a week for 20 minutes. This exercises the long muscles, stimulates the heart and lungs, and promotes restful sleep.

Rest. The body needs rest to work efficiently. Make sure you get enough sleep. Being tired can cause you to make errors resulting in injury to your client.

Hazards to Health

Listed below are three habits that are bad for your body and promote illness.

Smoking. There is nothing positive that can be said about the use of tobacco in any form. Smoking or chewing tobacco—or inhaling snuff—is very harmful to the body's tissues. It can cause cancer of the lung, lip, tongue, mouth, and throat. Secondhand smoke causes the same effects in the nonsmoker. Your agency prohibits smoking while on duty. If you smoke on your off-duty hours, others can smell the odor of smoke. It gets into your hair and clothing. It is often offensive to nonsmokers. For the sake of yourself and others, DO NOT USE TOBACCO.

Alcohol. Alcohol is the most popular and most often abused drug. Even a little alcohol—one drink—can dull the senses. It can reduce judgment and limit the ability to function efficiently. Reporting to work under the influence of alcohol or drinking on the job are causes for immediate dismissal. DO NOT RISK YOUR CAREER AND YOUR LIFE BY ABUSING ALCOHOL.

Drug or Substance Abuse. Drug abuse is a serious medical and social problem. Many people are destroyed by abusing legal and illegal drugs. As a home care aide, you may be caring for a client who is taking drugs prescribed by the doctor. These drugs are for the client's use ONLY. You must never take a drug that has not been prescribed for you. Do not share your prescription drugs with another person.

Reporting to work while abusing legal or illegal drugs may also result in immediate dismissal. Your abuse of drugs impairs your ability to provide safe, competent care. You may be charged and convicted of drug abuse. This results in loss of certification and loss of any future employment in a health career. DO NOT RISK YOUR CAREER AND YOUR LIFE BY ABUSING DRUGS.

More information about drug abuse is found in Chapter 21.

Having a Positive Attitude. In your experiences of life, you have met people who are friendly, willing to help, and genuinely concerned about you. Their behavior shows that they are worthy of your trust. They demonstrate positive attitudes about themselves and others. You have also met those who do not have these qualities. These people have negative attitudes that show, by their behaviors, that they are not friendly, caring, or concerned about you. Actions do speak louder than words!

As a home care aide, your positive attitude will show in the following behaviors (Figure 2-6).

- Arriving on time, ready to work
- Being cheerful—smiling

Confident

Dependable

Cheerful

Knows Limitations

Skillfull/Competent

Enthusiastic

Well Groomed

Cooperative

Follows Agency Rules

Respectful

Courteous

Honest

Kind/Caring

Flexible

Fig 2-6 Qualities of a successful home care aide.

- Being aware of your client's and family's needs, likes, and dislikes
- Being willing to adjust your routine to meet their needs
- Being able to understand another point of view
- Being able to accept others' behaviors that may not be familiar to you

Being Concerned for Others

As a home care aide, you are not only concerned about your client's welfare, but also for your agency, client's family, and others. Listed below are important points that show this concern.

- Call your agency if you will be late or absent.
- Do not make personal telephone calls or send text messages from your client's home.
- Do not give your home or cell phone number to the client.
- Leave your personal problems at home.
- Refer questions about the tasks you perform to your supervisor.
- Do not make private arrangements with your client for service.
- Respect the privacy of your client and the family members.
- Do not sit down and watch television.
- Keep information you receive about client and family matters confidential.
- Do not play the client's radio or use your own electronic device with earphones.
- Do not bring others, including children, to the client's home.
- Do not encourage familiarity with your client or the family members.
- Do not get personally involved with your client, the family, or neighbors.
- Do not drive the client in any car—yours or theirs—without agency permission.
- Keep yourself busy elsewhere in the home when visitors arrive.
- Do not expect or accept tips.
- Do not lend or borrow money.
- Do not purchase items from the client or sell anything to the client.
- Treat others as you would want them to treat you.
- Remember, you are a guest in your client's home.

PERFORMING YOUR DUTIES PROPERLY

Your training program will prepare you to provide safe, competent care to your clients. As a home care aide, you will perform activities under the direction of a nurse supervisor. Your responsibilities will involve care of your client and the home environment. DO NOT PERFORM ANY PROCEDURES THAT YOU HAVE NOT BEEN TAUGHT. DO NOT PERFORM ANY DUTIES THAT YOUR SUPERVISOR HAS NOT LISTED IN THE CARE PLAN.

The following are examples of some of the duties you will learn to perform:

Care of the Client
Assisting with bathing
Assisting with personal grooming
Assisting with dressing
Helping with feeding
Assisting with walking
Collecting specimens
Recording and reporting information

Care of the Client's Home Environment
Maintaining a clean home
Performing light housekeeping tasks
Assisting with meal preparation

Preparing meals
Laundering the client's clothes
Purchasing food
Cleaning equipment

WORKING AS PART OF THE TEAM

The team is only as good as each of its members. Most of the time, you will be working alone in the client's home; therefore, you are the team's representative. How you work with the client and family will tell them how well the team functions. Your attitude and behavior are very important in giving a positive impression of the home care team. Remember, you play a vital role on the team.

SCOPE OF PRACTICE

As you work in home care, you will be faced with decisions about what is right and what is wrong, about what is correct behavior and what is not. Many times, you will need to decide what you can do and what you cannot do—you must determine the behavior that is appropriate for you within the scope of your education.

Regulations regarding the responsibilities and limitations of the home care aide are established and enforced by an agency of the state government. It may be the Department of Health, the Board of Nursing, or the Department of Consumer Affairs—it will vary from state to state. These agencies carefully define the scope of practice (what you are permitted to do for clients AND what you are not permitted to do) for home care aides. You will learn the responsibilities and limitations specific to home care aides in your state as a part of your training program.

As a home care aide, you are legally responsible (liable) for your actions at all times. What you do can lead to a lawsuit if others are injured or harmed. At times, you may be directed to do something that is not within the scope of your responsibility. Your supervisor may tell you that it is "OK" to do what is asked because he or she will assume the responsibility. If something goes wrong, your supervisor may indeed be held responsible, but you will not be relieved of any personal liability. Families, too, may ask you to do something that is outside of your scope of practice. They will tell you that it is "OK" for you to perform an act that you know is not permitted. REMEMBER, YOU ARE ALWAYS LIABLE FOR YOUR OWN ACTIONS AT ALL TIMES—NO MATTER WHAT ANYONE MAY TELL YOU. Do only what you are permitted to do according to the regulations that govern home care aides and your agency policy.

CHAPTER SUMMARY

- Home care is an important health care industry.
- Many types of clients are served, from the very young to the very old.
- Most people prefer to be cared for in their own homes.
- Home care is less expensive than hospital care.
- Several types of agencies provide home care; these services are paid through state and federal programs, private insurance, and clients and their families.
- The case manager of the agency coordinates the services and activities of the home care team.
- You, the home care aide, are an important member of the team.
- The agency, your client, and family members expect you to look and act professional. They expect you to perform your duties properly and work as part of the team.

STUDY QUESTIONS

1. List three benefits of home care.
2. Describe four types of clients who receive home care.
3. How do clients pay for home care?
4. List five duties and responsibilities of a home care aide.
5. Describe three services that are available in your community to assist clients at home.
6. Identify the home care team member who performs the following activities:
   a. Teaches crutch walking
   b. Provides breathing treatments
   c. Coordinates the activities of the home care team
   d. Provides spiritual consolation
   e. Helps the family with finances
7. List six qualities you must have to be a good team member and a successful home care aide.

Developing Effective Communication Skills

OBJECTIVES

After you read this chapter, you will be able to:

1. Define communication.
2. Explain the importance of clear communication in home care.
3. Describe the types of communication.
4. Identify three barriers to effective communication.
5. List five ways to improve listening skills.
6. Use guidelines for good communication with others.
7. Explain the rights and responsibilities of both client and agency.
8. Demonstrate three methods for effective communication with visually-impaired and hearing-impaired clients.
9. Describe the role ethics plays in communicating with the home care team, your client, and the family.

KEY TERMS

Advance directive Document that indicates a client's wishes about health care

Bias(es) To like or dislike someone or something without a good reason; prejudice

Communication Sharing of thoughts, information, and opinions with others

Confidentiality Something written or spoken in confidence; in secret (in private)

Disability Physical, mental, or emotional condition that interferes with abilities to carry out activities of daily living

Ethics Code of behavior or conduct

Grievance A wrong, considered as grounds for a formal complaint

Nonverbal communication Communication without the use of words

Prejudice Having or forming a preconceived judgment or opinion without fair reasons

Surrogate One who is appointed to act for another

Verbal communication Communication using the spoken or written word

Communication is the sharing of thoughts, information, and opinions with others. This may be done from one person to another on a face-to-face basis, or it may be done in a group setting, such as a teacher and a class of students. Other times, communication occurs through books, newspapers, television, radio, telephone, music, movies, art, sign language, and computer. All around us there is a constant demand for our attention, a constant wish to communicate with us.

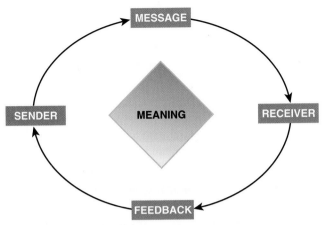

Fig 3-1 The four parts of communication.

Fig 3-2 Talking (verbal communication) and touch (nonverbal communication) are part of this family visit.

COMMUNICATION PROCESS

The process of communication involves four parts: a sender and a receiver, the message, and feedback (Figure 3-1). The sender is the person who begins the communication—the first speaker. The receiver is the person to whom the message is sent. The message is the actual expression of the thought, information, or opinion. Feedback is the return of information from the receiver to the sender. Feedback is used to tell whether the communication was successful.

EXAMPLE

a. Sender: Rosina Chavez, home care aide
b. Receiver: Mrs. Stevens, client
c. Message: "Goodbye, I'll be back tomorrow at the same time. Please sign my time sheet."
   Meaning: The home care aide is finished working for the day and will return tomorrow at the agreed-on time.
d. Feedback: Mrs. Stevens says, "Thank you. I'll see you tomorrow," and signs Rosina's time sheet.

IMPORTANCE

IN HOME CARE, COMMUNICATION IS THE LINK BETWEEN YOU, THE CLIENT, AND THE AGENCY. YOU HAVE TO BE CERTAIN THAT YOUR MESSAGE HAS BEEN RECEIVED AND UNDERSTOOD EXACTLY AS YOU MEANT IT TO BE RECEIVED. That is why feedback is an important part of the process. We must be able to say what we mean clearly and without confusion. By sharing accurate information and observations with the home care team, the aide helps the client receive better care.

TYPES OF COMMUNICATION

There are many methods of communication, such as radio, TV, telephone, books, and others. But all of these can be placed into one of two classifications: verbal communication or nonverbal communication (Figure 3-2).

VERBAL COMMUNICATION

COMMUNICATION USING THE SPOKEN OR WRITTEN WORD IS KNOWN AS VERBAL COMMUNICATION. WE ARE MOST FAMILIAR WITH SPEAKING; WE DO IT ALL THE TIME. COMMUNICATING WITH CLIENTS IS NOT THE SAME AS A CASUAL CONVERSATION WITH FRIENDS; IT IS AN IMPORTANT PART OF HEALTH CARE. USE SIMPLE WORDS AND SPEAK CLEARLY AND A LITTLE MORE SLOWLY THAN IN EVERYDAY CONVERSATION. DO NOT USE "SLANG" WORDS. REMEMBER THAT THE TONE OF YOUR VOICE AND YOUR EXPRESSION CAN AFFECT THE MEANING OF THE MESSAGE. The words "good morning" do not change when you say them, but their meaning may change depending on how you use your voice to say those words.

Written communication is usually considered a part of verbal communication because words are included. Written communication is discussed in Chapter 6. A few general rules apply to written messages. They must be legible, spelling must be correct, and the information must be accurate.

NONVERBAL COMMUNICATION

Nonverbal communication is the exchange of information without words (Figure 3-3). Both positive and negative messages may be sent even when nothing is said. In fact, sometimes saying nothing (silence) can become the message. Silence can be positive, as a hug, or it can be negative, as when angry people do not speak to each other.

Fig 3-3 Young people know the meaning without using words.

Other examples of nonverbal communication include personal appearance, facial expression, gestures, posture, types of food we eat, and the way we eat our meals. All of these combine to send powerful messages to others. Also, many of these are determined by cultural background—our own and our client's.

When verbal and nonverbal communications are combined, the sender can emphasize a point and make the message clearer. For example, the aide holds the time sheet and a pen while asking the client to sign it. Sometimes, combining verbal and nonverbal communication can be confusing when the words tell you one thing but the actions tell you another. For example, it is hard to believe a client who tells you that everything is "okay" and is sobbing into a tissue at the same time. Two different messages are being sent. It is up to you to find out which is correct.

BARRIERS TO COMMUNICATION

Barriers or blocks to communication occur when something acts as a wall between one or more of the four parts of communication. Then the message just cannot get through. There are many barriers to communication. The more common ones are discussed in this section.

BIAS AND PREJUDICE

Preconceived ideas, biases, prejudice, "mind already made up," "only one way to do it"—these are clearly barriers to communication. When all we see is a person's color, age, sex, or disability, we are unable to accept that person's ideas, opinions, or thoughts. Sex bias is often a problem. Male home care aides may be asked why they are doing a "woman's job." Clients sometimes wonder out loud how "such a tiny little girl" is going to be able to get grandpa out of bed. You can remind people that, in health care, there are no jobs reserved for men or women. Also, you can let your client's family know (in a respectful manner) that you have learned the skills of the job. Once the client and family get to know you as a competent, caring aide, they will come to rely on your assistance and forget their initial preconceived ideas. We have closed the door to communication when we fail to see each person as an individual of worth.

We all have some preconceived ideas, biases, and prejudices. Be aware of them. Then, set them aside to provide client care. When clients request and receive care from an agency, they also agree to put aside bias and prejudice to receive the care they need at home.

LANGUAGE, CULTURE, AND ETHNIC DIVERSITY

The population of the United States is made up of people from all over the world. You may work in homes where the culture is quite different from yours (Figure 3-4). The approach to sickness, healing, death, dying, and religious consolation may be unfamiliar to you. Perhaps no one in the household speaks English or any other language that you know. The ideal situation would be to have a home care aide of the same culture in the home, but this is not always possible. The next best thing to do is to find a person who can help you. Discuss the situation with your supervisor, who can assist you in finding a neighbor, friend, or another relative who will act as an interpreter. Also, try to learn as much about that culture as possible; it will enrich your life and help you become a more sensitive caregiver (Table 3-1).

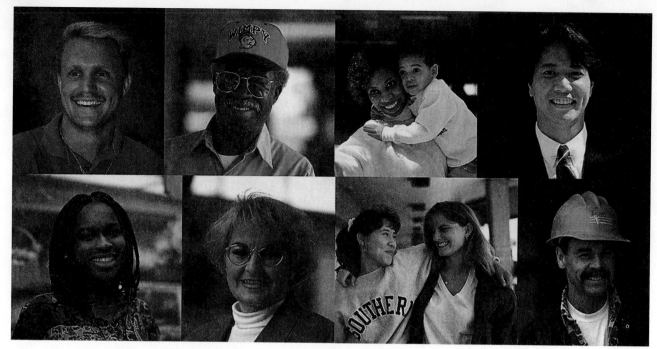

Fig 3-4 Ethnic and cultural diversity makes home care challenging and rewarding.

TABLE 3-1	Understanding Other Cultures
BEHAVIOR	**CULTURE**
Eye contact	Many people of Haitian and Asian backgrounds believe that having direct eye contact is a sign of disrespect.
	African Americans prefer direct eye contact.
Displaying emotion	Northern Europeans, Russians, and Asians usually do not show strangers emotions of grief, anger, or sadness.
	Latinos, Arabs, and African Americans tend to show their emotions more openly.
Handshake	Most cultures prefer firm handshakes.
	Native Americans prefer a light handshake.
	In some cultures, handshakes between men and women are inappropriate.
Privacy	Most people need privacy during toileting and bathing.
	Most cultures prefer physical examinations by members of the same sex.
	People of the Islamic faith need privacy during prayer times (at least five times a day).
Pain	Showing signs of pain to strangers is unacceptable to people from Japan.
	Those of English, German, and Irish backgrounds often "grin and bear" the pain instead of talking about it.
	In other cultures, people are very verbal in expressing pain—sometimes moaning and screaming.

SEXUAL HARASSMENT

Unfortunately, you may work in a home where the client or family member may demand sexual favors from you. Even though you perform your duties in a professional manner and in no way indicate any romantic interest in this person, the harasser will not stop bothering you and may become sexually aggressive. This is a situation in

Fig 3-5 Communication devices make it possible for disabled persons to reach out to those around them. (Courtesy of Enabling Devices/Toys for Special Children, Hastings, NY.)

which no effective communication is occurring, and it is a situation that is unsafe for you. No employer expects you to work under these conditions. Report the situation to your supervisor immediately.

ILLNESS, PAIN, AND MEDICATIONS

It is hard to communicate clearly when one is sick. All of your client's energy and attention may be focused on the illness and getting well. Sometimes clients are too weak or too sick to talk. Quiet, nonverbal communication and asking questions that can be answered with one word may be appropriate. Some illnesses cause an inability to speak, hear, or understand on a temporary or permanent basis. See Chapters 7 and 22 for details on working with ill people.

DISABILITIES

Certain disabilities, such as blindness, deafness, aphasia (the inability to speak), and brain damage, can create barriers to communication. See Chapter 7 for more details on disabilities. Individuals with disabilities may communicate by using hand signals and eye movements. Sometimes clients use special devices to communicate, such as computers or pointers (Figure 3-5). You will need to adjust to your client's special needs. If you are having trouble communicating, see if the family can help you. Discuss any communication problems with your supervisor.

COMMUNICATING WITH AGENCY PERSONNEL

AS THE EYES AND EARS OF THE TEAM, YOU WILL BE EXPECTED TO REPORT ANY PROBLEMS OR CHANGES TO YOUR SUPERVISOR.

Report what you observe with your senses.
- Eyes: What you see
- Nose: What you smell
- Ears: What you hear
- Touch: What you feel

DO NOT REPORT WHAT YOU THINK HAPPENED OR YOU THOUGHT YOU SAW. BE FACTUAL. GIVE YOUR SUPERVISOR THE FACTS, NOT YOUR OPINIONS (Box 3-1).

> **BOX 3-1   Report to Your Supervisor**
>
> Some things to report to your supervisor:
> - A change in the client's physical condition
> - A change in the client's emotional or mental condition
> - Signs of injury, neglect, or abuse (see Chapters 19, 20, and 21)
> - A change in the home environment that may be hazardous for the client and family
> - You do not understand a procedure or task
> - Problems with medications
> - You are unsure of how to proceed with your assignment
> - The client/family asks you to do something that is not your responsibility
> - You feel unsafe in the client's home
> - The client tells you things that concern you

COMMUNICATING WITH YOUR CLIENT AND FAMILY MEMBERS

RESPECT FOR THE CLIENT AND FAMILY

Effective communication starts with the following basic principle: respect for the client and family as human beings. Each person, the sender of the message and the receiver, brings with him or her characteristics that are unique. Physical, emotional, mental, social, and spiritual aspects make up who we are. Try to accept each individual as a person of worth. Listen to what they have to say. Be respectful. Do not "write off" what another person has to say as meaningless and not worth listening to.

LISTENING

LISTENING IS AN ESSENTIAL PART OF THE COMMUNICATION PROCESS. The message being sent is much like a football that must be caught for a pass to be completed. So, too, the message must be caught (received) and understood for effective communication to take place. Good listening is essential to receiving and understanding the message being sent.

GOOD LISTENING INVOLVES THE USE OF EYES, EARS, AND FEELINGS. IT TAKES ENERGY, CONCENTRATION, AND EFFORT TO BE A GOOD LISTENER. The first step in developing and/or improving listening skills is to decide that you want to become a better listener. This means that you will devote your full attention to the other person (the speaker [the sender]). It is difficult to be a listener. The following are some suggestions to improve listening skills.

1. Be quiet. Pay attention to what the other person is saying.
2. Stop all other activities. Focus on the speaker.
3. Listen to the entire message.
4. Do not interrupt the speaker. Let the speaker finish, even if it takes a long time.
5. Do not try to think of a response while another is speaking.
6. Keep confidences. Keep private matters private unless the information shared is essential for client care, health, or well-being.
7. Practice listening skills (Box 3-2).

A LEARNED SKILL

Communication is a skill that improves with practice. As your skill increases, you will be able to speak more clearly and to send and receive more accurate messages. You will also be more sensitive to the nonverbal messages you are sending and receiving from the client and family.

BOX 3-2   Listening Skills

- Concentrate; LISTENING IS HARD WORK.
- Take time to listen.
- Be patient; let the sender complete the message, even if it takes a lot of time.
- Do not interrupt; let the speaker finish.
- Get feedback; give feedback.
- If you do not understand, do not let the person continue; say, "Would you please tell me again? I do not understand what you just said."
- Observe body language and facial expression.
- Listen to the tone of the sender's voice.
- Do not think about how you will respond before the person has finished talking; use quiet time to mentally summarize main ideas.
- Focus your attention on what is being said, not on what you will say later.
- Show interest, and use nonverbal communication to demonstrate your interest.
- Give the speaker your full attention. Sit with the client, when possible, to encourage him or her to talk.
- Listen for feelings.
- Ask questions that will encourage the speaker to continue.
- Do not be afraid of silence; observe, ask the client to tell you more, and ask the client how he or she feels about what he or she is discussing.
- Do not finish sentences that the speaker begins.
- Do not jump to conclusions by assuming that you know exactly what your client means.
- Be aware of your own feelings and point of view.
- Listen with an open mind; try to hear everything, not just what you want to hear; avoid selective hearing.

Rosina comes to Mrs. Stevens' house to weigh her and to record and report the findings. She talks with Mrs. Stevens to see how things are going. There are many verbal communication techniques, but a few will be used more often than others. Five examples follow.

1. Use open-ended questions that may be answered with an explanation, instead of closed questions that can only be answered by a "yes" or "no" response.
   Closed question:
   Rosina: "Did you eat all of your breakfast?"
   Mrs. Stevens: "No."
   Open-ended question:
   Rosina: "What did you eat for breakfast?"
   Mrs. Stevens: "Nothing. I was too sick to eat."
2. Restate the message to let the client know you heard what is being said. This encourages further communication.
   Rosina: "You were sick this morning and didn't eat any breakfast."
   Mrs. Stevens: "That's right. After I took my pain pill, I felt like I was going to throw up, so I didn't have anything to eat."
3. Ask for clarification so the message can be clearly understood.
   Rosina: "I am not sure I understand. You say that after you took your pain medicine, you were too sick to eat breakfast and you felt like you were going to throw up?"
   Mrs. Stevens: "Yes. Every time I take that darned medicine, it makes me feel like throwing up. That's why I hate to take it, even though it eases the pain."
4. Summarize what you have been hearing.
   Rosina: "This sounds like a problem to me."
   Mrs. Stevens: "It sure is. I've been putting up with it for a week."

BOX 3-3   **Communication Guidelines**

- Introduce yourself on the first visit to the client's home.
- Find out the name your client prefers to be called.
- Reduce the amount of background noise (turn off the television, radio), if possible.
- Get the client's attention, face the client, and make eye contact (unless this is culturally inappropriate).
- Think about what you will say; organize your thoughts.
- Show interest.
- Explain procedures.
- Use nonverbal communication—a touch on the shoulder, a smile, or hold the client's hand.
- Be polite, courteous, respectful, and considerate.
- Do not talk down to the client.
- Avoid words that may have another meaning.
- Do not use slang, obscene words, or gestures.
- Do not discuss religion, politics, or sex.
- Dirty jokes and sarcastic humor are inappropriate.
- Learn the meaning of new words you hear and that the client may use.
- Let the client finish what is being said.
- Be a good listener.
- Say what you mean.
- Use family and/or friends to translate when necessary.
- Use a normal tone of voice—DO NOT SHOUT.
- Speak slowly.
- Speak clearly and distinctly.
- Use words that both you and your client or family member understand.
- Avoid the use of technical or medical terms.
- Use as few words as necessary to convey the message—BE CONCISE.
- Do not mumble or whisper.
- Listen to the client's feedback; ask the client to repeat what you said, so you can determine the effectiveness of the communication.
- If you do not understand what your client has said, say so; do not be afraid to say, "I don't understand what you are telling me." Or restate, "Are you telling me …?"
- Smile; use your sense of humor.
- Practice, practice, practice using these guidelines.
  With your family
  With your friends
  With your classmates

---

5. Share information with the client.

Rosina: "I'm going to call my supervisor about this. Maybe there is something that can be done to take care of this problem. What do you think about that?"

Mrs. Stevens: "Sounds good to me. I hope I don't have to put up with this much longer."

Practice these techniques with your friends and family. Box 3-3 contains a list of guidelines to enhance communication.

COMMUNICATING WITH HEARING-IMPAIRED CLIENTS

In addition to their illnesses, many of your clients or their family members experience difficulty in hearing. Some wear hearing aids; others do not. Communicating with the hearing impaired is a challenge for members of the home care team. The client's record should show what methods team members use to communicate successfully. If you find a technique that works for you, record it so that others can use it, too. In addition to the guidelines outlined in Box 3-3, the following are suggestions for communicating with the hearing impaired.

- Reduce background noise of household appliances (e.g., fans, dishwasher, television, radio).
- Be sure your face is clearly visible; this will help those who lip-read.
- Lower the tone of your voice.
- Do not exaggerate your speech by mouthing the words.
- Introduce the topic, and use a visual aid, if possible.
- Use short, simple sentences.
- Rephrase the sentence if it is not understood.
- Pause before changing the topic.
- Keep a pad and pencil ready so that the person can communicate in writing, if possible.
- Try to speak to the side where better hearing occurs, if known.
- Be patient; show by your body language that you are supportive.

COMMUNICATING WITH VISUALLY-IMPAIRED CLIENTS

If your client is visually impaired, the following tips will help you to communicate more effectively.

- Provide adequate light.
- Check glasses, if worn, to be sure they are clean, are in good repair, and fit properly.
- Reduce glare from exposed light bulbs or waxed floors.
- Provide aids to communication, such as magnifying glasses.
- Stand directly in front of the client when communicating; side vision may be poor.
- Say the person's name before you start the conversation.
- Speak in a normal tone of voice.
- Touch the client on the hand or shoulder to get and keep attention.

PROTECTING PERSONAL HEALTH INFORMATION

In 1996, the federal government issued national standards to protect the use and disclosure of an individual's personal health information (Health Insurance Portability and Accountability Act; HIPAA). It also set standards for people to understand their rights to privacy of health information and to control how this information is to be used by health care agencies. The goal is to assure that a person's health information is properly protected while allowing the use of this information by health care agencies that is necessary to provide high-quality health care. Home care agencies and their employees are required to adhere to HIPAA regulations. Your employer will explain how these regulations apply to you. Each client will receive a copy of the HIPAA policies.

THE CLIENT'S BILL OF RIGHTS

This document explains the rights and responsibilities of the client (Table 3-2). If the client cannot understand the information, a representative (family member or surrogate) acts for the client.

TABLE 3-2   The Client's Bill of Rights

CLIENT'S RIGHTS	CLIENT'S RESPONSIBILITIES
AGENCY STAFF	
Receive care without regard to race, color, national origin, religion, age, or disability.	Accept agency staff without regard to race, color, national origin, religion, age, or disability.
Be treated with respect and dignity by agency staff.	Be considerate and respectful of agency staff.
Receive information about the types of team members who will provide care and the number of visits to be made.	Notify the agency when an appointment cannot be kept.
Obtain the name of the supervisor and the agency telephone number.	Notify the agency of any problems or dissatisfaction with care.
Request a change in staff to provide home care.	Notify, in advance, of intention to terminate the agency's services.
Receive advance notice of transfer or discharge.	
CLIENT'S PROPERTY	
Have property treated with respect and consideration.	Store valuables in a safe place.
	Provide a safe home environment where care can be given.
CARRYING OUT THE PLAN OF CARE	
Be fully informed, in writing and in advance, about the care and treatment to be given. This includes any changes in care or treatment.	Remain under a doctor's care while receiving services of the agency.
	Provide the agency with an accurate and complete health history.
Participate in developing and revising the plan of care or service.	Sign required release and consent forms.
Be fully informed about the expected plan of care or service.	Participate in developing and revising the plan of care or service.
Refuse treatment, medication, or other services.	Cooperate with your doctor and agency staff.
Be fully informed about the expected outcomes of refusing treatment, medications, or other services.	Notify the agency when changing doctors.
Accept the results that come from refusing treatment, medication, or other services.	
Be informed about completing an **advance directive**.	Provide a copy of the advance directive, if it exists.
PAYMENT FOR SERVICES	
Know, ahead of time, charges for services and payment policies, if responsible for payment.	Provide agency with all requested financial and insurance records.
Be informed, in advance, about any changes in service charges or payment policies.	Pay for services according to plan for payment.
	Notify the agency when changing insurance.
OTHER	
Receive a copy of the agency's policies and procedures.	Follow the procedures outlined.
Be informed about the agency's procedure to voice **grievances** about care or lack of respect, without fear of harmful results.	Follow the grievance procedure in a timely manner.
Be assured of **confidentiality** of all records and information related to care, including financial records.	
Be informed about the name, address, and telephone number of the state agency that regulates home care.	File a complaint with the state agency, if necessary.

There are two parts: (1) what the client has a right to expect from the agency and its members and (2) what action the client agrees to take.

A copy of the document is given to the client and family by the agency. It is reviewed with them, and questions about the statements are explained.

CODE OF BEHAVIOR

Each profession has a code of behavior to follow. This code of behavior is called ethics. Ethics are standards to follow in your behavior toward others. The way you act and react to others also has an effect on you. You have chosen to be a home care aide because you like people and want to give them the kind of care you would want to receive. By setting high standards of conduct for yourself, you are contributing to quality home care services for clients.

Home care agencies have policy and procedure manuals that include the code of behavior expected for each employee in performing day-to-day activities on the job. Your agency also has a Client's Bill of Rights similar to the one shown in Table 3-2. It contains standards of behavior for the home care team to follow.

During your orientation to the agency, supervisory staff will discuss the ethical behavior expected of all of its employees. Some important behaviors include confidentiality and honesty. Behaviors to avoid will also be discussed.

CONFIDENTIALITY

While having dinner at home with her husband, Rosina says that she had another client assigned to her today. "My client lives on a small farm outside of town. It was great to see the baby calves in the field as I was driving up the road." Her husband says, "It must be good to get out of town and see the country, but, can't someone else, who lives closer, be given this assignment? What's wrong with this person, anyway?" "Oh, honey, you know that I never discuss my clients' conditions—they're confidential. Besides, I'm really looking forward to this assignment. My supervisor, Mrs. Quick, trusts me to do the job," says Rosina.

As a home care professional, you will receive information about the client and family that is to be treated as private or confidential. You will also observe situations in the home that must be shared only with your supervisor during meetings of the home care team. YOU SHOW YOUR RESPECT FOR THE CLIENT AND FAMILY BY NOT DISCUSSING ANY INFORMATION RELATED TO THE WORK ASSIGNMENT WITH YOUR OWN FAMILY, FRIENDS, OR OTHER CLIENTS. THIS IS FORBIDDEN BY FEDERAL LAW. INFORMATION YOU OBTAIN BY READING THE CLIENT'S CARE RECORD MUST ALSO BE KEPT CONFIDENTIAL.

Failure to keep information confidential is unprofessional behavior. This includes sharing information with others through social networking, such as Facebook and Twitter. You risk losing your job, your certification, and the opportunity for any future employment in the health care field.

HONESTY

You will experience situations in the home in which the client or family member may ask you to give them information about the client's condition that you know you are not allowed to give. Be honest. Do not lie by saying, "I don't know." This may give the impression that you do not know what you are doing. Tell the truth; say, "I really can't answer that question, but I'll ask my supervisor to contact you." Be honest with your client and family at all times. If you do not know the answer to a question, say so. Remember, you are not expected to know all of the answers all of the time. Your response may be, "I don't know, but I'll discuss it with my supervisor and get back to you." If you say this, make sure to do what you said you would do. By your actions, you are telling others that you are honest and reliable.

BEHAVIORS TO AVOID

Six behaviors to avoid when communicating with your client and family are as follows:
1. Giving advice
2. Making judgments
3. Giving false reassurances about your client's physical or emotional condition
4. Focusing on yourself
5. Discussing your own problems and concerns
6. Discussing topics that are controversial, such as religion and politics
   Other things to avoid are accepting gifts or tips. Do not smoke or drink alcohol "on the job," even with your clients. You should not eat your client's food or eat your lunch in their home unless you have a "live-in" job that was arranged through your agency.
   Clients may ask you to do things that are not permitted, such as the following examples.
- "Pick up a six-pack of beer for me on the way over here next time. I'll pay you back when you come on Wednesday."
- "Come back from 4 to 6 PM and make my dinner. I'll pay you more per hour than your agency. They don't need to know anything about this, you know; we'll have a private arrangement."
- "Oh, yes, take home a piece of jewelry. You are so nice to me. I feel like you are a member of my family. I want you to have something special from me."
- "Here, would you like to buy this television? You can have it cheap."
   These requests must be refused for several reasons.
1. You are not permitted to use your own money for clients. When shopping for a client, you may purchase items according to the care plan. If alcohol or tobacco is on the shopping list, obtain an "OK" from your supervisor before buying these items.
2. When you "come back" or work for the client "privately," you do not have the backing of the home care team. You stand alone and accept all the responsibility if something goes wrong and you or the client are harmed or injured. Some state regulating agencies forbid home care aides to practice privately. They must be employed by an agency and work in the client's home under the supervision of a nurse or therapist.
3. Many clients forget that they have given a gift or sold something to those working in their home. When they discover a "missing" item, clients may accuse the home care aide of stealing that object.
   There may be a time when you would like to give your client a special gift for a birthday or a holiday. This is a wonderful idea, but it can be very expensive if you give something to every client. There are many gifts that you can give that do not cost anything, such as helping to write a letter; reading a story; giving a special manicure; helping clients to put on a special dress shirt and a tie; sitting and listening to stories of the "good old days"; and sharing a good joke, a hearty laugh, big smile, and a hug. Home care aides usually cannot afford to give gifts to clients, but they can give something even more special—a bit of their time, attention, and love.

CHAPTER SUMMARY

- Communication is an important skill for the home care aide to develop.
- Clear, accurate communication is necessary so that you can share information and ideas with the client, the family, and your agency.
- There are four parts to the communication process: the sender, the receiver, the message, and feedback.

- Many barriers interfere with clear communication, and there are special techniques to encourage effective communication with clients.
- Guides to ethical behavior are found in your agency's policies and procedures manual and the Client's Bill of Rights.

STUDY QUESTIONS

1. Define communication.
2. Draw and label a diagram showing the parts of the communication process.
3. List three reasons for clear communication.
4. Give three examples of verbal and nonverbal communication.
5. List three barriers to communication.
6. Demonstrate three ways to communicate with
   a. Hearing-impaired people
   b. Visually-impaired people
7. What would you do in the following situations?
   a. You meet several other home care aides at the local restaurant for lunch. They ask how your client is doing.
   b. Your client says that money is missing from her purse.
   c. The client asks you if he is going to die.
   d. You are caring for two senior citizens in the same apartment building. One client asks you what is wrong with her neighbor.
   e. Your client has several friends who visit regularly. They go into his room, lock the door, and stay for about an hour. You suspect that they are using illegal drugs.
   f. Your client is going to celebrate his 85th birthday. You want to give him a special gift.
8. Read your agency's Client's Bill of Rights. Identify the rights of the client and the rights of the agency. Identify the responsibilities of the client and the agency. Explain these in your own words.

Understanding Your Client's Needs

OBJECTIVES

After you read this chapter, you will be able to:

1. Discuss basic human needs.
2. Describe three types of families.
3. Explain the importance of the family in society.
4. Discuss the role of the home care aide in helping clients meet their needs.
5. List three principles of growth and development.
6. Discuss each stage of development, and identify three characteristics of each.
7. Identify three ways of meeting the client's needs in each developmental stage.

KEY TERMS

Basic need Requirement for survival
Peers People who are one's equals
Physiological Pertaining to the normal functioning of the body
Primary caregiver A person who provides most of the care early in one's life

Self-actualization State of reaching one's full potential and being able to cope with problems
Self-esteem Thinking and feeling good about yourself
Sibling A brother or sister

NEED—how often do we use that word? How many times have we said,
"What do we need from the market?"
"I need a new shirt."
"I need a car."
"I need a dress to wear to the wedding."
   Over and over, we use the word *need*. Most often, when we say *need*, we are talking about what we want rather than what we need.

BASIC HUMAN NEEDS

Just what, then, is meant by the term *need*? **Basic need** is defined as a requirement for survival. The psychologist Abraham Maslow described the basic human needs and used a pyramid shape to illustrate them (Figure 4-1). At the base of the pyramid is

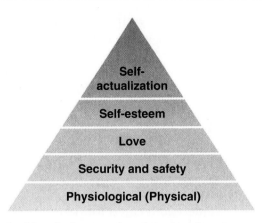

Fig 4-1 Basic needs as described by Abraham Maslow. (From Maslow AH, Frager RD, Fadiman J: Motivation and personality, ed 3. Reprinted by permission of Pearson Education, Upper Saddle River, NJ.)

listed physiological (or physical) needs. These needs must be met first before any of the others.

PHYSICAL NEEDS

Physical needs include the following:
1. Breathing/oxygen
2. Food/nutrition/water
3. Activity/rest/sleep
4. Elimination of body waste
5. Avoidance of pain
6. Personal hygiene
7. Sexuality

IT IS IMPORTANT TO BE AWARE OF THESE NEEDS BECAUSE THEY MUST BE TAKEN CARE OF BEFORE ANY OTHERS. A person cannot feel loved or give love if he or she is starving. If the most important need is food, then this need takes priority over all the others. Only after this physical need is met can other needs be met. When people cannot take care of their own basic needs for survival, others must help. For children, it is the primary caregiver—mother, father, grandparent—who meets their basic needs. For sick people, the family may provide for the basic needs. Many times, it is the home care aide who will provide for basic physical needs.

SAFETY AND SECURITY

Safety and security can be provided by
1. Accident prevention
2. Safe surroundings
3. Religion

Safety is a common concern for most people. "Is my neighborhood a safe place?" "How can fire be prevented?" "Is my seat belt buckled?" All of these questions concern safety. You, the home care aide, are responsible for the safety and security of the client, the client's belongings, and yourself. You will find that safety and accident prevention are stressed throughout the text.

Religion is a very personal set of beliefs, special to the client. As a part of the client's Bill of Rights, religious beliefs are respected. The aide's personal beliefs are just that—personal. What you believe is meaningful to you may not be helpful to clients in meeting their own needs. If necessary, your agency and/or the client's family may contact the appropriate clergy to assist your client.

LOVE

Love includes
1. Communication
2. Affection
3. Social relationships/friends/companions
4. Identity
5. Belonging and being cared for

We all need to feel loved, wanted, and cared for. We all need some relationship with others—even if it is only with one other person. For many lonely clients, the home care aide fulfills the client's need for love and belonging.

SELF-ESTEEM

Self-esteem includes thinking and feeling good about yourself. It also includes the feeling that others, too, think well of you. Self-esteem is not dependent upon a person's wealth, type of employment, or social contacts. It is an inner feeling of self-worth. While parents, relatives, friends, and coworkers may help encourage or hinder the building of a person's self-esteem, it is our own perception of self-worth that matters.

SELF-ACTUALIZATION

Maslow's fifth level of basic human needs is self-actualization. This is defined as the state of reaching your full potential and being able to cope with problems. Not everyone achieves self-actualization because the other needs, which are lower on the pyramid, have not been met.

How well needs are met affects our sense of well-being and our mental health. Most healthy adults are able to meet their own needs, along with the help of their family and friends.

THE FAMILY

In the past, the United States was primarily a farming society. Many people lived in rural areas, and the family took care of all their needs. Family members worked side by side to ensure their survival. Today, few American families live on farms or in rural areas. Most people are employed outside of the home, and, with the exception of family-owned businesses, family members usually do not work side by side.

THE CHANGING FAMILY

As society changed, families changed, too, but some things have remained constant. For example, most of us belong to a nuclear family—that family into which we were born or adopted. We also may belong to a family of procreation: the family we have started.

The word *family* has many meanings. Some are
• A group of people who are related and may or may not live under the same roof
• A group of people who live in the same home
• A circle of friends and relatives who love you
• A group of people who live together and share a past and a future

Fig 4-2 The changing family.

In addition to many definitions of the word *family*, there are several types of family structures. When you think of the word *family*, a certain image may come to mind. Do you "see" a mother, father, and two children? This is often thought of as the typical American family, the "intact family." But you may have had a different image come to mind—perhaps a widowed grandmother who is raising two young grandchildren. This, too, is an example of a family. In fact, there is NO typical family. There are so many varieties that it is hard to put them into categories; some examples of family patterns are found in Figure 4-2.

Families today are more mobile than in the past. Families who have lived in the same home in the same community for generations are the exception. Today, families may move "up" from a starter home or "down" into a retirement home. Some families are homeless, moving from shelter to shelter. Gone are the days when three generations routinely lived under one roof. The extended family (e.g., grandparents, aunts, uncles, cousins) is scattered all over the country and perhaps even all over the world.

IMPORTANCE IN SOCIETY

The family is the most important structure in society. Within this unit, children are born and reared. Here we learn to love, play, and express our feelings. Our culture and traditions are passed on from generation to generation. Families teach about manners, morals, religion, beliefs, prejudices, hates, and fears. Sometimes family members have so much anger and hate that they abuse themselves or others in the home. Further information about abuse is found in Chapters 19, 20, and 21.

Psychologists say that one person affects the lives of at least eight others for better or worse, and that each one of them will affect the lives of eight more. In other words, the family has a tremendous influence on its members and on society.

HELPING CLIENTS TO MEET THEIR NEEDS

Families continue to meet many of their own needs, but some organizations and agencies have been created to help when needed. For example, day care centers meet the needs of young children when their parents are at work or school. Home health agencies provide home care when families require help to care for sick members. Meals On

Wheels programs help homebound persons to have daily hot meals and good nutrition.

As the home care aide, you will follow the care plan established by the home care team to meet your client's individual needs. WHEN WORKING WITH A CLIENT, YOU MAY DISCOVER THAT HE OR SHE HAS ADDITIONAL UNMET NEEDS. NOTIFY YOUR SUPERVISOR WHEN YOU IDENTIFY UNMET CLIENT NEEDS. For example, your client tells you that she has not been able to sleep ever since she was discharged from the hospital 10 days ago. She is very tired and does not want to get out of bed. The care plan may be changed to meet the client's physical need for rest and sleep.

The family will also have needs, and, of course, you, too, have personal needs. However, your role is to care for the client. That is why you are in the home. The client's needs come first. Sometimes family members will ask you to take care of their needs, such as babysitting a grandchild at the same time you are supposed to be caring for the grandfather. If your responsibility is to assist the client with personal care, bathing, grooming, and dressing, how can you also supervise an active 2-year-old? Tell the family politely that the care of the sick person comes first. Also, report the situation to your supervisor, who can explain your role and responsibilities to the family members. If the family requires additional help, such as child day care, the agency may assist by making a referral.

When a person's needs are unmet, many difficult emotions arise, including anger, frustration, fear, and stress. Your client may have these feelings, which are quite common during illness (see Chapter 7). You may experience these feelings, too.

YOUR NEEDS VERSUS THE NEEDS OF YOUR CLIENT

As a home care aide, you will be prepared to recognize and meet the needs of your client. Your needs are important, too, and you must remember to take care of them. HOWEVER, WHEN YOU ARE AT WORK, TAKE GREAT CARE TO SEE THAT YOUR NEEDS DO NOT BECOME MORE IMPORTANT THAN THOSE OF YOUR CLIENT. Of course, there may be times when personal problems may make it difficult for you to give proper client care. If this happens, discuss the situation with your supervisor. Perhaps you need a day off or another assignment.

If your own needs are not being met, you will not be able to care for someone else. Sometimes a client may make you feel angry, frustrated, or resentful, but we all get those feelings from time to time. However, you must not forget the client's needs and focus on your own. Consider the following situations.

- Is it quicker, easier, and less messy to feed the client instead of letting him feed himself and gain some independence? Whose need is being met?
- It is a beautiful spring day, and you decide to take your client outside in the wheelchair. You really want her to go outside, but she does not want to go. She refuses to get into the wheelchair and is angry with you. Whose needs are being met? Are you angry and frustrated? Do you feel useless?
- Your client refuses to eat saying, "Why should I eat? I'm going to die anyway." You become frustrated and angry and feel guilty. Whose need is being met?

In each case, the need of the home care aide has become more important than the client's need. This can cause unpleasant emotions for you and the client. It is important to recognize these feelings and discuss them with your supervisor.

HOW WE GROW AND DEVELOP

Just as a knowledge of basic needs is important, so, too, is an understanding about how people grow and develop. Knowing what is normal for the various stages of development will help you understand how disease and illness are affecting your client. It will also help you modify your care based on the client's stage in the life cycle.

The five principles of growth and development are as follows.

PRINCIPLE 1

There are many factors that influence the way we grow and develop.

Genes

Our physical appearance is determined by genes, which are a part of our body cells. These genes, from our mother and father, contain codes that determine bone structure, facial features, and the color of eyes, hair, and skin. The statement, "You look just like your Grandma Burns," is true because of the physical characteristics inherited from the family. Genes also contain codes that transmit inherited (hereditary) diseases.

The Primary Caregiver

The person who assumes the major responsibility for care early in our lives plays a very important role in how we grow and develop. This person is called the *primary caregiver.* This is the one who provides for our basic human needs by bathing and feeding us, kissing and hugging us, and talking and playing with us.

In the nuclear family structure, the mother usually assumes the role of primary caregiver. In other families, the biological mother may give up the infant for adoption or get a job shortly after the infant's birth. In these situations, the primary caregiver may be the adoptive parent or the infant's father, grandmother, aunt, other relative, or guardian. Sometimes, the family will hire a person to act as the substitute mother or "nanny." In other situations, the "family" consists of the staff of the institution caring for an abandoned child.

There is no "typical caregiver" in today's society. The primary caregiver may be male or female, married or single, gay or lesbian, older or younger. He or she provides the physical, emotional, and social needs of the infant and child. How successful the caregiver is in meeting these needs has a great effect on the child's future. As we grow older, peers, teachers, other relatives, and friends contribute to our development, but it is the primary caregiver, early in our lives, who plays the critical role.

Nutrition

The quantity and quality of the food we eat certainly influence our growth and development. Even before birth, what the mother eats, drinks, and breathes has an effect on the unborn child. Poorly nourished infants and children are likely to grow and develop more slowly, be prone to illness, and have more infectious diseases.

The Environment

Where we live and with whom and what we receive and how we receive it affect our growth and development. The ideal environment
- Provides for the basic human needs of the person
- Reflects a loving and caring relationship among all family members
- Allows each member to make mistakes, to be corrected or disciplined with love, and to learn from mistakes

Fig 4-3 A loving environment is essential for all of us to grow.

- Permits each person to grow and develop as a unique human being
- Shows that members are accepted for who they are rather than what they can do for others

PRINCIPLE 2

What we experience early in life provides the basis for our growth and development in later years.

A well-nourished infant who receives love and affection in a caring environment has an excellent foundation for the next stage of growth and development. If, however, the infant is poorly nourished, physical growth will be seriously affected. If emotional nourishment—love and affection in a caring atmosphere—is absent or severely lacking, emotional and social growth and development will also be severely affected. A child who is loved learns to love and accept oneself and others, too (Figure 4-3).

PRINCIPLE 3

Growth occurs in a logical pattern.

Physical growth and development start at the head and progress to the feet. For example, an infant is first able to raise his or her head before learning to control the shoulders; he or she first learns to crawl and then to walk. This is called the "head to toe principle." Growth is also symmetrical, meaning that the right side of the body grows at the same rate as the left side. Even though the stages of growth and development are the same for everyone, each person grows at his or her own pace. For example, some infants are able to walk when they are 9 months old, whereas others may not be walking until they are 14 months old. Children will grow at different paces, even those in the same family. As an example, one child might be outgoing and talkative, whereas his or her sibling at the same age was quiet and subdued. In a large family, the youngest child may not begin to talk as early as the older children because needs are being met without having to speak. The rate at which a person grows and develops depends a great deal on the environment and the life experiences of that individual.

PRINCIPLE 4

We must complete one stage of growth and development before going on to the next.

As we grow and develop, we must first learn how to perform simple tasks before we can learn more difficult tasks. For example, Tommy must learn to walk before he can learn to run. Tamika must learn how to hold a pencil before she can learn how to write. Because each stage of growth and development builds on the skills learned in earlier stages, no stage can be skipped. For example, it is impossible for a child to skip the adolescent stage and go right to adulthood.

PRINCIPLE 5

Physical growth is usually completed at around 21 years of age, but we continue to grow emotionally, socially, and intellectually throughout our lives.

Bone growth stops at around 21 years of age, but our hair and nails continue to grow. New blood cells are produced as the old ones are destroyed. When injury occurs, new cells and tissues are produced so that healing can take place.

In each stage of growth and development listed here, there are tasks to be accomplished that help to make life meaningful and worthwhile. The experiences of life and how we respond to them influence the way we grow emotionally, socially, and intellectually. Although formal education in school may end at a certain time, we continue to expand our knowledge by communicating with others, reading, and learning from other experiences of everyday life. Growing socially, emotionally, and intellectually is a lifetime process.

STAGES OF NORMAL GROWTH AND DEVELOPMENT

Listed are the seven major stages of human growth and development, key characteristics of each stage, and some guides for meeting your client's needs during each stage. Additional information is found in Chapters 7, 10, 19, 20, and 22.

STAGE 1: INFANCY (TOTAL DEPENDENCY—LEARNING TO TRUST)
Age: Birth to 1 Year
Characteristics. The infant learns to survive outside the mother's uterus. The infant
- Triples birth weight
- Learns to control head
- Sits and grasps objects
- Learns to coordinate arms and legs by crawling
- Takes first step or even walks
- Develops the ability to speak first word and talk

Infancy is the period of the greatest growth and development of all stages (Figure 4-4).

Meeting the Infant's Needs. All of the infant's needs are provided by the caregiver. When caring for the infant, the home care aide
- Provides a safe environment to prevent injury
- Meets the infant's needs for food, sleep, and warmth
- Holds, cuddles, and talks to the infant
- Provides a "world" that is dependable, loving, comfortable, and consistent

The infant develops a sense of trust when this kind of environment exists.

STAGE 2: TODDLER (BEGINNING TO EXERT INDEPENDENCE—"MINE")
Age: 1 to 3 Years
Characteristics. This is a period of endless activity—getting into everything. The toddler
- Becomes more coordinated: walking, reaching, and eating
- Develops new skills: climbing and mastering basics of toilet training
- Does not understand danger; is accident prone as a result of curiosity

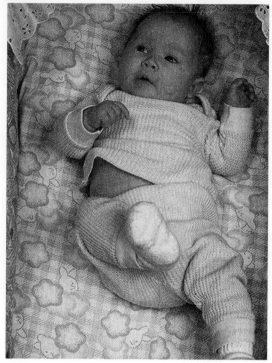

Fig 4-4 Infancy is a time of great growth and change.

Fig 4-5 Fear of separation from the primary caregiver is eventually overcome.

- Seeks attention and approval
- Has temper tantrums as a reaction to discipline, and develops self-will
- Plays alone, then plays alongside other children
  The toddler begins to tolerate separation from the caregiver (Figure 4-5).
  Meeting the Toddler's Needs. When caring for the toddler, the home care aide
- Maintains a safe environment by eliminating hazards
- Praises the toddler to reinforce safe behavior
- Is consistent when enforcing rules
- Sits down, if possible, when talking to the toddler
- Reinforces toilet training techniques provided by the primary caregiver
- Handles temper tantrums as discussed in Chapter 20

STAGE 3: PRESCHOOL (ENERGETIC AND CURIOUS—"WHY?")

Age: 3 to 5 Years
  Characteristics. This is a period of almost endless energy. The preschooler
- Has better control of complex muscular movements: running, jumping, and climbing
- Is eager to learn—always asking, "Why?"
- Imitates adults and other children
- May have imaginary playmates
- Learns to get along with more people
- Plays cooperatively with others
- Washes and dresses self
- Prints own name and draws pictures
- Becomes curious about sex differences
- Has rituals that are important, especially at bedtime
  The preschooler tolerates separation from the primary caregiver (Figure 4-6).

Fig 4-6 The preschooler is full of energy and eager to learn.

Meeting the Preschool Client's Needs. When caring for the preschool child, the home care aide

- Maintains the rules of conduct already set in the home
- Uses positive suggestions
- Avoids the use of "Don't"
- Is consistent and clear when describing acceptable behavior
- Answers questions truthfully
- Follows the ritual for nap time and bedtime

STAGE 4: SCHOOL (DECREASING DEPENDENCE ON FAMILY—LEARNING FROM SCHOOL AND PEERS)

Age: 6 to 12 Years

Characteristics. This is a period of slow but steady physical growth. At around 12 years of age, a rapid growth spurt indicates the transition to adolescence. The school-age child

- Is active and physically strong
- Enjoys being outdoors and playing with friends
- Participates in sport activities and has an attitude of fearlessness (is at risk for injuries)
- Moves out from family members to seek other relationships (the "gang" becomes important)
- Develops basic skills: reading, writing, and mathematics
- Likes to solve problems; likes challenges

Meeting the School-Age Client's Needs. When caring for the school-age child, the home care aide

- Maintains the rules of behavior already established in the home
- Continues to provide a safe home environment with supervision
- Reinforces rules set for bedtime; adequate rest and sleep are very important
- Provides adequate nutrition

Fig 4-7 Making friends and forming new relationships is important to the school-age child.

Fig 4-8 Adolescents go through many changes on their way to adulthood. (From Sorrentino SA, Remmert LN: *Mosby's textbook for nursing assistants*, ed 8, St. Louis, 2012, Mosby.)

- Encourages safety-conscious behavior
- Reinforces responsible behavior when performing assigned chores
- Honors the child's right to privacy
- Provides opportunities for the child to make choices in the care routine
- Encourages communication of feelings and emotions
- Is honest when answering questions

During this period, the school-age child develops a sense of conscience, morals, and values (Figure 4-7).

STAGE 5: ADOLESCENCE (THE YEARS OF CONFLICTS AND ADJUSTMENTS—ESTABLISHING INDEPENDENCE)

Age: 12 to 18 Years

Characteristics. This is the second major period of rapid physical growth. In addition, there are many emotional and social changes. The adolescent

- Develops sexual characteristics that may cause embarrassment
- Has intense loyalty to his or her peer group, which provides a sense of belonging
- Experiences mood swings and extremes in behavior
- Interacts with the opposite sex
- Wants to be independent, but still has a need for dependence on the family

At the end of this stage, adolescents usually achieve emotional independence from parents and move into preparation for adult life: career and family (Figure 4-8).

Meeting the Adolescent's Needs. When caring for the adolescent, the home care aide

- Maintains the rules already set in the home
- Respects the right to privacy
- Continues to reinforce safety-conscious behavior
- Provides opportunities for the client to make choices in the care routine
- Answers questions honestly

Fig 4-9 Adults must take responsibility for themselves.

- Reinforces limits already established for rest and sleep
- Remains calm if unacceptable behavior occurs; is firm in reinforcing the rules of acceptable behavior
- Encourages communication of feelings and emotions

STAGE 6: ADULTHOOD (ESTABLISHING AND MAINTAINING A MEANINGFUL LIFE)

Age: 18 to 65 Years

Characteristics. Physical development is complete, while social and emotional development continues (Figure 4-9). The adult
- Accepts self and body image
- Establishes an intimate bond with another through marriage or as a close friend of the opposite or same sex
- Works in a career that is satisfying and provides financial independence
- Becomes involved in community activities
- Enjoys an active social life with friends
- Establishes and maintains a home
- Decides whether to have a child (children), and if so, carries out the parenting role
- Copes with the stresses of living in a positive way
- Cares for parents and/or grandchildren, if needed
  Toward the middle and end of this stage, most adults accept and adjust to the physical and emotional changes that occur in middle life.

Meeting the Adult Client's Needs. When caring for the adult, the home care aide
- Assists the client to maintain independence during activities of daily living for as long as possible
- Provides opportunities for the client to make choices in the care routine

Fig 4-10 The older adult faces many changes and challenges.

- Encourages active involvement in family life and the household routine for as long as possible
- Encourages communication of feelings and emotions

STAGE 7: OLDER ADULTHOOD (ADJUSTING TO CHANGE AND MAINTAINING INDEPENDENCE)

Age: 65 to 100-Plus Years

Characteristics. This is a period of many changes: physical, emotional, and social. The older adult

- Adjusts to and accepts the many changes that occur
- Adjusts to retirement and the lifestyle changes that result from a reduced income
- Adjusts to decreasing health and physical strength
- Accepts and adjusts to the death of spouse, relatives, and friends; may learn to live alone following the death of a loved one
- Adjusts to the reality of one's own death

Most older adults learn to accept themselves as aging and find meaning in life (Figure 4-10).

Meeting the Older Client's Needs. When caring for the older adult, the home care aide

- Maintains a clutter-free environment to prevent accidents—safety is very important (see Chapter 8)
- Uses the strategies discussed in Chapter 3 to communicate with visually- and hearing-impaired clients, if necessary
- Provides extra time for the client to accomplish tasks
- Allows the client to do as much as possible, even though it takes more time
  See Chapter 19 for more information about caring for older clients.

CHAPTER SUMMARY

- Everyone has basic human needs.
- Physical needs must be met first.
- There are five levels of basic needs.
- There are many types of family patterns.
- The family is the most important structure in society.
- Organizations and agencies help families to meet needs.
- Knowledge of growth and development will be helpful to you in meeting the client's needs.

- There are five principles of growth and development.
- There are seven stages in human growth and development.
- Knowing what is normal for each stage will help you to understand how disease and illness affects your client.

STUDY QUESTIONS

1. List five basic needs and define each.
2. Define the word "family" using your own family as an example. Is your definition different from those in the text?
3. Explain the importance of the family in society.
4. Describe the five principles of growth and development.

5. Describe three characteristics of the following stages and how the home care aide can meet the needs of clients in these stages:
   a. Toddler
   b. Adulthood
   c. Older adulthood

5

Understanding How the Body Works

OBJECTIVES

After you read this chapter, you will be able to:

1. Describe how the body is organized.
2. List the body systems, and give the general functions of each.
3. Identify the important parts of each body system and their functions.
4. Discuss how the body systems work together.

KEY TERMS

Atrophy Decrease in size or wasting away of tissue

Body structure(s) Construction and arrangement of cells, tissues, organs, and organ systems

Carbon dioxide Gas that is eliminated from the lungs during exhalation

Contract To become smaller and tighter

Diastole Relaxation of the heart muscle that causes its chambers to fill with blood

Digestion Complete physical and chemical breakdown of food

Embryo Stage of human development during the first 2 months of pregnancy

Endocrine Glands that secrete hormones directly into the bloodstream

Exocrine Glands that secrete substances into a duct

Feces Formed body waste that is discharged from the bowels

Fetus Stage of human development from the third month of pregnancy to birth

Function(s) Action(s) performed by any structure

Hormones Chemicals produced by endocrine glands

Menarche First menstrual period

Menopause Permanent end of menstruation

Metabolism Burning of food to produce heat and energy in the body

Microscope Instrument for viewing objects that cannot be seen with the naked eye

Oxygen Gas that is essential for life

Peristalsis Rhythmic involuntary movement that occurs in hollow tubes of the body

Pigment Coloring matter in the body

Secrete/Secretion Release of a substance that serves a special function in the body

Semen Fluid containing sperm

Sphincters Rings of voluntary and involuntary muscles that surround external and internal body openings

Sterile Free of living organisms

Systole Contraction of the heart muscle that causes blood to leave the heart

Urinate Process of eliminating urine

To meet your client's physical needs, you must understand how the human body works. This knowledge is the foundation for working with sick people and will help you to understand your client's illness and treatment plan.

The home care aide uses a basic understanding of body structures and their functions when giving personal care. For example, Brigid Kennedy is recovering from a broken hip. The home care aide knows that the injury may have caused damage to other body tissues—blood vessels, muscles, nerves, and skin. The home care aide also knows that most of the body systems will be involved in recovery, because they work together to maintain health and to promote recovery.

ORGANIZATION OF THE HUMAN BODY

CELLS

The cell is the basic functioning unit of the body. Cells are the smallest structures of all living things. They carry out many complicated activities. The human body is composed of trillions of cells that are so small they can be seen only through a microscope (Figure 5-1).

TISSUES, MEMBRANES, AND GLANDS

Tissues

Cells that have a similar structure and function are joined together to make tissues. For example, individual muscle cells are joined together to form muscle tissue. There are four types of tissue in the human body.
1. *Muscle tissue* is able to contract.
2. *Nerve tissue* sends and receives messages between the body and the brain.
3. *Connective tissue* connects and supports other parts of the body.
4. *Epithelial tissue* covers the body (skin) and lines the body cavities and openings.

Membranes

Epithelial and connective tissue may also be arranged into large sheets called *membranes*. These structures cover body organs or line body cavities. Major types of membranes include:
1. *Mucous membrane* produces mucus and lines all openings to the outside of the body (e.g., mouth, nose, reproductive organs).
2. *Serous membrane* lubricates and protects internal organs and body cavities.
3. *Cutaneous membrane* (skin) covers the entire body.

Fig 5-1 Example of cell types.

Glands

Glands are groups of specialized cells that manufacture and secrete substances into the body. Exocrine glands secrete substances into a duct, such as sweat glands. Endocrine glands secrete hormones directly into the bloodstream and are called *ductless glands,* such as the thyroid gland, which secretes hormones to regulate body metabolism.

ORGANS

Organs are made up of several different types of tissue that work together to perform a specific function. They are far more complex than tissues. For example, the mouth is the first organ of the digestive system. It contains many different types of tissue that work together to begin food breakdown.

ORGAN SYSTEMS

An organ system is made up of many different organs that work together to perform a specific function. Systems are more complex than tissues or organs. For example, the digestive system contains many organs, and it is responsible for nutrition and elimination.

There are many organ systems. All of the systems work together and depend on one another for proper body functioning. The major organ systems are:
1. *Integumentary system* protects the body from injury.
2. *Skeletomuscular system* provides support, protection, and movement.
3. *Nervous system and senses* send and receive electrical messages and coordinate all body functions.
4. *Endocrine system* produces hormones that regulate body functions.
5. *Circulatory and lymphatic system* transports blood and tissue fluid throughout the body and fights infection.
6. *Respiratory system* takes in oxygen and removes carbon dioxide from the body.
7. *Digestive system* is responsible for nutrition and for the elimination of body waste.
8. *Urinary system* filters all of the blood to remove dissolved waste and excess water.
9. *Reproductive system* is responsible for the production of offspring.

POINTS TO REMEMBER

- Cells are the smallest functioning unit of the body.
- Cells of similar structure and function are organized into tissues.
- Organs are made up of several types of tissues in one structure.
- Organ (body) systems are made up of many organs that perform a specific function (Figure 5-2).

BODY CAVITIES

The organs of the various body systems are arranged in spaces within the body called *body cavities.* There are five major cavities (Figure 5-3).
1. *Cranial cavity* is the space inside the skull. It contains the brain.
2. *Spinal cavity* is the space inside the spinal column. It contains the spinal cord.
3. *Thoracic cavity* is the space inside the chest. It contains the heart, lungs, trachea (windpipe), and esophagus. This cavity is separated from the abdominal cavity by the diaphragm, a large, dome-shaped muscle.
4. *Abdominal cavity* is the space below the thoracic cavity. It contains the stomach, most of the intestines, liver, gallbladder, and other organs.

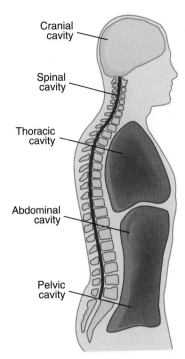

Fig 5-2 Body organization. The circulatory system is used as an example.

Fig 5-3 Body cavities.

5. *Pelvic cavity* is the lower portion of the abdominal cavity. It is surrounded by the hip bones. It contains the bladder, uterus, part of the large intestine, and rectum.

INTEGUMENTARY SYSTEM

Purpose: Covers the entire body and protects internal structures from damage by harmful invaders or substances; regulates body heat; relays body sensations; manufactures vitamin D for healthy bones; and holds in body fluids (Figure 5-4).

IMPORTANT PARTS

Skin contains pigment, blood vessels, nerve endings, fatty tissue, sweat glands, oil glands, and wax glands.

Hair covers the skin to protect the skin, eyes, ears, nasal passages, and external sex organs.

Nails protect sensitive tips of the fingers and toes from injury.

POINTS TO REMEMBER

- The skin is the body's first line of defense against injury.
- The skin's color and condition can be an indication of the general health of the body.
- Fatty tissue acts as insulation to keep in body heat.
- Healthy skin is essential for a healthy body.
- Sweat glands secrete sweat to cool the body.
- Skin breaks down very easily in some locations when a sick person becomes unable to move easily.
- Skin is nourished from the inside with a good diet and plenty of fluids.

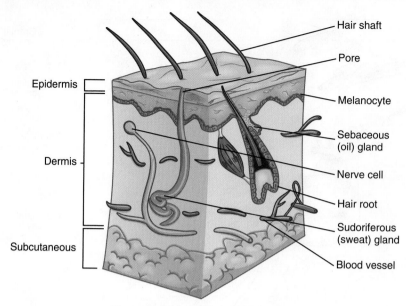

Fig 5-4 Microscopic view of the skin.

DO YOU KNOW?

- More money is spent on the care of skin, hair, and nails than on medical care of diseases.
- Exposure to ultraviolet radiation from the sun or a tanning bed can cause severe sun damage, even cancer.
- Skin is always covered with germs. Washing with soap and water is an effective method of preventing the spread of infection.
- Skin is the largest organ of the body.

SKELETOMUSCULAR SYSTEM

Purpose: Acts as a framework to support the body; produces movement; maintains posture; and protects delicate internal organs (Figures 5-5 and 5-6).

IMPORTANT PARTS

Long bones of the arms and legs allow for movement and manufacture blood cells.
Short bones of the hands, wrists, ankles, and toes allow for fine movements.
Flat bones of the ribs, skull, and pelvis protect delicate organs.
Irregular bones of the spinal column allow for bending and easy movement.
Joints are places where bones are joined together.
Muscles are attached to bones and cause movement to occur. Voluntary muscles are ones that we control. Involuntary muscles are ones that we cannot control, such as the heart muscle and those in internal organs.
Ligaments are tough fibrous bands that bind together joints.
Tendons are tough elastic bands that connect muscles to bones.
Cartilage is tough smooth tissue at bone ends that permits easy movement at the joints.

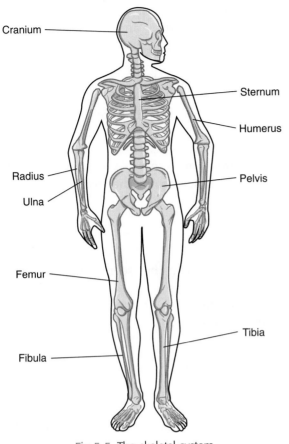

Cranium

Sternum

Humerus

Radius

Ulna

Pelvis

Femur

Tibia

Fibula

Fig 5-5 The skeletal system.

Muscle

Tendon

Ligament

Fig 5-6 The muscular system.

Ball and socket

Hinge

Pivot

Fig 5-7 Types of joints.

THE PROCESS OF MOVEMENT

Movement occurs when voluntary muscles, attached to bones, contract and relax, causing a change in the joint. These muscles work in pairs. When one contracts, the other relaxes, pulling the bone and moving the joint. Ball-and-socket joints located in the shoulder and hip produce circular movements. Hinge joints of the elbow, knee, fingers, and toes allow movement in two directions: bending and straightening. Pivot joints such as the skull on the neck permit rotation of the head from side to side (Figure 5-7). The brain controls movement of all muscles in the body.

POINTS TO REMEMBER

- Healthy bones and muscles require foods that is rich in vitamins and minerals.
- Bone growth stops in early adulthood.
- Bone marrow manufactures blood cells.

- There are 206 bones and more than 600 muscles in the body.
- Large, strong muscles in arms and legs are used for lifting and moving.
- Thin layers of muscles in the abdomen and back should be used for posture, not for strength.
- *Muscle tone* refers to the readiness of a muscle to contract.
- Exercise is essential to keep muscles healthy.
- When muscles are not used, they shrink (atrophy) and joints become stiff.
- Lack of movement is a major cause of muscle atrophy in sick people.
- Rings of voluntary and involuntary muscles called sphincters surround external body openings or openings in internal structures. For example, voluntary sphincters surround the eye and mouth; an involuntary sphincter joins the stomach and small intestine.

DO YOU KNOW?

- The smallest bones are in the inner ear and can be seen only through a microscope.
- The femur (thigh bone) is the longest and strongest bone in the body.
- Body heat is produced when voluntary muscles move.
- More facial muscles are used to frown than to smile.

NERVOUS SYSTEM

Purpose: Controls and regulates the activities of all body systems to keep them functioning properly. The nervous system is made up of two parts: the central nervous system and the senses, which include sight, hearing, touch, taste, and smell (Figure 5-8).

CENTRAL NERVOUS SYSTEM

Important Parts

Brain contains centers that control movement, speech, sensation, learning, vision, taste, emotion, thought, alertness, balance, breathing, heartbeat, and blood pressure. It sends and receives messages to and from other parts of the body.

Spinal cord is the passageway for messages going to and away from the brain.

Nerves send and receive messages for sensation and control of voluntary and involuntary muscles.

The Process of Sending and Receiving Messages

The nervous system is made up of millions of nerve cells called *neurons* (Figure 5-9). Bundles of neurons are called *nerves*. Some nerves carry messages from the body to the spinal cord. The spinal cord then passes the message to the brain. The brain receives the message and responds. It sends the message to the spinal cord. Then, other nerves carry the response back to the body. We move because nerves stimulate muscles to work.

For some activities, we can control nerve function, such as moving arms and legs. For other body activities, we cannot control nerve function, such as regulating our heartbeat. A *reflex* is a rapid involuntary response to messages from nerve endings, such as pulling a finger away from a flame.

Points to Remember

- The nervous system is like a giant computer that regulates all body functions.
- The brain and spinal cord are protected by bones and a special cushioning fluid.

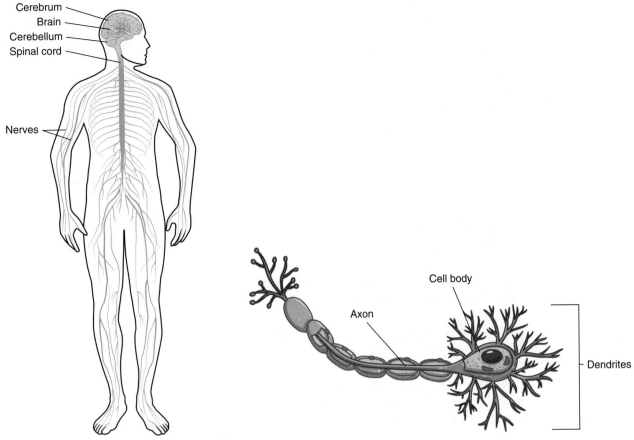

Fig 5-8 The nervous system.

Fig 5-9 The neuron.

- The nervous system must have sufficient amounts of oxygen and food to function properly.
- Permanent brain damage will occur if the brain is without oxygen for more than 7 minutes.
- Damaged nerve tissue takes a long time to repair; sometimes it never does.

Do You Know?
- Some neurons can be almost 3 feet long.
- Scientists are conducting research to better understand the functioning of the nervous system.

THE SENSES

The senses (sight, sound, touch, taste, and smell) are important parts of the nervous system. They receive and send information about the world around us to the brain. The brain in turn uses this information to help control the activities and functions of the body.

Important Parts

Nerve endings in the skin receive messages of pain, heat, cold, pressure, and touch. Those in the nose and tongue receive messages of smell and taste. Nerve endings in the mouth and stomach receive messages of thirst and hunger.

Eyes and *ears* receive messages of light and sound.

Points to Remember
- To learn about and interact with our environment, we need sense organs to receive information, nerves to transmit the information, and a functioning brain to interpret the information.
- The senses include sight, hearing, touch, taste, pain, smell, pressure, balance, temperature, position, and others.
- The brain uses information from the senses to maintain normal body functioning in an ever-changing environment.

Do You Know?
- The senses provide information to protect the body from harm caused by external forces (e.g., heat, cold, pressure, sun).
- The senses help us to take in new information and to learn new things.
- The senses help us to enjoy our world.

Eyes
Purpose: Receive light rays that focus and transmit images through the nerves to the sight center of the brain (Figure 5-10).

Important Parts
Cornea is the transparent part of the outer layer that protects the eye.
Pupil controls the amount of light entering the eye.
Lens bends the light rays to focus on the retina.
Retina contains special nerve endings for sight.
Tear glands produce tears to keep the eye moist.
Lids and lashes protect the eye from injury.

The Process of Vision. Light enters the eye through the cornea and passes through the pupil to the lens. The light rays are bent by the lens to focus on nerve endings of

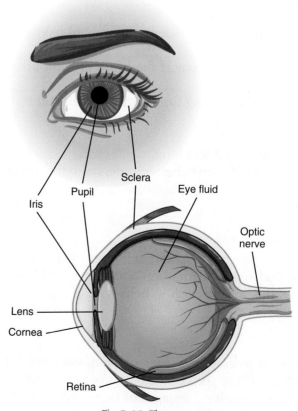

Fig 5-10 The eye.

the retina. The nerve endings send this information through the optic nerve to the sight center in the brain.

Points to Remember

- The eye is very delicate and protected from damage by tears, eyelids, and eyelashes.
- Eye injury and infection can lead to blindness.
- Germs can enter the eye from dirty hands, soiled washcloths, and cosmetics.

Do You Know?

- The iris is a circular, colored muscle that automatically controls the size of the pupil to adjust the amount of light coming into the eye.
- Color is seen when light is present.
- A cloudy lens is a condition known as a *cataract*.

Ears

Purpose: Receive and send sound through nerves to the hearing center of the brain (Figure 5-11).

Important Parts

Outer ear catches sound waves and sends them to the middle ear.

Eardrum, between the outer and middle ear, receives vibrations and sends them to the middle ear.

Middle ear contains three tiny bones that receive vibrations from the eardrum and send them to the inner ear.

Inner ear contains nerve endings for hearing and balance that send sound through nerves to the brain.

The Process of Hearing. Sound waves enter the outer ear, causing vibrations that travel through the eardrum to the bones in the middle ear. The nerve endings in the inner ear pick up these sound waves and send them to the hearing center of the brain.

The Process of Balance. Structures in the inner ear sense the position and changes in position of the head. These messages are sent to the brain.

Points to Remember

- The auditory canal leads directly to the delicate eardrum; nothing should be placed in this area (e.g., no cotton swabs, hair pins, pencils, fingernails).
- Damage to the eardrum may cause hearing loss.

Do You Know?

- The ear receives a wide range of sounds all at once, which occurs when listening to music. At the same time, we understand each separate sound (e.g., drum, keyboard, voice, guitar).

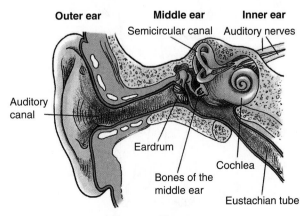

Fig 5-11 The ear.

- The eustachian (auditory) tube connects the throat to the middle ear; it equalizes the pressure within the ear and throat, but it can also transport infections from the throat to the middle ear.
- The middle and inner ear are located in the temporal bones of the skull.
- Wax in the outer ear canal protects the area and should not be removed.

ENDOCRINE SYSTEM

Purpose: Produces and secretes hormones from ductless glands. These hormones contain chemical messages and are responsible for human growth and development. They also control the activities of other systems, such as the reproductive system (Figure 5-12). Part of the brain (the hypothalamus) links the nervous system and the endocrine system.

IMPORTANT PARTS

Pituitary gland produces many important hormones that affect the functioning of several body systems.

Thyroid gland regulates the way food is used to provide energy.

Pancreas produces insulin in special cells of this organ. Insulin helps to break down sugar to give needed energy.

Andrenal glands produce several hormones that help the body to cope with stress. They also affect kidney function and blood pressure.

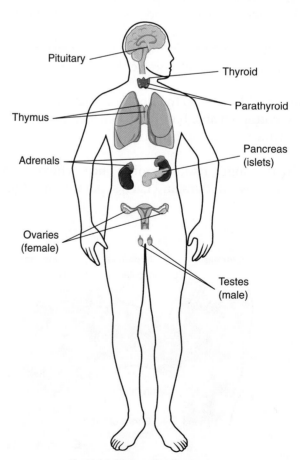

Fig 5-12 The endocrine system.

Ovaries produce the female sex hormones responsible for sexual development and reproduction.

Testes produce the male sex hormone responsible for sexual development and reproduction.

POINTS TO REMEMBER

- Hormones are chemicals that are produced by glands.
- Hormones enter the bloodstream and regulate many important functions in our bodies.
- Hormones influence all systems of the body.
- There are 15 endocrine glands; their total weight is less than ½ pound, yet they have a powerful influence on all systems of the body.

DO YOU KNOW?

- Replacement hormones can be used for those missing in humans.
- Hormones influence our emotions and feelings.

CIRCULATORY SYSTEM

Purpose: Delivers food and oxygen to all cells of the body, and transports each cell's waste products to the organs responsible for removing waste (Figure 5-13).

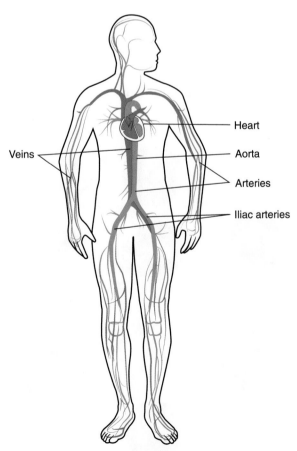

Heart

Veins

Aorta

Arteries

Iliac arteries

Fig 5-13 The circulatory system.

IMPORTANT PARTS

Blood, a thick red fluid, carries nutrients and oxygen to each cell of the body.

Blood vessels, called *arteries, capillaries,* and *veins,* are tubes that carry the blood to all parts of the body.

Capillaries are tiny tubes that connect the smallest arteries with the smallest veins and supply cells with nutrients and oxygen and remove waste.

Heart, a hollow and very muscular organ, pumps blood through the blood vessels.

THE PROCESS OF CIRCULATION—THE MOVEMENT OF BLOOD

When the heart contracts, blood that is rich in oxygen is forced into the arteries. The arteries branch out to serve all parts of the body. The smallest arteries join with capillaries. This is where nutrients, oxygen, and other substances carried by the blood are passed to the cells of the body. The cells in turn pass waste products and carbon dioxide back to the capillaries. The smallest veins join larger veins to carry the blood back to the heart. Next, the blood goes to the lungs to exchange carbon dioxide with oxygen, and the process begins again (Figure 5-14).

The Heartbeat

There are two parts to one beat: contracting and resting. When the heart muscle contracts, blood is forced out of the heart (systole). When the heart muscle rests, blood fills the chambers of the heart (diastole).

The Pulse

As blood is pumped from the heart, you can feel the beat in the arteries. This is called the *pulse.*

POINTS TO REMEMBER

- Blood distributes the oxygen we breathe, nutrients from the food we eat, and other substances to the body cells. Waste products enter the blood, too, and are sent to other systems to be removed from the body.

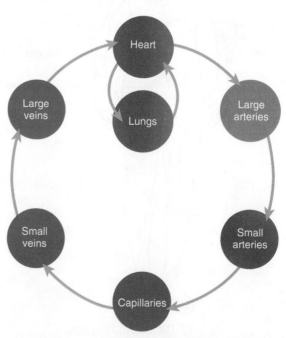

Fig 5-14 The process of circulation.

- Blood vessels transport blood to all parts of the body.
- The action of the heart causes blood to move throughout the body in a continuous circle.
- A heartbeat consists of two parts: contracting and resting.
- The circulatory system affects all systems of the body.

DO YOU KNOW?

- The heart is an amazing organ that pumps 1000 gallons of blood per day; it beats about 100,000 times per day and rests only between each beat.
- There are 60,000 miles of blood vessels in the human body.

LYMPHATIC SYSTEM

Purpose: Removes excess fluids from tissues and returns them to the blood. It also filters germs and other harmful substances from the blood. This system helps to protect the body by manufacturing substances that destroy germs causing infection. The lymphatic system and the circulatory system work together to help keep the body's fluids in proper balance (Figure 5-15).

IMPORTANT PARTS

Lymph, a colorless fluid, carries water and protein from the tissues to the circulatory system.

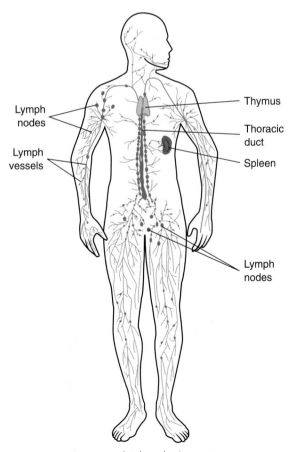

Fig 5-15 The lymphatic system.

Lymph vessels, similar in structure to veins, carry lymph to large veins that go to the heart.

Lymph nodes, small sphere-shaped bodies, act as filters by keeping germs and other substances from spreading throughout the body.

Spleen, the largest lymph organ of the body, manufactures white blood cells to fight infection.

POINTS TO REMEMBER

* Lymph vessels return excess tissue fluid to the circulatory system.
* The accumulation of lymph in the tissues is called *edema.*
* Lymph nodes act as the body's defense against infection; they trap infectious organisms and prevent them from traveling to other parts of the body.

DO YOU KNOW?

* About 600 lymph nodes protect the body by filtering out harmful products.
* Tonsils and adenoids are made of lymphatic tissue and filter out germs from the air we breathe.

RESPIRATORY SYSTEM

Purpose: Carries oxygen to all of the body's cells and eliminates carbon dioxide from the body. It is lined with mucous membrane. The system is divided into two parts: upper and lower respiratory tracts (Figure 5-16).

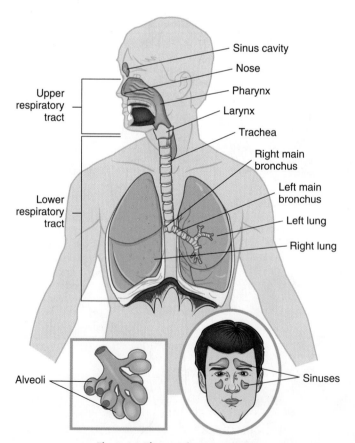

Fig 5-16 The respiratory system.

IMPORTANT PARTS

Upper respiratory tract contains the nose, sinus cavities, throat, eustachian tubes, larynx (voice box), epiglottis, and trachea (windpipe).

Lower respiratory tract contains tubes leading to the lungs, called the right and left *bronchi.* The lungs (large, spongy, cone-shaped organs) contain tiny air sacs called *alveoli.*

PROCESS OF RESPIRATION

There are two parts to the process of respiration: inhalation and exhalation.

Inhalation

When we breathe in (inhale), the chest expands, and the diaphragm, a dome-shaped muscle, pushes down to allow more room for the lungs to expand. Air containing oxygen enters the nose, sinus cavities, and throat, where it is warmed and moistened. These organs help to filter out harmful organisms and prevent them from entering other parts of the respiratory system. Next, air continues through the larynx to the trachea. The trachea transports the air to the lower respiratory tract. Tiny hairs in the trachea prevent dust and other materials from entering the lungs. Extensions of the trachea, tubes called the *right* and *left bronchi,* transport air to each lung. Branches of these tubes carry air to all parts of the lungs. At the ends of the smallest branches are the alveoli. Capillaries from the circulatory system surround the alveoli. Oxygen is exchanged for carbon dioxide between the alveoli and the capillaries.

Exhalation

When we breathe out (exhale), the diaphragm again becomes dome shaped and helps to force air, filled with carbon dioxide, from the lungs. Air is forced from the organs of the lower respiratory tract and through the organs of the upper respiratory tract to the outside.

POINTS TO REMEMBER

- The entire respiratory system is lined with delicate mucous membrane.
- Mucous membranes are the body's natural defense against germs.
- The respiratory and circulatory systems work closely together.
- The exchange of oxygen for carbon dioxide occurs in the lungs between the alveoli and capillaries.
- All cells need oxygen to survive.
- The cough reflex helps to remove material from the upper and lower respiratory tracts.
- When we swallow, the epiglottis closes to prevent food from entering the trachea.
- As air rushes over the vocal cords in the larynx during exhaling, the cords vibrate and allow speech to occur.

DO YOU KNOW?

- It takes 12 pounds of air to totally fill a person's healthy lungs.
- There are hundreds of millions of alveoli in the lungs; if they could be spread out, they would take up an area 25 times the surface of your skin.

DIGESTIVE (GASTROINTESTINAL [GI]) SYSTEM

Purpose: Breaks down the food we eat into nutrients that can be used by the body's cells (Figure 5-17).

IMPORTANT PARTS

Upper digestive tract contains the mouth, pharynx, esophagus, and stomach.
Small intestine connects the stomach to the large intestine.
Large intestine (colon) connects the small intestine to the end of the digestive system.
Other organs, such as the liver, gallbladder, and pancreas, assist with the breakdown of
    food into nutrients.

PROCESS OF DIGESTION AND ABSORPTION

Digestion starts in the mouth, where food is chewed (physical digestion) and saliva helps to moisten and break down food. The moistened food is swallowed and then goes through the esophagus to the stomach. The stomach produces chemicals called *enzymes* that continue to break down the food (chemical digestion). The action of stomach muscles causes the contents to churn. The stomach contents now enter the small intestine. Bile from the liver and gallbladder enters the small intestine. Juices from the pancreas also enter the small intestine. These chemicals break down the food to a liquid form. Capillaries in the small intestine absorb the nutrients and distribute them into the bloodstream to nourish each cell in the body. The amazing process of digestion and absorption of food is completed in the small intestine.

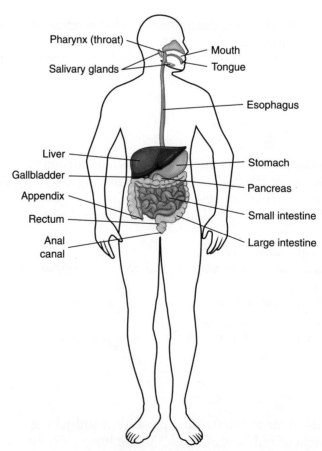

Fig 5-17 The digestive system.

PROCESS OF ELIMINATING SOLID WASTE

Water and waste products of digestion enter the large intestine. As this mixture travels through the tube, much of the water is reabsorbed into the body. When waste products reach the lower part of the intestine, they become formed and are called feces. Feces are stored in the rectum, and water from them continues to be reabsorbed.

The process of ridding the body of feces is complex and involves the digestive, muscular, and nervous systems. The muscular walls of the large intestine contain nerves. When the rectum becomes full of feces, nerves send a message to the brain. They tell us that it is time to have a bowel movement (BM). Peristalsis causes the feces to move; the internal and external anal sphincters of the anus open, and feces are eliminated from the body.

POINTS TO REMEMBER

- The digestive system is one continuous tube.
- Mucous membrane lines the entire system (about 26 feet or 8 meters long), from mouth to anus.
- Digestion begins in the mouth and is completed in the small intestine.
- Food and fluid travel through this system by peristaltic action.
- Water is reabsorbed in the large intestine.
- Waste products are stored and eliminated by the large intestine.
- When feces remain in the large intestine and are not eliminated, they become hard and are difficult to pass (constipation).

DO YOU KNOW?

- Organs of the digestive system manufacture over 8 quarts of fluid in 24 hours to carry out digestive system functions.
- The liver produces bile that is stored in the gallbladder; bile helps to digest fatty foods.

URINARY SYSTEM

Purpose: Filters out waste products from the blood and removes them from the body in the form of urine (Figure 5-18).

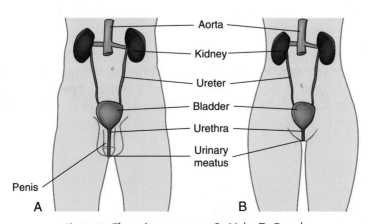

Fig 5-18 The urinary system. **A,** Male. **B,** Female.

IMPORTANT PARTS

Kidneys (two) filter out liquid waste products in the blood.
Ureters (two) are tubes that connect the kidneys to the bladder.
Bladder receives urine from the ureters and stores it.
Urethra is a tube that connects the bladder to the outside.
The end of the urethra is called the urinary meatus.

PROCESS OF ELIMINATING LIQUID WASTE (URINATION)

Kidneys are constantly producing urine. Urine drips from the kidneys through the ureters to the bladder for storage. The muscular walls of the bladder contain nerves. When the muscles have stretched due to the fullness of the bladder, nerves send a message to the brain. They tell us that it is time to get rid of the urine; it is time to urinate. Nerves also send messages to the bladder muscles to contract. Then urine passes from the bladder through the urethra to the outside.

The entire urinary system of a normal person is free of germs. It is sterile, like the blood and the circulatory system. Urine, which is a product of filtered blood, is also sterile. It becomes unsterile only when it comes in contact with the outside of the body.

POINTS TO REMEMBER

- The urinary system maintains a balance between fluids taken in and fluids removed in the form of urine.
- Increased fluids taken in means more urine being produced; what goes in must come out! Adequate fluids are essential for health.
- Urine is made up of water and other waste products that are no longer needed by the body.
- The bladder stores urine.
- Urination is a complicated process that involves the urinary system, the muscular system, and the nervous system.

DO YOU KNOW?

- Every 20 minutes, the kidneys filter all of the body's blood (5 to 6 quarts).
- The body is composed of 40% solids and 60% fluids (Figure 5-19).
- Fluids are located inside and outside the cell and in the blood.

REPRODUCTIVE SYSTEM

MALE

Purpose: Continues the human race by manufacturing the male sex hormone (testosterone) and sperm (the male reproductive cell). When sperm is united with the female reproductive cell, human reproduction takes place. This system is closely related to the urinary system because urine and sperm are carried by the same tube (Figure 5-20).

Important Parts
   Internal
Testes (two) produce sperm and the male sex hormone, testosterone.
Spermatic cord is a tube that connects the testes to the urethra and transports sperm.

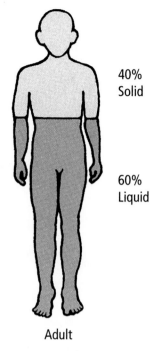

40%
Solid

60%
Liquid

Adult

Fig 5-19 Body composition.

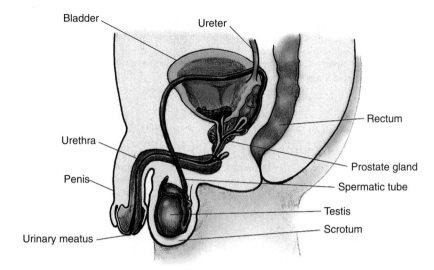

Fig 5-20 The male reproductive system.

Prostate gland surrounds the urethra below the bladder and secretes fluid to help sperm to travel.
External
Penis is the male sex organ that ejects semen. Urine is also eliminated through the penis.
Scrotum is a sac suspended behind and on either side of the penis that contains the testes.

Points to Remember
• The male reproductive system and the urinary system are closely linked to each other.
• Sperm cannot be produced in the heat of the body; they require a cooler place: the scrotum.

Do You Know?
• Male genes determine the sex of the baby.
• Men manufacture sperm well into older adulthood.

FEMALE

Purpose: Continues the human race by producing female sex hormones and ovum, the female reproductive cell. When the ovum is united with the sperm, human reproduction takes place (Figures 5-21 and 5-22).

Important Parts
Internal
Ovaries (two) produce female sex hormones and release eggs, or ova, from puberty to menopause.
Fallopian tubes (two) transport ova from the ovaries to the uterus. The union of sperm and ovum takes place here.

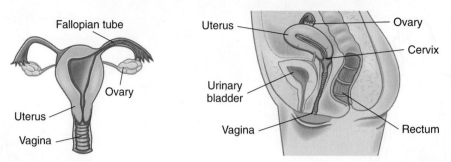

Fig 5-21 The female reproductive system: internal structures.

Fig 5-22 The female reproductive system: external structures.

Uterus provides nourishment and protection for growth of the fetus during pregnancy. If pregnancy does not occur, the lining is shed during menstruation.

Vagina is the birth canal and organ of sexual intercourse. Products of menstruation are removed through this canal.

External

Genitalia contains the labia (large and small lips) that protect the inner organs of the system.

Perineum is the area between the vagina and anus that provides support for the organs in the pelvis. It stretches during childbirth.

Breasts (two) produce milk after childbirth to nourish the infant.

Process of Menstruation

The beginning of the menstrual cycle, or menarche, is the most obvious sign of physical maturity in the female. With the onset of puberty, at around 12 years of age, the body begins to produce and release hormones that allow pregnancy to occur. Each month, hormones prepare the uterus for pregnancy by developing a thick lining of blood tissue. If pregnancy does not occur, the lining breaks up and is shed through the vagina. This process, known as *menstruation,* occurs about every 28 days for 30 to 40 years. Around 45 to 52 years of age, the production of hormones that cause menstruation will slowly decrease and eventually stop. This is called menopause.

Pregnancy

Each month, an ovary releases a mature egg (ovum) into one of the fallopian tubes. If this ovum is fertilized by a sperm, pregnancy occurs (conception). The fertilized ovum, now called an embryo, begins to grow as it travels through the fallopian tube on its way to the uterus. As mentioned earlier, hormones have prepared the uterus for pregnancy by lining it with a thick layer of tissue. Once the embryo reaches the uterus, it attaches itself to the lining to grow and be nourished. The body continues to produce hormones throughout the pregnancy that make sure that the growing embryo (later called a fetus) receives proper nourishment and has a safe place to grow. Hormones also play a role in starting labor, during childbirth, and in the adjustment to the non-pregnant state.

Points to Remember
A delicate balance of hormones controls the following.
- Menstruation
- Conception
- Growth of the fetus
- Childbirth
- Period after childbirth
- Menopause

Do You Know?
- A baby girl is born with 60,000 to 80,000 ova in her ovaries.
- The uterus, a very muscular organ, can expand from the size of a small pear to a size that holds a 7-pound or larger baby.

CHAPTER SUMMARY

- The body is organized from the smallest structure, the cell, to groups of organs called *organ systems*.
- All body systems are connected and depend on each other to function properly.
- Internal organs are contained within five body cavities.
- Each body system has unique functions.
- The body systems and their functions are as follows.
  1. *Integumentary system* protects the body from injury.
  2. *Skeletomuscular system* provides support, protection, and movement.
  3. *Nervous system* and senses send and receive electrical messages and coordinate all body functions.
  4. *Endocrine system* produces hormones that regulate body functions.
  5. *Circulatory and lymphatic system* transports blood and tissue fluid throughout the body and fights infection.
  6. *Respiratory system* takes in oxygen and removes carbon dioxide from the body.
  7. *Digestive system* is responsible for nutrition and elimination of body waste.
  8. *Urinary system* filters all the blood to remove dissolved waste and excess water.
  9. *Reproductive system* is responsible for the production of offspring.

STUDY QUESTIONS

1. Define and give one example of each of the following.
   a. Tissue
   b. Gland
   c. Membrane
   d. Organ
   e. Organ system
   f. Cavity
2. List the body systems, their function(s), and three important parts of each system.
3. Explain the following, and tell what systems are involved.
   a. Urination
   b. Movement
   c. Absorption of nutrients
   d. Breathing

6

Observing, Reporting, and Recording

OBJECTIVES

After you read this chapter, you will be able to:

1. Discuss three purposes of the client care record.
2. Discuss the responsibilities of the home care aide to accurately observe, record, and report information about the client, family, and home environment.
3. Describe the three types of observation methods.
4. Discuss the responsibilities of the home care aide to accurately observe, record, and report information about the client's pain.
5. List five general rules for recording information on the client's care record.
6. Describe five points to remember when calling your supervisor to report your client's condition.
7. Identify the meanings of 10 of each of the following used in medical terminology: prefixes, suffixes, word roots, and abbreviations.
8. Discuss the steps in reporting and recording an incident.

KEY TERMS

Care record Permanent written record of a client's progress during illness and rehabilitation; also contains information about client care

Chart To record in writing information on the client's record

Document To describe in writing observations or action taken; also called *recording* or *charting*

Incident Unexpected event

Observe/Observation Act of watching carefully and attentively

Prefix Word part that is attached to the beginning of the word root to modify its meaning

Suffix Word part that is attached to the end of the word root to modify its meaning

Word root Word part that is the core of the term; contains the basic meaning of the word

Anna Petrova has been visiting her client, Mr. Smirnoff, for 6 months. Twice a week, she gives him a shower, straightens his bedroom, and makes a lunch before leaving for her next assignment. Mr. Smirnoff lives alone and uses a walker to get around his small apartment.

The care plan indicates that he has poor circulation in his legs. Yesterday, while giving the shower, Anna noticed a reddened area the size of a quarter and hot to touch on the heel of his left foot. When she asked him about it, he said it was sore, especially when he put on his shoe. Anna recorded her observations on the agency's care record form and notified her supervisor, who in turn contacted the physician. "Because of Mrs. Petrova's accurate observations and prompt reporting, I was able to start treatment immediately to avoid serious complications," said the physician.

In addition to following the client's care plan carefully, three of the most important responsibilities of the home care aide are observing, reporting, and recording information accurately. The home care team relies on you to be an excellent observer of the client, family, and home environment. BECAUSE YOU SPEND MORE TIME WITH THE CLIENT THAN DO OTHER HOME CARE TEAM MEMBERS, YOU ARE THE VITAL COMMUNICATION LINK BETWEEN WHAT OCCURS IN THE HOME AND WHAT INFORMATION IS KNOWN BY THE AGENCY STAFF (Figure 6-1).

Throughout the book, there is highlighting to show examples of observing, recording, and reporting:

- **Observe:** Watch carefully and attentively.
- **Record:** Write what you observe using your agency's form.
- **Report:** Use the telephone to call your supervisor about what you observed.

Whenever you see this highlighting, it means that it is important to observe, record, and report the information accurately and completely.

The word *observe* means to watch carefully and attentively. This is a way of gathering information about something. In Chapter 3, general principles of communication were discussed. People communicate in various ways: verbal, nonverbal, and written. Just as communication is a continuous process, observation also must be a process that is constantly in use.

During the first visit, you will be gathering new information about your client, the client's family, and the home environment. Then, with each visit, you will build on this information by observing any changes in your client, the client's family, and the home environment.

OBSERVING THE CLIENT

When you observe your client, you will be using your senses to gather information on your client's condition.

There are three types of observations: objective, subjective, and vital signs.

Fig 6-1 The home care aide—a vital link.

OBJECTIVE

The *objective* method of observation means that you are using one or more of the body senses to gather information.
Sight: Seeing the bruise on the client's arm
Sound: Hearing two family members argue about financial problems
Smell: Smelling the odor of spoiled food in the refrigerator
Touch: Touching the client's hot skin

SUBJECTIVE

Another way of obtaining information is called the *subjective* method. This means that someone tells you information that you cannot observe. For example, your client says that he has a dull pain in the right shoulder and is dizzy, or a family member tells you that the client has been very depressed.

VITAL SIGNS

Vital signs include four important indicators about the body's condition. They are temperature, pulse, respirations, and blood pressure. Vital signs are discussed in detail, including procedures, in Chapter 17.

You will use all three methods of gathering information. For clients who are infants, children, and others who are not able to tell you about their symptoms, your powers of observation are especially important. Developing your observation skills takes time and practice. As you continue in your career as a home care aide, your observation skills will sharpen and improve.

OBSERVING PAIN

Pain or discomfort means feeling sore, aching, or hurting. Pain is unpleasant and may cause distress and suffering. It is a signal from the body that something is wrong. Because the client's pain is subjective, another person cannot observe it. Pain can be described only by the person who is feeling it. It is important to listen to the client's complaints of pain and to pay careful attention to what he or she is describing.

There are several types of pain.

- Acute pain is severe and lasts for a short period of time (usually no longer than 6 months). For example, pain after an injury (broken leg) disappears when the injury heals.
- Chronic pain lasts for a long period of time (longer than 6 months). It may be mild to severe and may come and go. Arthritis is a disease that causes chronic pain.
- Phantom pain is felt in a body part that is no longer present, such as a leg that has been amputated (see Chapter 22).

Many of your clients will experience pain. If this is an ongoing problem, the care plan will tell how to help your client. PAIN RELIEF AND PREVENTION ARE "RIGHTS" OF THE CLIENT, AND IT IS THE RESPONSIBILITY OF THE AGENCY STAFF TO RESPOND QUICKLY TO REPORTS OF PAIN. THEREFORE, PAIN IS ALWAYS REPORTED TO YOUR SUPERVISOR.

The client is the **ONLY** person who can describe his or her pain. Your agency will provide a form that will help your client explain what he or she is feeling. This self-assessment tool helps the client to determine the severity of the pain. Some questions that help clients talk about their pain are found in Box 6-1.

BOX 6-1 Client's Self-Assessment of Pain

- Where is your pain?
- When did it start?
- What does it feel like?
- How bad is it?
- How often do you have the pain? Is it there all the time?
- How long does it last?
- Does it stop you from doing your usual activities? Which ones?
- What makes your pain worse?
- What makes your pain better?
- What have you tried to relieve your pain? Does it help? What does not help?

BOX 6-2 Words Used to Describe Pain

Aching	Miserable	Sore
Burning	Nagging	Squeezing
Cramping	Numb	Tender
Crushing	Piercing	Throbbing
Dull	Pressure	Tiring
Exhausting	Sharp	Unbearable
Gnawing	Shooting	Viselike

Sometimes clients are unable to find the right words to describe their pain. Your agency may provide a list of words or a pain-rating scale for clients to use (Box 6-2 and Figure 6-2). Clients are asked to perform these self-assessments on a regular schedule, according to the care plan. The home care aide provides assistance as necessary and reports the client's complaints of pain to the supervisor. This is important because there are many barriers that prevent clients from reporting their pain (Box 6-3). In addition, some physical symptoms may accompany pain (Box 6-4). However, some clients may look happy, be smiling, and be telling jokes while complaining of pain. PAIN IS WHAT THE CLIENT SAYS IT IS—NOT WHAT YOU THINK IT IS. ALWAYS TAKE COMPLAINTS OF PAIN SERIOUSLY—AND REPORT THEM TO YOUR SUPERVISOR.

The nursing supervisor will assess the client's pain and determine the proper type of pain relief in cooperation with the physician, client, family, and home care team. There are many methods of pain relief, such as a change in position, use of medications and applications of heat and cold, use of music, and meditation. Pain relief is provided according to the client care plan, and the results are recorded and reported. If relief measures are not effective, notify your supervisor.

OBSERVATION GUIDELINES

Listed in Box 6-5 (see pp. 81-82) are guidelines to help you perform a head-to-toe observation of the client.

0	1	2	3	4	5
No Hurt	Hurts Little Bit	Hurts Little More	Hurts Even More	Hurts Whole Lot	Hurts Worst

A

Brief word instructions: Point to each face using the words to describe the pain intensity. Ask the person to choose face that best describes own pain and record the appropriate number.

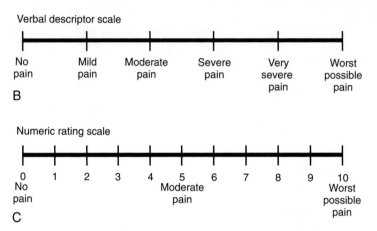

Verbal descriptor scale

No pain — Mild pain — Moderate pain — Severe pain — Very severe pain — Worst possible pain

B

Numeric rating scale

0 1 2 3 4 5 6 7 8 9 10
No pain — Moderate pain — Worst possible pain

C

Fig 6-2 Pain-rating scales. (**A,** Wong-Baker Faces Pain Rating Scale. From Hockenberry MJ, Wilson D: *Wong's nursing care of infants and children,* ed 9, St. Louis, 2011, Mosby; **B** and **C,** from U.S. Department of Health and Human Services, 1992, *Clinical practice guideline: acute pain management: operative or medical procedures and trauma* [AHCPR Publication No. 92-0032], Rockville, MD, 1992, Agency for Health Care Policy and Research.)

BOX 6-3 | **Barriers to Reporting Pain**

CLIENT BELIEFS
- Should "be good" and not complain
- Should "put up with the pain" and "offer it up for sins"
- Should be "strong"—"real" men do not complain about pain
- Pain is a normal part of the aging process

CULTURAL INFLUENCES
- Pain reactions vary with different cultures and religions
- Asians, Russians, Germans, and Armenians tend to be stoic and reluctant to discuss pain
- In some cultures, women have been taught to be quiet and to attract as little attention as possible, including not complaining about pain

COMMUNICATION PROBLEMS
- Inability to speak due to illness
- Non–English-speaking client
- Young children whose language skills are not fully developed
- People with mental illness or dementia (see Chapters 21 and 22)

| **BOX 6-4** | **Other Signs and Symptoms That May Accompany Pain** |

- Anger
- Constipation
- Crying
- Depression
- Diarrhea
- Dizziness
- Facial expression: Wincing
- Groaning
- Headache
- Increase in temperature, pulse, respirations, and blood pressure

- Lying very still, refusing to move
- Moaning
- Nausea
- Pale skin
- Perspiration
- Restlessness
- Rubbing painful area
- Screaming
- Suicidal feelings
- Very quiet
- Vomiting

| **BOX 6-5** | **Guidelines for Head-to-Toe Observation** |

I. Overall appearance
  A. Consciousness

Alert	Drowsy
Confused	Slow to react
Does not react	Listless

  B. Grooming

| Clean | Untidy |
| Dirty | Odor |

  C. Skin

Pale	Red
Yellow	Bruises
Clammy	Rashes
Dry	Open sores
Rough	Scaly patches

  D. Mood

Cheerful	Demanding
Withdrawn	Agitated
Anxious	Irritable
Sullen	Angry
Hostile	Sad

II. Head to toe
  A. Head and neck
    1. Hair and scalp

Clean	Dirty
Matted	Dry
Oily	Sores
Dandruff	

    2. Eyes

Bright	Glassy
Red	Discharge
Sensitive to light	Sees poorly
Sees well	Blind
Dull	

    3. Ears

Discharge	Difficulty hearing
Pain	Deaf
Hears well	

    4. Nose

| Dry | Bleeding |
| Discharge | Stopped up |

    5. Mouth

Odor	Condition of
Bluish or pale	teeth/dentures
lips	Difficulty
Discharge	swallowing
Sores	Gums: red,
Difficulty chewing	bleeding

    6. Speech

Normal for	Difficulty talking
individual	Unable to speak
Slurred	

    7. Breath

Slow	Difficulty breathing
Painful	Rapid
Coughing	Noisy

    8. Neck

Swelling	Pain
Difficulty	
swallowing	

  B. Arms, Wrists, Hands, and Fingers

Bruises	Cold
Cuts	Pale or bluish
Rashes	fingernails
Swelling	

    1. Movement

Easy	Twitching
Difficult	No movement:
Painful	one side or
Shaking	both sides

    2. Strength
      Weakness: general or one-sided
      Difficulty holding objects
      Loss of strength

Continued

BOX 6-5	Guidelines for Head-to-Toe Observation—cont'd

3. Feeling
   Numbness   Pain
   Tingling sensation
C. Chest and abdomen
   Bruises   Swelling
   Cuts   Pain
   Rashes
   1. Breasts
      Lumps   Irritation of skin
      Discharge from   under breast
         nipple   Pain
      Soreness
D. Pubic area
   Bruises   Swelling
   Cuts   Pain
   Rashes   Lumps
   1. Female
      Vaginal discharge
         Odor   Color
         Swelling in
            groin area
      Menstruation
         Odor   Pain
         Large amount   Blood clots
   2. Male: penis and scrotum
      Discharge   Pain
      Odor   Swelling in groin
      Swelling   area
      Lumps
E. Legs, ankles, feet, and toes
   Bruises   Pain
   Cuts   Bluish or discolored
   Rashes   toenails
   Swelling   Sores
   1. Movement
      Easy   Shaking
      Difficult   Twitching
      Painful   No movement
   2. Strength
      Weakness   Loss of strength
   3. Feeling
      Numbness   Pain
      Tingling

F. Upper and lower back and buttocks
   Bruises   Redness
   Sores   Pain
   Scaly patches   Swelling
   Dry skin
III. Other
   A. Activities of daily living (ADL)
      Performs ADL without assistance
      Performs ADL with assistance
      Cannot perform ADL
      Personal Care: Bathing, hair care, brushing
      teeth, shaving
      Toileting: Toilet, commode, urinal, bedpan
      Eating: In bed, in room, in kitchen, in other
      area
      Moving: Sitting, standing, walking
   B. Appetite
      Fluids   Drinks
      Thirsty   Eats
      Foods   Poor
   C. Elimination
      1. Urine
         Pale or red   Painful urination
         Dark amber   Difficulty urinating
         Odor   Frequent urination
         Small amount   Incontinence
         Large amount
      2. Feces
         Black, tarry   Difficulty with
         Frequent bowel   bowel
            movements   movements
         Clay-colored   Watery
         Incontinence   Odor
         Diarrhea   Painful bowel
         Bloody   movements
   D. Equipment needed by the client
      Wheelchair   Commode
      Walker   Cane
      Oxygen   Hospital bed
      Catheter   Mechanical lift
   E. Pain
      Dull   Aching
      Location   Severe
      Stabbing   Comes and goes

THE CLIENT'S CARE RECORD

EVERY CLIENT HAS A CARE RECORD. THIS IS A PERMANENT WRITTEN RECORD CONTAINING INFORMATION ABOUT THE CLIENT'S PROGRESS DURING ILLNESS AND REHABILITATION. The care record serves many purposes, as follows.

- To document the work done, the quality of care, and client progress according to the care plan
- For communication between team members
- As a basis for evaluating the plan of care and changing the plan accordingly
- To recall information at a later time, or if the client is discharged and then readmitted to agency services
- As a record for billing to obtain reimbursement for services

THE CARE RECORD IS ALSO A LEGAL DOCUMENT, AND ITS CONTENTS ARE CONFIDENTIAL. TO PROTECT THE CLIENT'S PRIVACY, MOST OF THE MEDICAL RECORD IS KEPT IN THE AGENCY OFFICES. (See Chapter 3 for information about confidential communications and the Client's Bill of Rights.)

Some part of the client record will be located in the home for your use. The particular type of form will vary from agency to agency, but you will use an assignment sheet (sometimes called a *client record* or *weekly/daily care record*) in the home. Most agencies require the home care aide to chart completed assignments on a checklist form. The checklist may be designed to record the care given in just 1 day, or it may cover a longer period of time (Figure 6-3).

RECORDING ON THE CLIENT'S RECORD

Document the tasks performed by initialing or checking off the appropriate area on the checklist. At the bottom of the list, or on the back of the form, there will be space for recording anything that does not fit into the usual daily routine. Always use this special area to record the following:

- Deviations from normal, as described in Box 6-5
- Medical emergencies, as described in Chapter 24
- Household emergencies, as described in Chapter 8
- Calls to supervisor, instructions followed, and results

Other forms that may be used in the home include the following:

- Identifying information record (e.g., client's name, address, telephone number, responsible person to call in an emergency) (Figure 6-4)
- Intake and output record (I&O sheet [see p. 274])
- Daily weight record

These records will be reviewed by your supervisor and returned to the agency offices when they are fully completed. New forms are available from your supervisor. Follow agency policy regarding confidentiality of records found in the client's home.

Other home care providers (e.g., therapists, nurses, social workers) will bring their own records to complete. These forms, too, will become a part of the client's record kept by the agency.

REMEMBER, THE CLIENT'S RECORD IS A LEGAL DOCUMENT THAT MAY BE USED AS EVIDENCE IN COURT. THEREFORE, IT IS IMPORTANT THAT YOUR CHARTING IS ACCURATE. RECORD WHAT YOU DID AND WHAT YOU OBSERVED. DO NOT RECORD WHAT YOU THOUGHT OR GUESSED OR HOW YOU FELT ABOUT YOUR WORK OR OBSERVATIONS. Be sure to follow the following basic rules for recording:

- Always record the correct date and time.
- Do not erase. Draw a line through your mistake; write "error" above it; place your initials and date next to the word *error;* and rewrite your entry.
- Always use blue or black ink. Do not use erasable or felt-tipped pens.
- Write legibly, or print the entry.
- Record telephone calls made to your supervisor.
- Use agency-approved abbreviations and medical terminology.
- Record only the facts.

WEEKLY CLIENT CARE RECORD

Client _____ Employee _____

Address _____ Title _____

City _____ State _____ Zip _____ Client or Account # _____

Phone (day) _____ (eve.) _____ Week Ending _____ / _____ / _____

Fill in the date for each day.

Write your initials in the box which corresponds to each task performed.

		DATE								
	DAY		Mon.	Tue.	Wed.	Th.	Fri.	Sat.	Sun.
	TIME ARRIVED								
PERSONAL CARE:									
Bath ☐ Bed ☐ Chair ☐ Shower ☐ Tub									
Perineal Care									
Hair ☐ Groom ☐ Shampoo									
Mouthcare ☐ Denture Care									
Shave									
Nail Care ☐ Clean ☐ File									
Foot Care									
Special Skin Care									
Dressing ☐ Assist ☐ Complete									
Toileting ☐ Bed Pan ☐ Commode ☐ BRP									
Other instructions: _____									
CLIENT ACTIVITIES: **Transfer Activity Instructions:** _____									
Assist with walking ☐ Cane ☐ Walker ☐ Crutches									
Assist with exercises ☐ ROM ☐ Other (specify)									
Wheelchair activities									
Other instructions: _____									
OTHER FUNCTIONS:									
Temp. ☐ Oral ☐ Rectal ☐ Underarm ☐ Ear									
Pulse									
Respirations									
Blood Pressure									
Weigh Client									
Record Intake/Output (use special form)									

Fig 6-3 Checklist—weekly client care record.

	Mon.	Tue.	Wed.	Th.	Fri.	Sat.	Sun.
OTHER FUNCTIONS:							
Prepare and serve meal/snack							
Special diet (Specify)							
Assist with feeding							
Medications reminder							
Stoma care							
Incontinent care							
Record bowel movements							
Change in condition (office was notified)							
Other instructions: _____							
HOUSEHOLD SERVICES:							
Change/make client's bed							
Clean client's room							
Clean bathroom							
Clean kitchen; wash dishes							
Vacuum, sweep, dust							
Client laundry							
Marketing							
Errands (specify) _____							
Other instructions: _____							
DEPARTURE TIME							
TOTAL HOURS							

I certify that the hours shown represent my true total hours worked.

Signature _____ Title _____ Date _____

Return form to Home Care Agency weekly.
Notify Home Care Agency if your client's condition has changed since your last visit.

Fig 6-3, cont'd

ABC HOME CARE AGENCY
Client Identification Record

Client Name _____

    Address _____

    _____

    Phone _____   Client or Account No. _____

    Religion _____   Age _____

    Place of Employment _____

        Occupation _____

        Social Security No. _____

Diagnosis _____

Date of Initial Service _____

Physician Name _____

    Phone _____

Pharmacy Name _____

    Phone _____

Advance Directive   Yes _____   No _____

Emergency Contact _____   Phone _____

HEALTH INSURANCE

    Primary Insurer _____

        Phone _____

    Secondary Insurer _____

        Phone _____

R.N. Signature _____   Date: _____

Fig 6-4 Identifying information record.

- Document the client's response to care.
- Record what the client tells you; use direct quotes; do not record what you think he or she told you.
- Be concise.
- Use correct spelling and proper English.
- Do not leave blank lines or empty spaces that someone else could fill in; print N/A (not applicable) in the space that is not used.
- Sign your initials or full name and title according to agency policy.

REPORTING TO THE AGENCY

The agency should be notified when you observe changes in the client's physical or mental condition. Also, report any client complaints about his or her physical condition or care. Report anything that seems unusual or out of the ordinary. Before you call, have a pen and paper ready so that you can write the instructions you receive.

When you call your supervisor to report information about your client, give the following information:

1. Your name
2. Client's name, address, and telephone number
3. Your observations, such as
   - What you saw: The client is crying.
   - What you heard the client say: "I feel sick to my stomach. I don't want to get up; let me sleep."
   - What you felt (to the touch): The client's skin is hot and dry.
   - What you smelled (if anything): A fruity odor to the breath.
4. How long the client has had the problem
5. How you handled the situation; if you were unable to follow the care plan, give the reason

IT IS YOUR RESPONSIBILITY TO FOLLOW THE CARE PLAN, RECORD THE CARE GIVEN, AND REPORT ANY CHANGES IN THE CLIENT'S CONDITION. IF YOU BELIEVE THAT THE CARE PLAN NEEDS TO BE CHANGED, NOTIFY YOUR SUPERVISOR AND RECORD YOUR FINDINGS ON THE CLIENT'S CARE RECORD. YOUR SUPERVISOR, CASE MANAGER, OR ANOTHER HEALTH PROFESSIONAL ARE THE ONLY PEOPLE WHO CAN CHANGE THE CARE PLAN.

INCIDENT REPORTS

As Anna Petrova was walking up the stairs to Mr. Smirnoff's apartment, she tripped and fell. She scraped her hands and knees on the concrete steps. They hurt, but she tried to ignore the discomfort while she cared for Mr. Smirnoff.

During the visit, Anna's hands and knees became stiff and swollen. The pain became worse. Before leaving Mr. Smirnoff's apartment, she decided to call Mrs. Quick, her supervisor, on her cell phone to explain the situation. Mrs. Quick told Anna to go to the emergency department at the local hospital to be checked. "You'll have to fill out an incident report when you return to the office, Anna. In the meantime, I'll notify your next client, Mr. Abrams, that you will not be coming this afternoon. I hope you'll be feeling better—talk to you later."

Sometimes an unexpected event (incident) occurs in the client's home or even in the agency offices. An incident usually involves an accident or injury. For example, you may fall and be injured; the client may fall; a visitor may fall—any one of a number of unusual events may happen. When anything of this nature occurs, notify your supervisor immediately and then fill out an *incident report form*. This special form is available from your supervisor. IT IS IMPORTANT TO RECORD INCIDENTS ACCORDING TO YOUR AGENCY POLICY TO PROTECT THE CLIENT, THE AGENCY, AND YOURSELF. COMPLETE THE INCIDENT REPORT AS SOON AFTER THE EVENT AS POSSIBLE, WHILE EVERYTHING IS FRESH IN YOUR MIND. Figure 6-5 shows a sample of an incident report form.

MEDICAL TERMINOLOGY

To record information correctly, you must understand the special language of medicine—medical terminology. A brief introduction to medical terminology follows.

Some medical terms are very old and originate from Latin or Greek words:
Humerus is from the Greek word for "upper arm bone."
Vertebra is from the Latin word for "one of the bones of the spine."

Some medical terms come from the names of the persons who discovered or described the medical condition. For example, Alzheimer's disease was named after Alois Alzheimer, a German neurologist born in 1864.

Another type of medical term is an acronym—a name formed from the first letters of several words, such as **AIDS** from *A*cquired *I*mmune *D*eficiency *S*yndrome.

WORD PARTS

Most medical terms are made up of several word parts. There are four components that may be found in medical terms, as follows.
1. Word roots
2. Suffixes
3. Prefixes
4. Combining vowels

Word Roots

One part of the medical term that is always present is the root. This is the word base to which other parts are attached. The root gives the basic meaning of the word. For example, in the word **microscope**, the root is **scope**. A **scope** is an instrument for viewing. In the term **arthritis**, the root is **arthr**, meaning **joint**.

Suffixes

A suffix is attached to the end of the word root to modify the word root. Suffixes are used to describe disease conditions, diagnostic tools and techniques, and various treatments. To understand or analyze a medical term, begin with the suffix. For example, in the term **arthritis**, the suffix **-itis** modifies the word root **arthr**. The suffix **-itis** means inflammation. Therefore, **arthr + itis = inflammation of the joint.**

Try it yourself. Analyze the term **dermatitis**. **Dermat** is the word root. It means **skin**, and **-itis** is the suffix, meaning **inflammation**. Therefore, **dermat + itis = inflammation of the skin.**

Prefixes

Other words may have a prefix attached to the beginning of a word root that will also modify the meaning of the word root. In the example **microscope**, the word root is

INCIDENT Home Care Agency REPORT

PERSON INVOLVED	(Last name)	(First name)	(Middle initial)	Adult ☐ Child ☐ Male ☐ Female ☐ Age _____

Address _____

| Date of incident/accident | Time of incident/accident | A.M. ☐ P.M. ☐ | Exact location of incident/accident | Bedroom ☐ Hallway ☐ Bathroom ☐ Other ☐ Specify _____ |

CLIENT ☐
List diagnosis if contributed to incident/accident:

Client's condition before incident/accident

Normal ☐ Confused ☐ Disoriented ☐ Sedated ☐ (Drug _____ Dose _____ Time _____) Other ☐ Specify _____

| Were bed rails ordered? Yes ☐ No ☐ | Were bed rails present? Yes ☐ No ☐ | If Yes, Up ☐ Down ☐ | Was height of bed adjustable? Yes ☐ No ☐ | If Yes, Up ☐ Down ☐ |

EMPLOYEE ☐

| Name | Job title | Length of time in this position |

VISITOR ☐
OTHER ☐

| Home address | Home phone |
| Occupation | Reason for presence |

Equipment involved ☐
Property involved ☐ Describe _____

Was person authorized to be at location of incident/accident? Yes ☐ No ☐

Describe exactly what happened; why it happened; what the causes were. If injury, state part of body injured. If property ot equipment damaged, describe damage.

_____
_____

Indicate on diagram location of injury:

Temp. _____ Pulse. _____ Resp. _____

B.P. _____

1. Laceration ☐

2. Hematoma ☐

3. Abrasion ☐

4. Burn ☐

5. Swelling ☐

6. None apparent ☐

7. Other (specify below) ☐

_____

LEVEL OF CONCIOUSNESS

_____
_____

Name of supervisor notified	Time of notification _____ A.M./P.M.	Time of responded _____ A.M./P.M.
Name and relationship of family member notified	Time of notification _____ A.M./P.M.	Time of responded _____ A.M./P.M.
Was person involved seen by a physician? Yes ☐ No ☐ If Yes, physician's name	Where	Date	Time	A.M. ☐ P.M. ☐
Was first aid administered? Yes ☐ No ☐ If Yes, type of provided by whom	Where	Date	Time	A.M. ☐ P.M. ☐
Was person involved taken to a hospital? Yes ☐ No ☐ If Yes, hospital name	By whom	Date	Time	A.M. ☐ P.M. ☐

| Name, title (if applicable), address & phone no.of witness(es) | Additional comments and/or steps taken to prevent recurrence: |

SIGNATURE/TITLE/DATE | **SIGNATURE/TITLE/DATE**

| Person preparing report | Case Manager |
| Supervisor | Administrator |

INCIDENT/ACCIDENT REPORT

Fig 6-5 Incident report form. (Modified from Briggs Corporation, Des Moines, Iowa.)

modified by the prefix **micro-**. The prefix **micro-** means **very small**. Therefore, **micro + scope = instrument for viewing something that is very small**. In the term **thermometer**, the prefix **thermo-** means **heat**, and the word root **meter** means **instrument to measure**. Therefore, **thermo + meter = instrument to measure heat**. Note that not all medical terms will have prefixes.

Combining Vowels

Combining vowels are used to connect roots to suffixes and roots to other roots. They make the words easier to say. The vowel that is used most often is **"o."** For example, to combine the word root **arthr** and the suffix **-scope**, it is necessary to add the combining vowel **o**. Therefore, **arthr + o + scope = arthroscope**, an instrument for examining the joints. Without the combining vowel, it would be very difficult to pronounce the term **arthroscope**. In fact, word roots are usually listed in their combining form, that is, with the combining vowel attached or in parentheses.

Here are a few rules to remember about combining vowels.

1. Use a combining vowel between word roots even if the root begins with a vowel.
2. Drop the combining vowel before a suffix that begins with a vowel.
   Example: **OSTE/O/ARTHR/ITIS**

OSTE/O is the combining form of the word root that means *bone.* The combining vowel is used between the word roots.

ARTHR/O is the combining form of the word root that means *joint.*

-ITIS is the suffix that means inflammation. Because it begins with the vowel *I,* the combining vowel is not used.

So, the term **osteoarthritis** means **inflammation of the bones and joints**.

Listed in Table 6-1 is a small sample of medical word components that, when combined, form terms commonly used in health care. A medical dictionary is a valuable resource for your use.

TABLE 6-1	**Medical Word Components**

WORD ROOT (COMBINING FORM)	MEANING	EXAMPLE OF USE
abdomin/o	abdomen	abdominal
arteri/o	artery	arteriosclerosis
arthr/o	joint	arthritis
ather/o	yellowish, fatty plaque; fatty substance	atherosclerosis
bronch/o	bronchial tubes	bronchitis
cardi/o	heart	cardiac
cerebr/o	cerebrum	cerebral
chem/o	chemical, drug	chemotherapy
col/o	bowel	colostomy
colon/o	bowel	colonoscopy
cyan/o	bluish color	cyanosis
cyst/o	urinary bladder	cystoscope
enter/o	intestines	enteritis
gastr/o	stomach	gastrostomy
glyc/o, glycos/o	sugar	glycosuria
hem/o, hem/a, hemat/o	blood	hemocyte
hepat/o	liver	hepatitis
mast/o	breast	mastectomy
nephr/o	kidney	nephritis

TABLE 6-1	Medical Word Components—cont'd

WORD ROOT (COMBINING FORM)	MEANING	EXAMPLE OF USE
neur/o	nerve	neuralgia
oste/o	bone	osteoporosis
phleb/o	vein	phlebitis
pneumon/o	lung, air	pneumonia
rect/o	rectum	rectal
therm/o	heat	thermometer
thromb/o	blood clot	thrombophlebitis
trache/o	trachea	tracheostomy
ur/o	urine, urinary tract, voiding	uremia
urethr/o	urethra	urethral
urin/o	urine	urinalysis
vascul/o	blood vessel	vascular

SUFFIX

-algia	pain	neuralgia
-ectomy	surgical removal	tonsillectomy
-emesis	vomiting	hematemesis
-emia	blood condition	uremia
-itis	inflammation	hepatitis
-meter	measuring instrument	thermometer
-osis	abnormal condition	cyanosis
-pnea	breathing	apnea
-rrhage, -rrhagia	excessive flow	hemorrhage
-stomy,	new opening	colostomy
-tomy	cutting, incision	tracheotomy
-uria	urine, urination	hematuria

PREFIX

a-, an-	without	apnea
ab-	away from	abduct
ad-	toward	adduction
dys-	painful, difficult	dysuria
hyper-	over, above, excessive	hyperglycemia
hypo-	under, below normal	hypoglycemia
micro-	small	microscope
post-	after	postoperative
pre-	before	preoperative
trans-	across	transurethral

ABBREVIATIONS

Many medical phrases and word combinations are used repeatedly. To save time and space in written communication, abbreviations are used. Some abbreviations are standard (i.e., in common use and understood by health care workers). However, some agencies will use abbreviations that are exclusive to that employer. Ask your supervisor if your agency has such a list.

TABLE 6-2 Abbreviations

ABBREVIATION	MEANING	ABBREVIATION	MEANING
abd	abdomen	OOB	out of bed
a.c.	before meals	OT	occupational therapy
ADL	activities of daily living	pc	after meals
ad lib	as desired	po	by mouth
AM	morning	PM	evening
bid	twice a day	prn	as required
BP	blood pressure	PROM	passive range of motion
BRP	bathroom privileges	PT	physical therapy
$\bar{c}$	with	qid	four times a day
CA	cancer	qs	sufficient quantity, as
cc	cubic centimeter		much as necessary
c/o	complains of	ROM	range of motion
h or hr	hour	$\bar{s}$	without
hs	hour of sleep (bedtime)	SOB	shortness of breath
H_2O	water	tbsp	tablespoon
I&O	intake and output	tid	three times a day
IV	intravenous	TPR	temperature, pulse,
meds	medications		respirations
mL	milliliter	tsp	teaspoon
N/A	not applicable	w/c	wheelchair
NPO	nothing by mouth	wt	weight
O_2	oxygen		

IF YOU DO NOT KNOW WHETHER AN ABBREVIATION IS ACCEPTABLE, YOU SHOULD WRITE THE COMPLETE PHRASE SO THE RECORD IS ACCURATE AND EASILY UNDERSTOOD. Listed in Table 6-2 are some abbreviations in common use.

CHAPTER SUMMARY

- Observing, reporting, and recording information accurately are important responsibilities of the home care aide.
- The home care aide is a vital communication link between the home and the agency.
- There are three types of observation methods: objective, subjective, and vital signs.
- Pain is an important symptom that must be accurately reported to your supervisor.
- Observations are recorded on the client's care record.

- All client records are legal documents. Their contents are confidential.
- Follow the general rules for recording information on the client's care record.
- Notify the agency when changes in the client's physical or mental condition or behavior are observed.
- When calling your supervisor, give precise and accurate information.
- Follow agency policy regarding telephone communications and incident reports.
- Medical terminology is the special language used by health care workers.

STUDY QUESTIONS

1. Why do agencies keep client records?
2. What is meant by
   a. Subjective observations? Give three examples.
   b. Objective observations? Give three examples.
   c. Vital signs?
3. List five rules to be followed when recording information on the client's care record.
4. Immediately after lunch, your client vomits everything she ate and complains of sharp pains in her abdomen. With a classmate, gather more information about the client's pain and act out placing a telephone call to your supervisor. Document your observations and telephone call.
5. Identify the prefix, word root, and suffix, and give the meaning of the following words.
   a. Osteoarthritis
   b. Colostomy
   c. Thrombophlebitis
   d. Neuralgia
   e. Glycosuria
   f. Mastectomy
   g. Hyperglycemia
   h. Hepatitis
   i. Thermometer
   j. Gastrostomy
6. Write the meaning of the abbreviations shown in italics.
   a. *OOB tid*
   b. *NPO* from midnight
   c. Client must take *meds c̄* milk
   d. *OT* will perform *PROM* every other day
   e. Record *I&O* and *wt* daily
7. You have been giving Mr. Simons a shower, according to the care plan, for the past 4 weeks. Today, he says, "I haven't had a tub bath in months. I don't want a shower anymore. I just want to soak in the tub." You explain the reasons for giving him a shower, but he refuses. "I told you, 'NO'. Give me a tub bath!"
   What will you tell Mr. Simons?
   What will you do?
   Why?
8. You have been Athena Kotopolis' home care aide for 3 weeks. She always waits at the door for your visit and greets you with a big smile and a hug, saying, "It's so good to see you, my friend." Today, you ring the doorbell several times before Athena comes to the door. She looks afraid and does not let you enter, saying, "Who are you? I don't need any help—go away." You explain who you are, but she slams the door in your face.
   What action will you take?
   Why?

7

Working With Ill and Disabled Clients

OBJECTIVES

After you read this chapter, you will be able to:

1. Define the terms *health, acute illness, chronic illness,* and *disability.*
2. Identify three effects of illness on the family.
3. Identify five effects of illness on the client.
4. Recognize your feelings about illness and disability.

5. Discuss ways the home care aide can help the client and family cope with the effects of illness.
6. Explain the importance of formal and informal support systems to the client and family.

KEY TERMS

Anxiety A state of intense worry and/or fear
Assistive devices Equipment or other items to help clients perform activities of daily living more easily
Congenital Present at birth
Denial A refusal to admit the truth
Depression/Depressed A prolonged feeling of intense sadness
Genetic Inherited through the genes from mother and father

Grief Physical and emotional responses associated with extreme sorrow or loss
Health State of physical, mental, and social well-being
Illness State of being sick
Mourn Process of grieving caused by great personal loss
Prostheses Devices used by disabled people to replace a missing body part

You may have heard a conversation like the following.

Alice: "Ever since Helen first became sick a few months ago, she's been so worried about what will happen to her. She wonders how long the illness will last and how she will be able to care for herself."

Sarah: "Yes, and her daughter and son-in-law are concerned about the change in Helen. She used to be so outgoing and pleasant. Since her illness, she's become very irritable and doesn't even want to see her friends or relatives. That's really difficult for the family to understand."

This conversation is just one example of many ways people and their families react to illness. As a home care aide, you will work with a variety of clients with a range of illnesses and disabilities. Some may be short term; others may be life threatening or

Fig 7-1 The home care aide helps a mother at feeding time.

permanent. Some, such as a mother and her newborn child, will be healthy but need the special care a home care aide provides (Figure 7-1). Each client and family member will react differently to illness. IT IS IMPORTANT FOR YOU TO UNDERSTAND YOUR CLIENT'S REACTION TO ILLNESS BECAUSE IT WILL HELP YOU GIVE THE QUALITY CARE YOUR CLIENT NEEDS. IT WILL ALSO HELP YOU TO DEAL WITH THE CONCERNS THE FAMILY MAY HAVE ABOUT THE ILLNESS.

HEALTH AND ILLNESS

To understand what illness and disability mean, it is important to define the opposite: health.

Health means a state of physical, mental, and social well-being. It is not just the absence of disease. For example: Many people with arthritis take medicine each day and follow a special program of rest and activity. We say they are healthy because they are able to go about the routine of daily life without any problems.

Illness means the state of being sick or a change from the state of being healthy. We use the terms *disease* and *illness* to mean the same. There are two main types of illness—acute and chronic—that are based on the length and results of the illness and the type of care needed.

ACUTE ILLNESS

- Symptoms appear suddenly and may be severe.
- The illness lasts a short time; care is given at home or in the hospital.
- After illness, full function usually returns.
  Example: Common cold, sprained ankle, food poisoning

CHRONIC ILLNESS

- Symptoms do not subside; they may appear gradually or come and go.
- The illness lasts a long time, maybe a lifetime; care is given at home, in a rehabilitation center, or in a nursing home.

Fig 7-2 Disability may be permanent or temporary, as for this person.

- Permanent changes occur in the body with a decrease in the ability to function.
  Example: Diabetes, tuberculosis, Alzheimer's disease

DISABILITY

A person who cannot perform the normal activities of daily living is said to have a disability (Figure 7-2). This inability to function may
- Be temporary or permanent
- Affect the ability to function physically, mentally, or both
- Be caused by illness, injury, or other factors
  Disabilities are classified as the following:
- **Physical:** Resulting from illness or injury to one or more body systems.
  Example: Loss of an arm or leg
- **Emotional:** Resulting from mental illness or physical condition (more information about clients with emotional disabilities is found in Chapter 21).
  Example: Depression
- **Developmental:** Resulting from illness or injury occurring before, during, or after birth, or in early childhood. It also may be congenital or genetic. This type of disability affects the ability to grow and develop at a normal rate.
  Example: Cerebral palsy

EFFECTS OF ILLNESS ON THE FAMILY

Whether the illness is acute or chronic, or results in temporary or permanent disability, the client's family will be affected by changes that occur. Some typical effects on the family include changes in routine and income, worry and fear, disruption of plans, and

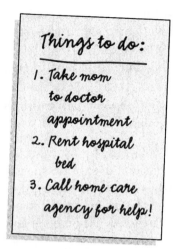

Fig 7-3 Illness may cause changes in routine.

changes in family members' responsibilities. ILLNESS IS NEVER CONVENIENT. ILLNESS DOES NOT GO ACCORDING TO A SET SCHEDULE, BUT IT DOES CAUSE CHANGES IN THE LIVES OF FAMILY MEMBERS.

CHANGES IN ROUTINE

One of the first responses the family may make to illness is to change the routines of everyday life. Meal times may have to be adjusted so that care can be given to the sick family member. Sometimes meals are "on your own," if all members are able to prepare for themselves. Shopping for groceries, cleaning the home, doing laundry—all of these routines may be affected by illness in the family. These changes can be especially upsetting to those who have established routines in their lives. Even weekly planned recreational activities may have to be postponed, such as bowling, playing cards at the neighbors, or going to the movies (Figure 7-3).

If the client is school age, the routines of school are broken. Playing with friends and learning in class are not possible. If the client is an adult and employed, the routine of going to work and being with others outside the family is changed. The caregiver, who is employed, may have to change the work schedule, take a leave of absence, or even quit his or her job. When routines are disrupted, most family members experience difficulties in adjusting to these changes.

CHANGES IN INCOME

When illness occurs, there is usually a loss of income and an increase in extra expenses. If the client has been the only one employed in the family, the loss of income may be a serious problem. In some cases, the savings of a lifetime can be spent in a short period of time.

WORRY AND FEARS

When one person in the family is ill, other family members are often quite worried. Sometimes their worries and fears make it difficult to concentrate on their jobs or their school work. They may also find it hard to talk about their worries, fears, and feelings. Some typical concerns include the following:

The unknown	How long will the illness last?
	What about the future?
	Will there be enough money?
	Will I be able to care for this family member?
Loss	Will there be permanent loss of function?
	Loss of income?
	Loss of companionship?
	Loss due to death?
Pain and suffering	Seeing loved one in pain
	Feelings of helplessness
Resentment	Too much extra work
	Additional burdens and not enough help
	Other family members not helping
	"Why me?"
Stress	Changes in family routines
	Additional responsibilities
	Learning to care for the family member
	Not enough time in the day
	Conflicts with other family members

DISRUPTION OF PLANS

Illness can also change priorities and future plans. Perhaps the family had planned a vacation away from home or an anniversary party where friends and relatives from out of town were expected. These plans may now have to be postponed or even cancelled. The effects of illness are felt by all those involved with the client and family.

ROLE CHANGES

The word *role* means the duties and responsibilities assumed by a person. When the role of the client, before the illness, was that of "breadwinner," another family member may have to find employment to pay the bills. If the mother or father is ill, perhaps the oldest child will become the substitute parent. Or grandparents may take on the additional responsibilities. Mother, father, spouse, partner, significant other, child, grandparent, or friend may assume substitute roles for the ill and disabled client.

Changes in roles can result in periods of adjustment for all family members, and relationships can become strained. Each family will cope with illness and disability in its own special way. In some instances, the family bonds become stronger as each member assumes a special role and adjusts to changes in the home. In other situations, adjustments are made with difficulty or not made at all. The bonds become weak and even break under the weight of family illness and disability.

ADAPTING TO THE NEED FOR A HOME CARE AIDE

In most instances, the family will welcome you into the home to care for the client. The family recognizes the special skills you have and will cooperate with you in every way. Sometimes, however, a family member might react to your visits differently. When this happens, do not take it personally.

Let's look at the case of Winston Campbell, who has been ill with a brain tumor for the past several months. As his condition worsened, his partner, Alex, took a leave of absence from his law firm to care for Winston. During a recent stay in the hospital, the doctor talked to both of them about the need for services of the local visiting nurse association, including professional nurse and home care aide support. Winston was agreeable, but Alex said, "I've been caring for Winston ever since he became ill. I'd rather continue to do it myself." After some discussion, Alex agreed to try the home care services.

When Mrs. Quick, the nurse supervisor, visited the home, she encouraged Alex to take time for himself while the home care aide was giving care. "It's important for you to get a change from caregiving while Ms. Randolph is here. She's one of our most experienced and competent personnel." He agreed, reluctantly.

For the first 2 weeks, Alex followed Betty Randolph wherever she went in the home to "make sure everything is done the way Winston wants it to be done. I know what he can and can't do. No one can give a bed bath as well as I do." Betty understood that Alex was concerned about his partner's care and the seriousness of his illness. Her confident manner in performing her tasks correctly went a long way in helping to build a sense of trust. Actions DO speak louder than words. Slowly, Alex developed confidence in Betty's ability to care for Winston. One day he said, "Betty, I thought I knew exactly what to do, but you've shown me some tips to make my job easier when you leave." Betty smiled and said, "Thanks, Alex. You've made my day!" Now, Alex leaves the home when Betty arrives and visits friends or goes shopping.

AS YOU PROGRESS IN YOUR CAREER, YOUR SUPERVISOR WILL HELP YOU TO RESPOND APPROPRIATELY TO SITUATIONS WHEN FAMILY MEMBERS ARE HAVING SOME DIFFICULTY ACCEPTING YOUR ROLE AS CAREGIVER. FAMILY STRESS, ANXIETY, AND WORRY CAN INTERFERE WITH A GOOD WORKING RELATIONSHIP AMONG THE CLIENT, FAMILY, AND HOME CARE AIDE.

REACTIONS OF THE CLIENT TO ILLNESS

Because each person is an individual, his or her emotions and reactions to illness will vary (Figure 7-4). The way each person responds depends on many things, including the following:

- Age
- Personality and attitude
- Prior physical condition
- Nature and length of condition or illness
- Family support
- Culture

You can play an important role in helping your client to deal with those feelings. Here are some of the common reactions to illness and/or disability.

DENIAL

Denial is a refusal to admit the truth. Sometimes clients use denial as a means of maintaining their emotional health because they cannot cope with what is happening to them. This helps reduce the discomfort that is felt by disturbing facts. For example, it is common for people to deny the fact that chest pain might come from a heart attack.

- Denial
- Withdrawal
- Anger
- Change in self-image
- Fear of over-dependence
- Dependence
- Spiritual distress
- Role changes

Fig 7-4 Client reactions to illness.

"It's just indigestion. I'll just take some medicine, and it will go away." These statements are typical of denial. The individual does not want to face the fact that he or she may have a life-threatening illness. "No, not me. The doctor must have made a mistake. It can't possibly be me." Sometimes this denial will cause a person to delay seeking needed medical treatment.

Your Role: Be caring and supportive. Do not force clients to "realize" they are truly sick. Allow them to come to terms with their illness in their own way. Have a positive attitude and follow the client's plan of care to the best of your ability. If you feel that your client's denial interferes with the care plan or is causing other problems, discuss this with your supervisor.

DEPRESSION

Illness can cause a person to feel **depressed**, sad, and uninterested in his or her surroundings and life. One can be so tired of being sick that there is no energy left for anything else. This feeling is understandable when the client is overwhelmed by all of the problems associated with illness. This type of depression is temporary and should subside as recovery progresses. However, there is always the risk that the depression may increase and the client may require psychiatric care. You must be alert for any indication that your client may be considering suicide (see Chapter 21).

Your Role: Have a positive attitude when caring for the client who feels depressed. Allow the person to express his or her feelings of sadness and loss because of the illness. Remind the client of any improvements that you have observed, such as increasing strength, appetite, or activity. Smile and be pleasant; do not become depressed yourself. On the other hand, do not minimize what the client is feeling.

ANGER

Anger is a common feeling associated with illness. Clients are angry because they are sick, and they may take that feeling out on their friends and families and sometimes the home care aide.

Anger can be demonstrated as impatience. The client is irritated with the caregiver or the doctor and is impatient about all the things that he or she has to "put up with."

Clients also express frustration because they are angry about their limitations, the slowness of their progress, and their inability to control the situation.

Your Role: Be calm and patient. Try not to become angry yourself. Remember, anger is a barrier to communication. You know you are doing your very best, even if nothing seems to please the client.

Keep in mind that the client is angry about being sick or disabled, not with you. Discuss the situation with your supervisor to gain a better understanding of your client's individual needs and problems.

DEPENDENCE AND OVERDEPENDENCE

During an illness, people are often dependent on others. When you have a cold, it is nice to have someone take care of you, tuck you into bed, and fluff your pillows. However, this brief period of dependency is enjoyable only because you know you will be better and back to normal in a few days. Some chronic illnesses cause the person to become progressively weaker and increasingly dependent on other people for care. Clients who value their independence will become very angry and frustrated when they are dependent.

Your Role: You can help clients to maintain their independence by offering choices and opportunities to try to do things on their own. Perhaps the only thing they can do is wash their face, and only if you prepare the washcloth. Still, it is important for the client to do so, no matter how long it takes. Be careful not to become frustrated and impatient when a client's self-care takes "too long." IT IS VERY DIFFICULT TO WATCH A CLIENT STRUGGLE IN AN ATTEMPT TO PERFORM SELF-CARE WHEN YOU KNOW THAT YOU COULD DO IT BETTER AND FASTER. REMEMBER THAT YOU ARE PROMOTING INDEPENDENCE—A GOAL OF CARE FOR ALL CLIENTS.

Some sick people become overly dependent, helpless, and demanding. Even if they are able to become independent, they do not choose to do so. They find excuses to avoid participation in their care. It seems to you that they enjoy their dependence and all the attention that goes with it. Be careful that you do not grow to resent this individual. Do not become angry and nasty. Do not judge your client's behavior as good or bad. Follow the care plan, and discuss your observations with your supervisor.

Encourage clients to be as independent as possible for as long as possible. Praise them for trying, and cheer their progress.

ANXIETY

Although illness itself does not cause anxiety, fears and worries often accompany illness. In addition to worries about money and family relationships, there are often unspoken worries.
- What if there is something else wrong?
- What kind of treatment is needed?
- Will my appearance change?
- Am I going to die?

Anxiety can be so severe that it can interfere with treatment. As with denial, anxiety and fear over "what the disease could be" may cause a person to delay seeking care. Or treatment may be refused altogether. Sometimes people become so anxious about their conditions that they build a wall of silence rather than discuss their worst fears.

Your Role: The home care aide can help the anxious client by carefully explaining as much as possible. If the client is afraid of falling, explain in detail how you will assist him or her to get out of bed and into a chair. There should be no surprises. Be calm and confident. Carry out personal care properly.

Also, prepare the client for any problems that may develop. For example, explain that many times clients feel faint and dizzy when they get out of bed. Explain what you will do to prevent this from happening and what you will do if the client experiences those symptoms. Knowing what to expect helps to put the client at ease.

WITHDRAWAL

When an illness is prolonged, painful, or disfiguring, the client may avoid contact with others. Family members and visitors are turned away because the client is too sick to tolerate other persons. Other causes of withdrawal may be the side effects of treatment, depression, or anxiety. Sometimes withdrawal is forced on clients when they are ignored or abandoned by family and friends.

Your Role: Your approach to the client will vary depending on the underlying cause of the withdrawal. Discuss the client's behavior with your supervisor. Schedule periods for rest and quiet. Perform your duties calmly and efficiently. Assist the client to readjust to socialization when possible. Telephone calls, e-mails, letters, and cards from family and friends can prevent some of the loneliness that accompanies withdrawal. "Be there" for your client. Be attentive to spoken and unspoken needs. Observe carefully any changes in condition, and report these to your supervisor. Make certain that basic physical needs for food, fluids, exercise, rest, and elimination are being met. If depression and withdrawal are both present, be alert for the risk of suicide (see Chapter 21).

ROLE CHANGE

No matter what the roles of the client before the illness, now there is a change. Clients may become angry and frustrated when they cannot perform their usual roles. Family members are busy trying to keep the household running, taking the client for treatment, or dealing with medical personnel and bills. They do not always have the time or energy for the client.

Your Role: The home care aide can encourage the client to participate in family discussions and activities. Arrange a schedule of care and rest periods that includes a special time for family activities. Clients need to be part of everyday family activities and decisions as much as possible.

CHANGE IN SELF-IMAGE

The way we see ourselves, our self-image, plays a very important role in how we react to the world around us. We all have an image in our mind of the perfect self, and we want the world to see us that way. When injury or illness causes a change in body image, the client may feel unattractive and worthless—even repulsive. Changes to body image can come in many forms.
• Loss of a limb by accident or through surgery
• Loss of hair from cancer treatment
• Scars from burns, cuts, or surgery
• Speech problems caused by stroke

Clients not only see themselves negatively, but they also believe that other persons do, too. Unfortunately, in some cases the client is correct.

Your Role: CONTINUE TO MEET THE CLIENT'S BASIC HUMAN NEEDS: PHYSICAL, PSYCHOLOGICAL, AND SELF-ESTEEM. ACCEPT THE CLIENT EXACTLY AS HE OR SHE IS, AND, IF YOU CANNOT DO THIS, PERHAPS

ANOTHER AIDE WOULD BE ABLE TO DO SO. DISCUSS THIS WITH YOUR SUPERVISOR.

Be especially aware of your nonverbal communications, such as facial expressions. Any sign of disgust or revulsion on the part of the aide will cause the client to sense your rejection and feel unaccepted by you. Be matter-of-fact about carrying out procedures that are distasteful to you. Allow the client to use denial by refusing to participate in care. Some clients will refuse to look at their surgical incision. Most will do so, eventually—when they are ready.   When denial interferes with care and progress toward the goals in the care plan, it must be reported to your supervisor.

Help clients to express their feelings about the body changes. Many clients will experience grief and will mourn what they have lost. Be a good listener. Grief causes many feelings, and it helps to talk with an understanding person.

Encourage clients to perform as much self-care as possible. This will promote independence and offer them some control. If assistive devices are needed, encourage their use. Help clients to dress in clothes that will minimize body changes and maximize appearance. Hair loss is easily covered by a wig, cap, or turban. Both men and women feel better when their hair and face are groomed. Assist clients to use prostheses, such as artificial limbs or mastectomy replacements.

Treat clients normally and encourage the family to do the same. Offer praise for their efforts in self-care and rehabilitation. Your respect and courtesy will help the client to feel worthwhile.

There are many support groups (discussed later in this chapter and throughout the text) for persons coping with changes in body image. Many people have been helped by these groups. Your supervisor can provide the client and family with information about specific support groups in your community.

SPIRITUAL DISTRESS

Within the life of every person is a belief system that relates to birth; life; suffering; pain; one's place in the world, universe, and eternity; and death. For many people, this includes an awareness and acceptance of a creator, supreme being, supernatural force(s), or spirit(s). When illness occurs, these beliefs may be challenged and questioned. This can cause great distress and discomfort. Clients may be angry with God (or whatever name they use) and avoid their religious practices. Others may seek religious consolation through prayer and meditation. Families and clients question the meaning of suffering, life, death, and what is to come. The choice of treatment or nontreatment can sometimes cause ethical and moral questions.

Your Role: How can the home care aide help? First, realize that belief systems are very personal. What has worked for you in a crisis situation might not be helpful for your client. Respect each person's right to his or her own beliefs, no matter how foreign they may seem to you. A spiritual advisor may be able to assist your client; a family member should be the one to call the appropriate advisor. If they do not know of any resource, your agency will be able to help them. Sometimes a spiritual advisor's visit is considered a sure sign of impending death. SPIRITUAL CONSOLATION IS FOR THE LIVING, AND MANY VIEW IT AS AN IMPORTANT COMPONENT OF HEALING. PROVIDE TIME AND PRIVACY FOR PRAYER, MEDITATION, SPIRITUAL READING, AND VISITS FROM SPIRITUAL ADVISORS. TRY TO SCHEDULE PERSONAL CARE AND ACTIVITIES OF DAILY LIVING SO THAT CLIENTS WILL HAVE THE PHYSICAL ENERGY TO MEET THEIR SPIRITUAL NEEDS.

PHYSICAL DISTRESS/PAIN

Each illness or injury has its own signs, symptoms, and effects on the physical condition of the client. The amount of physical distress a client experiences depends on the type and severity of the illness or injury. The person's prior physical condition will also play a part in how much distress a person feels and how quickly he or she recovers. For example, a young man in excellent shape may suffer less physical distress from a broken hip than an older man who already has severe arthritis.

Your Role: Carefully observe your client's physical condition and symptoms. Any changes should be reported. Each individual's care plan will tell you what to watch for. Be sure to record on the client's care record what you have discussed with your supervisor. If you have any questions about what to look for or you are unsure of your responsibilities, ask your supervisor so there will be no confusion.

SUPPORT SYSTEMS

Support systems are organizations that provide assistance in times of crisis and stress and help the client and/or family to make it through the tough times. These may be informal or formal.

INFORMAL SUPPORT SYSTEMS

Family members, neighbors, church groups, support groups, and senior citizens' clubs are examples of informal support systems. They respond when the need arises, and there is no charge for the service. For example, when Mrs. Jackson's sister became ill, the Sunday school class from her church sent meals to the home. This was a big help to Mrs. Jackson. It gave her more time to spend with her sister. Then there is Louis Roupp, who has a serious heart and lung disease. He uses oxygen and leaves his apartment only to go to the doctor. His many friends perform his marketing, laundry, and house cleaning. Because of his informal support system, Louis is able to be independent and remain in his own home.

Support Groups

In a support group, people in similar situations come together to discuss their problems with each other. Group meetings are conducted by a leader, usually a health professional or other qualified individual. There are groups for clients and/ or caregivers. Sharing similar concerns helps the client to cope with the day-to-day problems of living with illness. The client must travel to the support group meeting. Caregivers can talk with each other and a leader about the concerns of caring for a loved one on a day-to-day basis. Their frustrations, fears, and anxieties are discussed.

Example: Alcoholics Anonymous, Children of Aging Parents, and stroke clubs

Those who are familiar with the Internet will find many online support groups.

Example: Children of Aging Parents and cancer support groups

FORMAL SUPPORT SYSTEMS

Formal support systems are organized and structured and charge a fee for service (Figure 7-5).

Example: Your agency, Meals On Wheels, cleaning services, and shopping services

Fig 7-5 Formal support systems help a family to cope with unexpected illness or injury.

CHAPTER SUMMARY

- Health is a state of physical, mental, and social well-being, not just the absence of disease.
- Illness is described as acute or chronic.
- Disability is a lack of function and can be classified as physical, emotional, or developmental.
- Changes in roles, routines, loss of income, and disruption of plans can occur as a result of illness in the family.

- Clients experience many effects of illness, including denial, depression, anger, dependence, anxiety, withdrawal, role change, change in self-image, and spiritual and physical distress/pain.
- You have an important role in assisting the client and family to cope with the effects of illness and disability.
- Informal and formal support systems can help the client and family to cope with the effects of illness and disability.

STUDY QUESTIONS

1. Define the terms *health, illness, acute illness, chronic illness,* and *disability.*
2. Identify three effects of illness on the family.
3. List five reactions a client may have to illness. Discuss your role in each.

4. Identify two formal support systems available to clients in your community. Describe the services and costs.
5. Identify two informal support groups available to clients in your community. What do they offer, and how frequently do they meet?

8

Maintaining a Safe Environment

OBJECTIVES

After you read this chapter, you will be able to:

1. Identify 10 common hazards in the home.
2. Discuss 10 safety measures to prevent accidents in the home.
3. Identify clients at risk for accidents and injury in the home.
4. List the steps to be taken in case of fire.
5. Identify personal safety precautions for the home care aide.
6. Describe procedures to be followed in a household or weather-related emergency.

KEY TERMS

Combustible Capable of catching on fire and burning
Crisis A critical time
Emergency (emergencies) A serious situation that comes on suddenly and threatens life or well-being

Flammable Burns easily
Fracture Broken bone
Habit A repeated pattern of involuntary behavior or thought
Toxic Poisonous

Local newspaper stories tell of accidents in the home that could have been prevented. You probably have seen headlines similar to the following.

- EIGHT ROW HOMES DESTROYED BY FIRE—CARELESS SMOKING CAUSES 50 TO BE HOMELESS
- WOMAN ELECTROCUTED WHILE USING CURLING IRON IN BATHROOM
- 2-YEAR-OLD SCALDED WHILE PLAYING WITH HOT WATER FAUCETS

Most of us think that such accidents could never happen to our families. But they can happen! An *accident* is an unplanned and unforeseen event or circumstance. For example, a child runs and falls. Some accidents are caused by an act of nature, such as damage done by a hurricane, tornado, or earthquake. Unfortunately, many accidents are caused by carelessness, including

- Doing something we should not do, such as using a chair as a stepladder
- Not doing something we should do, such as not wearing a seat belt in the car

In many cases, it is impossible to know that an accident is about to happen. Sometimes it just seems to be fate—being at the wrong place at the wrong time. However, many accidents that occur in the home can be prevented. PREVENTING ACCIDENTS REQUIRES THE DEVELOPMENT OF A HABIT OF SAFETY AWARENESS ON THE JOB AND IN ONE'S PERSONAL LIFE. THROUGHOUT THE BOOK, PRINCIPLES OF SAFETY ARE GIVEN FOR EACH ACTIVITY YOU PERFORM AS A HOME CARE AIDE. MAINTAINING A SAFE ENVIRONMENT IS VERY IMPORTANT FOR YOUR CLIENT, THE FAMILY, AND YOURSELF!

BECOMING SAFETY CONSCIOUS

This chapter introduces you to safety-conscious behavior. Being "safety aware" never ends; it is a lifelong habit. It means that you
A—are **AWARE** of potentially unsafe conditions and always practice your skills safely
C—**CORRECT** the condition or notify the appropriate person
T—**TAKE** precautions to avoid future problems
   To be aware of potentially unsafe conditions means that we know what safety hazards are commonly found in the home. The following are typical hazards found in the home environment.

- Inadequate or dim lighting, especially near steps and stairs
- Clutter on the floor, steps, or stairs, such as toys or newspapers
- Frayed rugs or throw rugs that are not tacked down
- Defective electrical appliances, frayed electrical cords (Box 8-1)
- Several appliances plugged into one electrical outlet (Figure 8-1)
- Electrical and telephone cords in the path of traffic areas
- Wobbly stairs, handrails, and furniture
- Highly waxed floors
- Portable home heaters close to curtains, drapes, newspapers, bedding, or clothing (Box 8-2)
- Chairs or tables used as ladders
- Medicines, household cleaning fluids, and other chemicals within easy reach and in unmarked containers
- Incorrect tools used for household jobs

BOX 8-1   Equipment Safety

- Check all equipment before use by yourself or your client.
  Surfaces should be free of cracks, rough or sharp edges, and chips.
  Electrical cords should be intact, not frayed.
  Electrical plugs should be intact, not damaged.
  Bolts and screws should be tightened properly, not loose.
- Use appliances and equipment that are in proper working condition.
- Do not use damaged or defective equipment; if you get a shock while using an appliance or equipment, notify your supervisor.
- Do not allow your client to use damaged or defective equipment.
- When in doubt about operating equipment or the proper procedure for use, notify your supervisor for advice or direction.
- If an unusual noise or odor is present when operating appliance or equipment, turn it off immediately; notify your supervisor for further directions.
- Do not attempt to repair frayed electrical cords, appliances, or equipment.
- Do not cut off the "extra" prong of the three-pronged electrical plug so that it fits into a two-pronged receptacle.

Fig 8-1 Electrical outlets should not be overloaded like this.

BOX 8-2   Portable Home Heater Use

- Locate the heater away from curtains and drapes.
- Never use the heater as a drying rack or toaster or to heat food.
- Move the heater only when it is not being used.
- Never place the heater in a doorway to obstruct a passageway.
- Keep the heater away from water.
- If an extension cord is needed, use only a heavy-duty type.
- Freestanding electric heaters should have tip-over switches that shut off the current if the unit is knocked over.
- Use kerosene heaters only when approved by the local community.
- Do not touch a kerosene heater when it is operating.
- Use a protective screen in front of a portable heater if children or pets are near.
- Never use gasoline or any substitute fuel for a kerosene heater.
- Store kerosene outdoors in an approved container that is properly labeled.
- Install a smoke detector in any room where a heater is used.
- Turn off the heater when the room is unoccupied or when going to sleep.

- Oily rags, old newspapers, rubbish left in piles
- Sharp objects (knives, scissors) left unprotected, within easy reach
- Spilled liquids that were not removed immediately
- Lit cigarette, cigar, pipe, or candles left unattended
- Electrical appliances operated near water
- Electrical wiring under rugs
- Firearms unprotected and within easy reach
- Household pets underfoot

GENERAL RULES OF SAFETY IN THE HOME

The following are 10 basic rules for maintaining a safe home environment.
1. Provide adequate lighting, especially at steps, stairs, hallways, entrances, and uneven walking surfaces.
2. Maintain a clutter-free home (stairways; heavy traffic areas).
3. Remove frayed rugs and scatter rugs, if possible.
4. Have major gas, oil, coal, and electrical appliances (furnace, hot water heater, air conditioner) checked by a qualified person to ensure proper working order.
5. Clean up spills immediately, especially liquids and grease.
6. Store gasoline and kerosene in approved containers.

7. Keep windows in working order and screens in place.
8. Maintain clean but not highly polished floors, steps, and stairs.
9. Install smoke detectors on the ceiling of each level of the home.
Test every month. Replace batteries (long-life alkaline only) every 6 months. Install carbon monoxide detectors according to manufacturer's directions. Test every month. If batteries are used, replace batteries every 6 months.
10. Set hot water heater at 120° F (48° C) or lower to reduce burns due to scalding.

In addition to these 10 basic safety rules, each area in the home has its own special requirements to make it a safe place.

CLIENT'S BEDROOM

The bedroom is a place where falls often occur. Your role as a home care aide is to care for your client in an environment that is as safe as possible. The following are some helpful hints to make the bedroom as "fall proof" and safe as possible.
- Remove clutter from the floor and bedside.
- Arrange furniture to allow for free movement around the room.
- Provide a source of light (lamp) at or near the bedside.
- Provide a night light.
- Keep side rails up on the bed, if necessary.
- Position a hospital bed (if used) at the lowest possible height when care is not being given.
- Remove obstacles in the traffic pattern of the room.

If your client is a smoker, an extra smoke detector should be installed in the bedroom and any other area in which he or she spends time. WHEN SMOKING, THE CLIENT SHOULD ALWAYS BE SUPERVISED BECAUSE CARELESS SMOKING IS THE LEADING CAUSE OF FIRE DEATHS IN THE UNITED STATES.

BATHROOM

This area of the home can be the site of serious accidents because of the presence of electrical outlets, water, and slippery surfaces. Does the bathroom have
- Hot and cold water faucets correctly marked?
- Grab bars for the toilet, bathtub, and shower?
- Night light in place and operating?
- Nonskid mat in the shower and tub?
- Nonskid mat on the floor, if necessary?
- Soap in the dish and not in the tub?
- Electrical appliances (fan, shaver, hair dryer, curling iron) used away from water?
- Toilet secure to the floor?
- Toilet seat securely attached to the toilet?

KITCHEN

Many preventable accidents happen in the kitchen, especially burns and cuts. Make sure that
- Major kitchen appliances (stove, refrigerator, microwave oven) are in working order.
- Fire extinguisher is in working order and located near the stove.
- Small electrical appliances (e.g., toaster, coffee maker) are unplugged when not in use.
- Detergents, cleaning liquids, bleach, and so on, are stored separately (away from food) in clearly marked containers and out of the reach of children and confused clients.

- Items most frequently used are stored within easy reach.
- Pan handles are turned inward and out of children's reach when cooking.
- Pot holders are used, not towels or the corner of an apron.
- Loose, long sleeves are rolled back or fastened with pins or elastic bands when cooking.
- Knives and other objects are sharpened and stored properly.
- Stove or microwave oven is never left unattended while cooking.
- Flammable or combustible items (aerosol cans, gasoline, kerosene) are stored away from the stove or other sources of heat or sparks.
- Aerosol sprays are never used near open flames.
- Oven/stove is not used to heat the area.

OTHER AREAS OF THE HOME

The following are some additional guidelines for maintaining a safe environment in other areas of the home.

Living room	Keep air space between the TV/DVD and wall.
Garage	Store pesticides and fertilizers in well-marked containers out of children's reach.
	Recycle old newspapers and magazines frequently.
Basement	Remove oily rags. Provide a good light source. Keep steps and handrails in good repair.
Outside	Remove snow and ice from steps and walkways as soon as possible. Use kitty litter or commercially prepared substances to melt ice. Keep steps and handrails in good repair.

SPECIAL SAFETY CONSIDERATIONS

In addition to the common hazards and safety measures previously discussed, there are special considerations for older adults, children, and confused clients. The use of oxygen in the home increases the risk of fire. Smoking is an additional hazard.

OLDER ADULTS

The normal changes that are part of the aging process (Chapter 19) make older adults candidates for accidents. Because their bones may be brittle, a minor fall may cause a serious fracture. Slowed reaction time also puts them at risk for injury.

Falls are quite common and occur most frequently in the home. Many falls happen when the older adult trips over something. Little things, like unmended shoes, untied laces, floppy slippers, and loose drooping clothing, can cause a person to trip. Anything left on the floor, such as magazines, toys, electric cords, shoes, and clothing, can lead to a fall. THE HOME CARE AIDE HELPS TO PREVENT INJURY BY BEING ALERT TO POTENTIAL HAZARDS; THIS INCLUDES REMOVING CLUTTER AND ALERTING CLIENTS AND FAMILIES TO POTENTIALLY HAZARDOUS CONDITIONS.

CHILDREN

As children grow and develop, they begin to explore the world and to try out and learn new things. Children do not have a sense of caution or awareness of danger. They take many risks during their growing years. Accidents are the leading cause of death for children and adolescents. Hints for child safety are listed in Box 8-3.

BOX 8-3 | Hints for Child Safety

- Use care to prevent burns, drownings, bumps, cuts, and falls.
- Keep dangerous items out of children's reach; use products in child-resistant containers.
- Lock dangerous items in a secure place, out of children's sight and reach.
- Do not store dangerous items in a cabinet under the sink.
- Keep all thin plastic wrapping material (dry cleaner, produce, grocery, or trash bags) away from children.
- Never use thin plastic material to cover mattresses or pillows; the film can cling to a child's face and cause suffocation.
- Protect against electrical shocks; cover unused outlets with safety covers.
- Disconnect all electrical appliances when not in use.
- Keep children away from open windows to prevent falls. Screens will not keep a child from falling out; they are designed to keep insects out, not to keep children inside.
- Do not place furniture near windows; children may climb up to a window sill or seat.
- Keep window blind cords away from the child's crib or bed and out of the child's reach.

CONFUSED CLIENTS

Confused clients may not know their names, addresses, or telephone numbers. There is a great risk that they will leave the home and wander in the neighborhood, at any time of day or night and in any type of clothing. The following are some protective measures.

- Have recent, clear photographs of the client available.
- Have the client wear an ID bracelet or electronic device.
- Know where the client is at all times.
- Closely supervise the client in potentially dangerous situations (e.g., smoking, shaving, cooking, bathing).
- Attach bells to ring when outside doors are opened.
- Lock doors to basements, attics, and all stairways.
- Label doors to other rooms using word and picture signs.
- Put sharp objects, weapons, chemicals, and other harmful materials in a safe place. Information about confused clients is found in Chapter 21.

OXYGEN

OXYGEN IS NECESSARY FOR LIFE. WE NEED OXYGEN TO BURN OUR FOOD AND CONVERT IT INTO ENERGY. THERE MUST BE OXYGEN TO BUILD A FIRE, AND FUEL BURNS FASTER IN THE PRESENCE OF HIGHER CONCENTRATIONS OF OXYGEN. THEREFORE, THE USE OF OXYGEN (O_2) IN THE HOME POSES A GREAT RISK FOR FIRE. Follow the procedures for oxygen therapy (see Chapter 18) and all the safety guidelines discussed. Remember, there should NEVER be an open flame or spark-producing object near oxygen. No matches, lighters, cigarettes, pipes, electric razors, or pilot lights should be anywhere near the oxygen delivery system (Figure 8-2). Post "No Smoking" signs on the outsides of all doors into the home. Inside the home, place signs near the source of oxygen. Know how to turn off the oxygen and what to do in the event of fire.

SMOKING

Careless smoking is a major cause of home fires. An individual who falls asleep while smoking may not awaken to a smoke filled room, or be unable to leave the room

Fig 8-2 Never allow cigarettes, pipes, or fire-producing items in the same room with an oxygen delivery system!

without help. More people die from smoke inhalation than from burns. Smoke produced by burning household furnishings is toxic and interferes with breathing. Smoke detectors are a necessity in every home, especially where there is a smoker.

Smoking is risky behavior for the smoker and other family members, too. Some special safety rules include the following.

- **DO NOT SMOKE IN BED.**
- Use ample ash trays to prevent cigarette butts and ashes from falling on floor.
- Do not dispose of cigarette butts and ashes in the garbage; place them in a large covered metal container, and put the container outside for the embers to cool.
- Keep matches, lighters, and cigarettes out of the reach of children and confused persons.
- **MAKE SURE ALL SMOKE DETECTORS ARE WORKING; TEST EVERY MONTH, AND REPLACE BATTERIES EVERY 6 MONTHS.**

HOUSEHOLD EMERGENCY MEASURES AND PROCEDURES

Experts agree that people who prepare for emergencies cope better during the crisis and recover more quickly. The best way to reduce risk is to think ahead. The home care aide can assist the client and family to prepare for possible emergencies.

FIRE

Some causes of fire include the following.
- Smoking and matches
- Unattended lighted candles
- Misuse of electricity
- Defects in heating system
- Materials that ignite easily
- Improper trash disposal
- Improper cooking techniques
- Improper ventilation
- Improper use of aerosol cans (e.g., hair spray, cleaning fluids, paints)
  It takes three things to start a fire (Figure 8-3).
1. Fuel—any material that will burn
2. Source of heat—matches, flame, spark
3. Supply of oxygen—present in the air

Fig 8-3 A fire triangle.

BOX 8-4   Extinguishing a Small Enclosed Fire

GREASE OR FOOD FIRE
Cover pan with a lid; turn off burner.

MICROWAVE OVEN FIRE
Keep door closed; push STOP switch.

OVEN FIRE
Close oven door; turn off stove.

Fire can be prevented by removing any one of these three ingredients. Very tiny fires become big ones almost immediately.

Stove fires become kitchen fires, and kitchen fires become whole house fires (Box 8-4). An open, moving fire triples in size in 1 minute. Prevention is the key to fire safety. Most house fires occur between 8:00 PM and 8:00 AM. Therefore, a working smoke detector *must* be on the ceiling of every level of the home.

The first time you enter a client's home, look for an alternate exit.

Identify two escape routes from each room, just in case a fire starts. In a high-rise or apartment complex, find the fire alarm box so you will be aware of its location if needed.

THE NUMBER 1 RULE IN ANY FIRE IS GET OUT AND GET YOUR CLIENT OUT WITHOUT ANY DELAY. CALL 9-1-1 OR THE FIRE DEPARTMENT (Box 8-5). If you are in an apartment building, leave the unit and scream "FIRE" in the hallways. If there is a fire alarm system, use it. Never go back into the home for any reason. Follow the do's and don'ts listed as follows:

BOX 8-5 | Reporting a Fire

REMAIN CALM

Call 9-1-1 or the fire department

GIVE THE DISPATCHER

1. Your name
2. Your location (including building number, floor and apartment number, and nearest cross street)
3. Location of the fire
4. Telephone number you are calling from

Fire Escape Do's and Don'ts

Do

- Get out with your client as fast as you can.
- Notify the fire department immediately.
- Feel the door to see if it is hot. If it is cool, open it carefully, with your face turned away from door opening; slam the door if heat and smoke rush in.
- Use an alternate exit route when necessary.
- Keep doors closed to prevent smoke from entering the room.

Don't

- Use elevators—smoke rises; elevator shafts act as chimneys.
- Waste time trying to put out a fire.
- Run if your clothing is on fire. (Instead, *stop*, *drop down*, and *roll* to smother the flames.)
- Go back into a burning structure.

Smoke is dangerous. If you encounter smoke, use an alternate escape route. If you must exit through smoke, drop and crawl on your hands and knees to the nearest exit. Take your client with you in the same way, if possible. Cover nose and mouth with a damp cloth to ease breathing, but do not waste a lot of time with this detail. Remember the number 1 DO rule and GET OUT.

If you are unable to get out of the building, try to call 9-1-1 or the fire department and tell them where you are—building, floor, and apartment number. If the fire is outside of the apartment, close the door of the unit and block the bottom of the door with wet towels or blankets to keep the smoke out. Move your client away from the fire to a room with a window. Close the door to that room, blocking the bottom as before. Cover your nose and mouth with a damp cloth—and your client's, too. Hang a sheet, towel, or tablecloth in the window to alert the fire fighters of your location. Do not panic. Help will come.

One of the biggest problems in fire safety is the attitude that "it can't happen to me." But that is simply not true. Each year millions of home fires in the United States cause thousands of deaths and injuries. Being alert and prepared can save lives and prevent injury.

GAS LEAK

Natural gas and propane used for cooking and heating have no odor. The odor is added as a safety measure to detect leaking gas. When you smell gas in the home

- Ventilate the area—open windows and doors.
- Check to see if the pilot lights in the stove, oven, furnace, or hot water heater are on.

Fig 8-4 If the power goes out, check the electrical service panel to see if the circuit breaker needs to be switched on.

- Do not use anything that will produce a spark (turning on electric switches or thermostat, using matches) and cause an explosion.
- Call the gas company using a telephone away from the area in question (a tiny spark may be created by the telephone's electrical contacts).
If the odor is strong
- Leave the house.
- Call the gas company.

If the odor is outdoors, call the gas company. Emergency crews are on call at all times of day and night.

LOSS OF ELECTRICITY

A power loss in the home may be caused by an overload to the electrical system. In this case, a fuse may need to be replaced or the circuit breaker switched on. First, turn off all appliances (except the refrigerator), and check the electrical service panel or fuse box (Figure 8-4). Follow the instructions in Box 8-6 to restore power. This may be your responsibility, if no one else is available.

If the power does not come back on, call the electric company. The failure may involve several homes, the neighborhood, or a wider area. Notify your agency, and follow the instructions given. The extent and length of the power outage will determine the action to be taken.

PLUMBING PROBLEMS

Plumbing problems are a possibility in any home with running water. A little advance knowledge may help you to deal with a gushing pipe when necessary. Knowing where the water valves are located will save time if an emergency occurs. You should know the location of the main valve that controls the flow of water into the home. Also, find the controls to sinks, tubs, and toilets.

If a leak occurs, turn off the flow of water to the fixture. Once the leak has been stopped, the appropriate person (family member, building superintendent, custodian, etc.) must be notified so repairs can be made. Notify your agency regarding the problem.

> ## BOX 8-6 | Fuses and Circuit Breakers
>
> ### FUSES
>
> Fuses are protective devices that cut off the power if there is an overload or a short in the electrical system.
>
> Replacing a blown fuse is *not* usually the responsibility of the home care aide, but there may be a time when you will have to do it.
>
> CAUTION: DO NOT TOUCH THE MAIN ELECTRICAL PANEL IN THE HOME WHEN WATER IS PRESENT. CALL YOUR AGENCY FOR INSTRUCTIONS.
>
> ### REPLACING A FUSE
>
> 1. Locate the main electrical service panel, usually in the basement or utility room. Turn off the main switch, or pull it out before you start.
> 2. Look at fuses in the panel. Check the window of each fuse plug to see if the metal strip is broken or cloudy. A broken strip indicates an overload—too many appliances are in use at one time. Disconnect them. A clouded plug indicates a short circuit. The electricity is flowing from its normal path to objects that cannot handle the great amount of heat produced and may melt or catch fire (e.g., frayed electrical cord).
> 3. With one hand, unscrew the blown fuse and replace it with a new one with the same rating.
> 4. Restore the power.
>
> ### CIRCUIT BREAKERS
>
> Circuit breakers are heat-sensing switches that shut off the electrical power if the smallest imbalance occurs.
>
> CAUTION: DO NOT TOUCH THE MAIN ELECTRICAL PANEL IN THE HOME WHEN WATER IS PRESENT. CALL YOUR AGENCY FOR INSTRUCTIONS.
>
> ### CORRECTING A TRIPPED CIRCUIT BREAKER
>
> 1. Turn off all extra appliances and big electricity users.
> 2. Locate the main electrical service panel, usually in the basement or utility room. Turn off the main switch before you start.
> 3. Look at the breaker switch. It has three positions: "On," "Off," and tripped (middle position).
> 4. Switch the tripped breaker to the "Off" position, and then flip it to "On" again.
> 5. Restore the power.

NATURAL AND WEATHER-RELATED EMERGENCIES

Every area of the country experiences natural and weather-related emergencies. The television news reports deep snows in the northeast, hurricanes along the southeast coast, floods in the Plains states, earthquakes in the west, and tornadoes in the southern states. No part of the country is untouched by nature's elements. You and your client can be severely affected by these natural disasters.

Think ahead, prepare for the possibility of disasters, and know what to do if a disaster occurs.

* Prepare a disaster supply kit (Box 8-7) that is appropriate to your climate, seasons of the year, and past disasters.
* Have drills to prepare for possible emergencies (fire, tornado, earthquake).
* Keep in touch with your agency; they can relay information to your family and the client's family.
* Follow directions given by police and rescue workers; have the agency notified if you are evacuated.

BOX 8-7 Disaster Supply Kit

Keep the following in the closet nearest to the door used during evacuation:
- First aid kit
- Essential medications—protect from children
- Canned food and opener
- Bottled water
- Utensils for eating and drinking
- Extra clothing
- Rain wear, boots
- Blankets
- Battery-operated radio (extra batteries)
- Important telephone numbers
- Safety matches (waterproof container)
- Extra car keys
- Flashlight (extra batteries)
- Face mask
- Hand sanitizer
- Tissues or toilet paper

- Take care of your client's personal needs as best you can.
- Protect yourself and the client from injury.
- Keep a 2-week supply of prescription medications on hand during a "disaster time" (snow, hurricane, tornado season) and always in an earthquake zone.
- Stay tuned to your television or radio emergency broadcast system for updated news and emergency instructions.
- Water may be purified by boiling for 20 minutes.

EARTHQUAKE

- Learn how to turn off the main source of water, electricity, and gas.
- Look around each room, and decide where you can protect yourself from falling items.
- Position the client's bed away from anything that could fall on it during an earthquake (e.g., windows, mirrors, shelves, light fixtures).
- If an earthquake occurs, get under a heavy table or desk.

HURRICANE/FLOOD

- During wind and driving rain, move away from windows.
- Close blinds, drapes, and curtains.
- Stay in an interior protected room.
- Place fresh water in jugs, bottles, or buckets.
- Put possessions on a higher level.
- Prepare to evacuate when water rises rapidly.
- Call for help.
- Do not use the telephone during periods of thunder and lightning.
- Have flashlights, matches, or oil lamps ready for use.
- Move cars to a higher and drier location, if possible.
- Remain in contact with your agency, if possible.

BOX 8-8 Emergency Telephone Numbers

Local Emergency Number or 9-1-1 ( )_____–_____
Police ( )_____–_____
Fire Department ( )_____–_____
Ambulance ( )_____–_____
Doctor ( )_____–_____
Agency ( )_____–_____
Relative
    Home ( )_____–_____
    Work ( )_____–_____
Neighbor ( )_____–_____
Location of House _____
Nearest Cross Street _____
House Phone ( )_____–_____ and/or Cell Phone ( )_____–_____
Other Numbers
    Gas Company ( )_____–_____
    Electric Company ( )_____–_____
    Building Superintendent ( )_____–_____
    Landlord ( )_____–_____

SNOW/WINTER STORM

- Have sufficient amounts of food and medicine on hand.
- Have an extra blanket on hand.
- Prepare the car for winter travel, if necessary.
- Stay inside, keep warm, and keep the client warm.
- Be prepared for an electrical power failure (discussed earlier).
- Remain in contact with your agency.

TORNADO

- Decide ahead of time the place where you will go when there is a tornado warning.
- Listen for warnings on the television and radio.
- Stay away from windows.
- The lowest level is safest; stay inside, and go to the basement or an interior windowless room or closet.
- In all of the emergency situations discussed in this chapter, you will need a list of telephone numbers readily available (Box 8-8). Keep the list on the refrigerator door. Keep this list of telephone numbers with you at all times. Complete the list during your first visit to the client.

PERSONAL SAFETY OF THE HOME CARE AIDE

Home care aides work everywhere—in the city, suburbs, country, farms, and desert. You will probably travel alone to unfamiliar areas, and you must be alert to protect your own safety. Practice fire safety in your own home twice a year. Conduct EDITH (*Exit Drill In The Home*) with your family (Box 8-9).

BOX 8-9   EDITH Practice

EXIT DRILLS IN THE HOME

1. Everyone in bedrooms; doors closed.
2. One person sounds the alarm.
3. Each person tests the door to see if it is hot.
4. Pretend it is hot; use an alternate exit to escape.
5. Everyone meets at a designated spot. One person uses a prearranged telephone to notify the fire department.

LIST OF SAFETY DO'S AND DON'TS

In Client's Home

Do

- Follow all rules of home safety.
- Keep doors locked at all times.
- Check carefully before letting a stranger into the home; always ask for identification from anyone who comes to the door.
- Shout "I'll get it," even if you are alone.
- Hang up if you receive threatening telephone calls.
- Notify the agency and police about threatening calls; they will tell you what to do and what records to keep.
- Call your supervisor when you arrive and leave the client's home according to your agency's policies.

Don't

- Let strangers in to use the telephone, but offer to make a call for them if there is an emergency.
- Let strangers into a security entrance of an apartment building.
- Give information over the telephone to wrong number callers.
- Let strangers (wrong number callers) know that you are alone or that your client is sick or disabled.
- Stay, if you feel unsafe in the client's home; get out.

Driving

Do

- Use your seat belt at all times.
- Keep your car in good repair.
- Keep a cell phone handy, if available. Make sure the battery is fully charged.
- Make sure your spare tire is useable.
- Have enough gas in your car in case of a lengthy traffic jam or a detour; always keep your gas tank half full.
- Have money to buy gas.
- Plan your route; use well-traveled streets; avoid unsafe areas; "safety" of the neighborhood may change according to time of day.
- Let supervisor and a member of your family know your travel route.
- Know where police and fire stations are located in the client's neighborhood.
- Drive to the nearest police, fire, or well-lighted gas station if you are being followed.
- Keep doors locked and windows closed while driving.
- Park in a well-lighted area, and always lock car doors.
- Have your key ready to unlock the car door.
- Look around inside the car and back seat before entering.

Don't

- Keep your purse or valuables on the front passenger seat.
- Pick up hitchhikers.
- Stop to help another driver; call police on your cell phone.
- Get out of your car until you have checked your surroundings and feel that it is safe.
- Ask strangers for directions; instead, go to the police station, fire station, or gas station for assistance.
- Ever let a stranger into your car.
- Use your cell phone or send text messages while driving. Pull over to a safe place and stop before using the cell phone.

Car Trouble

Do

- Put on emergency flashers.
- Stay in the car; keep doors locked and windows rolled up.
- Use your cell phone, if available, to call for help.
- Place a "Call Police" sign in the window.
- Ask any person who stops to notify police.
- Ask any person in an unmarked police car and in street clothes for proper identification, or request a marked police vehicle.

Don't

- Leave the car and walk alone on a highway or unfamiliar area.
- Go in a stranger's car.

Public Transportation

Do

- Use busy, well-lighted bus, train, and subway stops.
- Wait where there are other people; stay near the group.
- Sit near the bus driver.

Don't

- Wait alone at a bus stop; try to go to a busier area.
- Get off if you feel unsafe; speak to the bus driver about your safety concerns.
- Talk to strangers; avoid eye contact.

Walking

Do

- Keep your cell phone within easy reach.
- Plan your route to use well-lighted streets.
- Plan the shortest, safest route possible.
- Walk in the street at night, facing oncoming traffic.
- Carry some money in your pocket.
- Carry a whistle or personal alarm.
- Keep house keys and car keys in your hand.
- Walk confidently like you know where you are going.
- Check with your police department to see if they offer programs on "street safety."
- Be aware of what is going on around you.

Don't

- Walk in alleys, deserted areas, or near buildings or bushes.
- Walk with strangers.
- Walk alone at night, if possible.
- Hitchhike or accept rides from strangers.

- Carry all your money in your purse or wallet.
- Carry a purse.

Arriving Home
Do
- Keep headlights on and car doors locked until you have checked the parking area or garage.
- Have your house key or apartment key in hand.
- Leave a light on before you leave home (indoor and outdoor).
- Ask the driver to wait until you are safely inside before leaving; use a prearranged signal to indicate that it is safe to leave.

Don't
- Go inside if something seems to be wrong. Instead, go to a safe place and call the police.
- Delay entering your home, especially at night.

CHAPTER SUMMARY

- A safe home environment is maintained by
   Being aware of potentially unsafe conditions.
   Correcting unsafe conditions or notifying the appropriate person.
   Taking precautions to avoid future problems.
- The home care aide must be alert to safety risks for client, family, and self.
- Home care aides need to know the general rules for maintaining a safe home.
- Older adults, children, and confused clients require special attention to prevent injury.

- Smoking is the number 1 cause of home fires.
- The use of oxygen in the home poses great risk for fire.
- Planning in advance for possible household emergencies helps you to handle them more effectively.
- The number 1 rule in any home fire is "Get out and get your client out without delay."
- Prepare ahead for natural and weather-related emergencies.
- Keep a list of emergency telephone numbers handy.

STUDY QUESTIONS

1. List 10 common hazards found in the home, and describe how you would correct them.
2. Identify two types of clients who would be at risk for accident/injury in the home. Describe three measures to take in preventing accidents for each type of client.
3. List steps to be taken in case of a fire.
4. What are five important safety precautions to take when traveling to and from a client's home?
5. What is the most common weather-related emergency in your area? What procedures would you take to protect yourself and your client?

9

Maintaining a Healthy Environment

OBJECTIVES

After you read this chapter, you will be able to:

1. Discuss the importance of a clean and well-maintained home environment to the client's health and safety.
2. Explain the role of the home care aide in maintaining a clean, healthy home environment and the usual tasks performed.
3. Select and use appropriate supplies for cleaning and maintaining the client's environment.
4. Perform basic tasks of cleaning and housekeeping of the client's immediate environment.
5. Know when to seek assistance from others, such as the agency and the client's family.
6. Teach others in the home to assist with the care of the client's environment.

KEY TERMS

Contamination Introduction of harmful organisms
Disinfect To destroy germs
Disinfectant Chemical that can be applied to objects to destroy germs

Ecologically Relating to the environment
Microorganisms Living plants or animals that can be seen only through a microscope

You may be asking yourself, "Why does a home care aide have to maintain a clean, healthy environment? Why doesn't the aide just care for the client who is sick?" These are good questions. Consider the following client situations.

- When Brigit Kennedy, 82 years of age, fell in the bathroom, she broke both her hip and her wrist. She had a surgical repair of her broken hip and has been discharged from the hospital to her home, where she is using a wheelchair. Brigit cannot bathe, clean, cook, or do her laundry without assistance. She lives alone in a senior citizen apartment complex and has a clothes washer and dryer. A widow for 20 years, she looks forward to visits from her daughter and three grandchildren.

"But my daughter doesn't have any time to take care of me. Thank goodness, I have you!" Anna Petrova helps Brigit with bathing, grooming, laundry, and basic housekeeping.

- Louis Roupp, 64 years of age, lives alone in a first-floor apartment in the city. Because of his heart disease, he is unable to leave his home and uses oxygen most of the time. He has no strength or energy for home maintenance, cleaning, laundry, or shopping. Russ Larson helps Louis with personal care and grooming. Once a week, Russ shops for food. Mr. Roupp receives one meal a day from the Meals On Wheels program. He also has assistance from a cleaning service.

- Lily Chiang, 29 years of age, is pregnant with twins. It has been a difficult pregnancy, and she is now confined to bed until she delivers in about 2 months. She says that her 4-year-old daughter, Elizabeth, "is a handful, but loves nursery school." Her husband's work as an engineer requires him to take frequent business trips out of state. "I'm lucky that my parents live nearby and can help." The Chiangs have a housecleaning service that does all of the heavy cleaning. Betty Randolph comes to Lily's home to help her bathe, to make the bed, and to straighten the bedroom. Lily's mother takes care of Elizabeth, so Betty can spend all of her visit caring for Lily.

- Father Kowalski, 72 years of age, had a stroke 6 weeks earlier. He has difficulty speaking and swallowing. "My right side is very weak, too," he says. Father lives on the second floor of the rectory of the church in a combination bedroom/sitting room. The bathroom is next to the bedroom. Victoria, the housekeeper, takes care of all meals and cleaning. Father looks forward to Rosina Chavez's visits. "She has a good sense of humor—she makes me laugh!" Rosina gets Father out of bed, assists him with personal care, makes the bed, and straightens the area as needed. The physical therapist and speech-language therapist each visit three times a week, too.

A CLEAN ENVIRONMENT IS IMPORTANT

Brigit, Louis, Lily, and Father Kowalski cannot assume full responsibility for themselves or their surroundings. They do not have the strength or the ability to perform their own personal care or their own housekeeping duties. When a person is sick or disabled, care of the home is often not done. The family may be too busy caring for the sick person, and home maintenance may not be possible. Yet, a clean environment is an important part of health care. Clutter, disorder, dirt, and odors are health and safety hazards. They increase the risk for infection, disease, and accidents that can interfere with the client's recovery.

You are responsible for maintaining a clean, safe, and healthy environment. This is accomplished in many ways.

1. Performing housekeeping duties, as listed in the work plan, while the client is sick or disabled.
2. Helping the client to assume increasing responsibility for maintaining a clean, healthy environment whenever possible.
3. Teaching disorganized families to develop and carry out plans for maintaining a safe home environment.
4. Helping with home management during a crisis situation (e.g., death and/or hospitalization of a primary caregiver, suspected child abuse, sick children) until a long-term plan can be developed.

RESPONSIBILITIES OF THE HOME CARE AIDE

Housekeeping responsibilities include care of the client's immediate environment, usually the bedroom and the bathroom. The work plan may call for some light cleaning throughout the house. If you use the kitchen, you will be expected to clean up after

---

BOX 9-1   In the Client's Home

- Be sensitive to attitudes of client and family regarding maintaining a clean, neat home.
- "Make do" with housecleaning products available.
- Do not ask the client to purchase products that you personally prefer.
- Always know the products you are using—READ THE LABEL.
- If unsure about the operation of an appliance, ask the family for instructions, read the "use and care" booklet from the manufacturer, or contact your supervisor.
- Do not operate equipment you are not familiar with.
- If changes are needed in placement of furniture and storage of cleaning equipment and supplies, discuss them with the client and family; give reasons why changes would help in housekeeping tasks.
- Encourage family members to help maintain a healthy home; when needed, teach the necessary skills.
- Teach the family, by example, how to maintain a healthy home.
- Learn how to improvise when cleaning materials or equipment are not available.
- Do not judge the client or family whose home is not up to your own personal standards of "good housekeeping."
- Do not make comments about "poor" housekeeping.
- Wear heavy-duty protective gloves for cleaning or using household cleaning liquids.
- Wash your hands immediately after performing household tasks.
- Ask your client for permission to open bureau (dresser) drawers to obtain items needed.
- Do not climb on chairs; use a sturdy step ladder.

---

yourself. Specific duties will be listed on the work plan developed by your supervisor, the client, and the family. These may include dusting, vacuuming, laundry, cleaning the kitchen, and washing the dishes. **IF THERE IS ANY QUESTION OR CONFUSION ABOUT YOUR DUTIES OR THE TIMING OF EACH JOB, CONTACT YOUR SUPERVISOR. DO NOT ARGUE WITH YOUR CLIENT ABOUT YOUR HOUSEKEEPING RESPONSIBILITIES.**

Caring for your client's environment is NOT the same as cleaning your own home. The client may want things done his or her way. Some clients may be frustrated because they must depend on you. Others may be embarrassed by all the mess in their home.

A note of caution: Not all homes are like your own home. Some will be better equipped, and, as in the case of Father Kowalski, there may be full-time household help. Other times, you may be working in an environment where the resources are limited. In urban areas, a single-room-occupancy (SRO) unit may have a shared bathroom, no kitchen, and no running water in the room. In rural areas, the toilet may be outdoors, and the water may come from a hand-operated pump. Be prepared to improvise, substitute, and "make do" when necessary (Box 9-1).

TYPES OF TASKS TO BE PERFORMED

The work plan (Figure 9-1) lists your responsibilities for maintaining the client's environment. Both your agency and client agreed on these services during the first visit from the case manager. Types of tasks to be performed vary according to each client's individual needs and can include any of the tasks listed below.

- *Client's bedroom:* Clean the immediate environment. Empty and clean the commode (Figure 9-2). Make the bed, and change and launder linens as necessary. Care for the client's personal laundry: hand wash in the sink, or machine wash in the client's home, the laundry room, or the laundromat. Dry laundry, and return it to its proper place. Empty the wastebasket.

ABC Home Care Agency
Home Care Aide Instructions

Client   Date   Case Manager/Supervisor

_____   _____   _____

Housekeeping Work Plan	Daily	Weekly
Bedroom		
Floor (clean/vacuum)	✓	
Dust	✓	
Make bed	✓	
Change bed linens (as needed)		✓
Empty wastebasket	✓	
Clean commode	✓	
Bathroom		
Floor (clean/vacuum)	✓	
Clean sink, tub, commode	✓	
Change bath linens (as needed)		✓
Empty wastebasket	✓	
Kitchen		
Floor (clean/vacuum)	✓	
Dishes – client's	✓	
Refrigerator		✓
Stove	✓	
Counter and sink	✓	
Remove trash	✓	
Other Areas		
Floor (clean/vacuum)		✓
Dust furniture		✓
Laundry		
Wash		
Client's personal laundry (as needed)	✓	✓
Bed and bath linens		✓

Fig 9-1 The work plan.

Fig 9-2 Cleaning the commode may be one of the home care aide's duties.

Fig 9-3 Cleaning the splashguard of a raised toilet seat.

- *Client's bathroom:* May be private or shared with other family members. It may be down the hall and shared by unrelated residents of the building. Clean the toilet and the raised toilet seat attachment daily (Figure 9-3). The tub and shower are cleaned after each use. In some situations, it may be necessary to clean them before your client uses them. Change and launder bath linens as necessary. Replace toilet tissue, soap, and facial tissue as needed. Empty the wastebasket.
- *Client's kitchen (or family kitchen):* Light cleaning of counter surfaces, dishes the client uses, and utensils and appliances you use to prepare the client's meals. Clean the refrigerator, if there is no one else to do so. Clean the sink and drain. Sweep the floor, and remove and discard trash.
- *Other areas:* Vacuum carpets, dust furniture, empty ashtrays, water plants, and discard trash.

DEVELOPING A WORK PLAN

Developing a work plan is important because your time in the client's home is limited. Your first priority is care of the client, so you are not able to spend a lot of time on housekeeping duties. Box 9-2 gives tips for organizing your cleaning time. One hour should be enough time to complete routine tasks. Big cleaning jobs are not your responsibility. Your agency will help the client contact a cleaning service for help in this area. Your work plan lists the jobs to be done, the schedule, and who will do each task. Typical responsibilities include the following:

EVERYDAY TASKS

- Washing dishes
- Cleaning the kitchen counters and sink
- Sweeping the kitchen floor
- Removing trash

BOX 9-2 **Rules of Organization**

- Have a cleaning plan; be flexible.
- Do each job correctly from top to bottom (except on walls), clean to dirty.
- Work around the room along the walls; come in the door, turn to the right, and begin cleaning; continue until you are back at the door again.
- Try to make work easier by taking fewer steps and using a larger broom or big sponge.
- Do not try to do everything in 1 day.
- Do the jobs that must be done daily, plus only one of the weekly jobs.
- Post a schedule of jobs and who will do each one (do not forget children).

- Making the bed
- Straightening rooms and removing clutter
- Cleaning the toilet, commode, and bathroom sink

WEEKLY TASKS

- Dusting and vacuuming the bedroom or client area
- Mopping the kitchen floor
- Cleaning the refrigerator
- Changing and laundering bed linens
- Watering plants

FOLLOW YOUR WORK PLAN AS CLOSELY AS POSSIBLE, BUT REMEMBER TO BE FLEXIBLE. YOUR CLIENT'S PERSONAL PHYSICAL NEEDS COME FIRST, AND SOMETIMES YOU WILL HAVE TO ADJUST YOUR PLAN OF WORK. If your client has soiled the bed linens, you must change them, even if it is not on your schedule for that day. Your client may need a bath, clean clothing, and his or her personal laundry done. A work plan is just that, a plan, and plans can always be changed when necessary.

Organize your work. Straighten up as you go along. Managers in a famous fast-food restaurant chain teach their employees this easy, time- and work-saving rule: CUAYG, that is, CLEAN UP AS YOU GO.

Do not take extra steps; do not make extra work for yourself. Work smarter, not harder.

Once you begin a task, finish what you are doing. Begin with the worst room first. Both the kitchen and bathroom require careful cleaning. Plan to clean the kitchen daily. Toilets and sinks should be **disinfected** daily. Follow the schedule listed earlier in the chapter if your agency does not provide one for you. Work around the room until you are finished.

Always work from the cleanest to the dirtiest area. For example, in the bathroom, begin with the mirror and finish with the floor. If the weather is pleasant, open windows and ventilate the room as you work, but do not expose your client to a draft or chill the home unnecessarily in cold weather.

MAINTAINING AN UNCLUTTERED ENVIRONMENT

One of the easiest ways to make a home look cleaner is to eliminate clutter. However, what may look like clutter to you can be treasure to your client. Do not throw away anything without discussing it with your client and receiving permission to discard the item. Ask permission from your client or your client's family member before opening bureau drawers to get needed items.

Some general rules for straightening up and reducing clutter are as follows:

- Carry a basket or bag to collect clutter and to redistribute items to their proper location.
- Remove scraps of paper, newspapers, and old magazines; recycle.
- Remove dead leaves from plants; discard old flowers.
- Empty ashtrays and wastebaskets.
- Put items in their proper place (e.g., books, shoes, clothing, toys, boots, tools).
- Clean countertops; put things away.
- Check dates on containers; discard and replace outdated items.
- Check under the bed, sofa, and chairs for clutter in hiding.

Clutter is a safety hazard and is a major cause of accidental falls in the home. A magazine on the floor is as slippery as ice, so protect your client by keeping the environment as free from clutter as possible. If you cannot discard it, try to arrange the clutter as neatly as possible and move it out of the way.

CLEANING EQUIPMENT AND SUPPLIES

Television and magazine advertisements lead us to believe that we need a special cleaner for each and every housekeeping job. Not true! There are some basic cleaning supplies and tools. There also are some "nice to have but not always necessary" things.

NECESSARY ITEMS

- **Dust cloths:** For dusting dry surfaces; wash in soapy water after each use; air-dry as they may retain flammable materials from the polishing chemicals.
- **Broom:** For sweeping hard-surfaced floors; shake into a large, moistened paper bag after each use; hang to store.
- **Sponge mop:** For wet cleaning hard-surfaced floors; wash and rinse after each use; stand upside down to dry; replace sponge when needed.
- **Scrub brush:** For rough surfaces; wash and rinse after each use; always dry brush with bristles down.
- **Bucket** (or two): For cleaning and rinsing solutions; rinse and dry after each use.
- **Sponges:** For washable surfaces; wash in soapy water and air-dry.
- **Toilet brush:** For cleaning the toilet bowl; rinse in cold water and store.
- **Dust pan and brush:** For gathering small amounts of dust from dry hard surfaces; wipe pan with damp cloth and shake brush into large, moistened bag after use.
- **Rubber gloves:** Heavy duty to protect hands from irritation; hang to air-dry.
- **Vacuum cleaner:** For cleaning carpets and upholstery. Follow manufacturer's instructions; empty frequently; replace filter/bags as needed; check to see that cord and plug are in good repair before each use.
- **Dishwashing supplies:** Cloths, brushes, detergent, scouring pads.
- **Cleaning agents**
  All purpose cleaners for floors, walls, counters, and other hard surfaces
  Detergents for laundry and dishwashing
  Cleansers for scrubbing
  Specialty cleaners for toilets, ovens, windows, tiles, and so on.
  Baking soda to clean the refrigerator, bathroom tiles, counter stains, as well as many other items
  White vinegar to clean toilets, commodes, tile, windows, mirrors, as well as many other items
  Disinfectants—chemicals used to destroy germs; some cleaning agents are also disinfectants. Bleach is a disinfectant that is used in certain situations (see Chapter 11).

The above items may be considered as necessary, but many homes may not have all of these supplies. When in doubt, ask your supervisor.

"NICE TO HAVE" BUT NOT NECESSARY SUPPLIES

- Floor dust mop for hard floors
- Floor polisher
- Carpet sweeper
- Automatic dishwasher, clothes washer and dryer

PRODUCT SAFETY: A HOUSEHOLD CONCERN

Incorrect use of cleaning agents can cause serious damage to the user, the surface to be cleaned, and the environment. Certain chemicals in cleaning products are thought to be ecologically dangerous.

The home safety hints that follow provide information that will help you to avoid endangering yourself, home surfaces, or the environment.

HOME SAFETY HINTS

- Know the surface you want cleaned. Know what it is made of. Is there an outer coating or finish over another material? Ask the client if there are special cleaners to be used or any cleaners to be avoided.
- Know the cleaner. Are you using the right cleaner for the surface? The right amount of cleaner? Are you giving it the right amount of time to do the job?
- **READ THE LABEL.** Do you know how to use the product safely? Do you understand all the directions? Are there any potentially dangerous ingredients?
- Pay special attention to food surfaces. Do not use home cleaning products to wash dishes. Keep food away from all cleaning sprays and liquids.
- NEVER MIX CLEANING AGENTS. FOR EXAMPLE, AVOID MIXING CLEANERS CONTAINING BLEACH (MOST SCOURING POWDERS) AND AMMONIA, BECAUSE THEY REACT TO CAUSE POISONOUS FUMES.
- Allow adequate ventilation when using cleaning agents. When cleaning closets or shower units, leave doors open for excess vapors to escape. Take the same precaution when using strong ammonia solutions.
- Keep aerosols away from heat. Aerosol cans are packed under pressure. Excess heat may cause them to explode. Never store them at temperatures higher than 120° F (49° C). Keep all aerosols away from hot pipes, radiators, stoves, and ovens. Never burn aerosol cans. Do not store cans in a car's glove compartment or trunk in the hot sun. Avoid spraying aerosols near an open flame.
- Separate food, personal care, and home care aerosols. This prevents using the wrong can by mistake.
- Keep spray cleaners away from the face and eyes. Certain products contain chemicals that could irritate the lungs if inhaled. The eyes may also be injured.
- Keep all cleaning agents out of the reach of children and away from animals. Many are poisonous if taken internally. Keep containers closed. Store out of children's reach. Whenever possible, buy products with safety caps.
- Purchase cleaning agents from a reliable source. These products will include information for proper use and safety. Reputable companies manufacture products that meet tough standards for durability and safety.

CLEANING THE BATHROOM

Unless the client has his or her own bathroom, most bathrooms are used by other family members. Sometimes a bathroom is shared by other residents of an apartment house. It is not your responsibility to clean the bathroom after use by family members or residents. It is your job to make sure the bathroom is clean after you or your client use it.

Keeping the bathroom clean is very important. Microorganisms grow and multiply rapidly in this area because there is moisture and warmth. Any materials used to clean the bathroom, such as brushes or sponges, should be used only in this area.

See the "How to" box below for daily tasks needed to keep the bathroom clean and free from harmful microorganisms.

CLEANING THE CLIENT'S LIVING AREA

If your client has limited mobility, he or she will probably spend a lot of time in one part of the home. This area should be clean and orderly. Items frequently used by the client must be within easy reach for the client's comfort. In many cases, it is the bedroom that will be used, but sometimes it is another area, such as the living room couch or chair. In addition to the general housekeeping tasks mentioned earlier, the following should be performed each day:

* Remove clutter, such as old newspapers, toys, and magazines.
* Place reading materials, reading glasses, television remote control, pen and paper, and so on, in a location that is convenient for the client and off the floor.

How to Clean the Bathroom

TASK	MATERIALS NEEDED	BE SURE TO
All surfaces	• Detergent and water • Disinfectant • White vinegar and water solution • Pail, soft rag, or sponge • Gloves	• Wipe toilet tank, sink, window sills, bathroom tiles, or washable wallpaper.
Mirror	• Glass cleaner or white vinegar and water solution • Paper towels or newspaper	• Clean so that mirror is not streaked.
Toilet bowl and seat	• Disinfectant and water • Toilet brush or sponge and pail • Gloves	• Wear gloves. • Clean thoroughly: under rim of toilet bowl, under and behind toilet seat, outside toilet bowl. • If used, clean plastic splash guard of raised toilet seat using a brush or sponge.
Tub or shower stall	• Detergent and water • Pail, soft rag, or sponge	• Clean tub or shower stall after each use by the client.
Points to Remember:	• Wear utility gloves when cleaning the bathroom. • Work from the cleanest area (mirrors) to the dirtiest (floor). • Clean the bathroom using a disinfectant. • Keep the area well ventilated and as dry as possible to prevent mildew from forming. • **DO NOT MIX AMMONIA WITH OTHER CLEANING AGENTS**—toxic fumes may result.	

How to Clean the Client's Living Area

TASK	MATERIALS NEEDED	BE SURE TO
Change bed linens	• Sheets • Pillow cases • Bedspread (optional) • Protective sheets or pads (optional) • Blankets	• Change at least once a week or more often if necessary. • Change immediately when soiled, damp, or wet.
Damp-dust surfaces Dust furniture	• Damp cloth	• Dust all surfaces once a week or more often if your client has allergies.
Damp-mop floor Vacuum rug Clean commode	• Damp mop • Vacuum cleaner • Disinfectant and water • Toilet brush or sponge • Pail • Gloves	• Damp-mop floor weekly. • Vacuum rug at least once a week. • Wear gloves. • Remove pail, and dispose of waste in toilet. • Clean commode with brush and pail. • Clean all surfaces of commode with disinfectant.
Check supply of toilet tissue, and replace as needed.	• Toilet tissue	• Place toilet tissue within easy reach of client and commode.
Points to Remember:	• Remove clutter each day to maintain a clean, safe home. • Vacuum or brush corners of chairs to remove crumbs or other pieces of food where client eats; sweep floor or vacuum rug as needed. • After cleaning, replace all personal items within easy reach of client. • Wear utility gloves when cleaning commode.	

- Wash the drinking cup and water pitcher; refill them with fresh water, and place them within easy reach.
- Tidy the bedside table.
- Empty the wastebasket.
- Replace items on the bedside table according to the client's wishes.
- Make the bed (see Chapter 13), and straighten bedding as needed.
- Damp-dust surfaces as needed.

See the "How to" box above for other tasks to be performed to maintain a clean, healthy environment in the living area.

MAINTAINING A CLEAN, ORDERLY KITCHEN

CLEANING THE KITCHEN

As a home care aide, you may have the responsibility to prepare and serve a meal to your client. Cleaning the kitchen after making a meal is also your job. The phrase *work smarter, not harder* is especially true. Develop a routine, and it will save you time and energy. Plan before you act. Sometimes the client's work plan calls for light cleaning in the kitchen. Typical tasks include washing dishes; cleaning the sink, countertops, and table; and discarding spoiled food from the refrigerator.

DISPOSING OF HOUSEHOLD WASTE

It is estimated that each person disposes of more than 1½ pounds of paper per day. Used cans, glass bottles, wrappers from candy and gum, plastic containers, and food scraps add to the list of household waste. If these items are not recycled or disposed of each day, the environment becomes cluttered and unhealthy in a very short time.

Most communities participate in recycling programs for newspapers, cartons, glass, plastic, and aluminum cans. There are special rules and regulations that apply to recyclable items. It is important that you know what kinds of items are to be recycled and how frequently they are picked up. Obtain this information from your client, the client's family member, or a local municipal government office.

Garbage, including food and fluids, must be discarded promptly to avoid odors and growth of organisms. Place garbage in a closed container lined with a plastic bag. Remove the plastic liner daily, tie it, place it in a larger closed container, and store outdoors. In an apartment complex, use the garbage chute.

Some clients will have a garbage disposal unit connected to the kitchen sink. This equipment grinds up food and empties it into the sewage system. By using the garbage disposal unit, food is removed quickly and efficiently. Although many food items can be removed by this method, some garbage (bones, fruit pits) will still need to be placed in containers and stored until it can be disposed. See the "How to" box below for tasks to be performed to keep the kitchen clean and free from harmful microorganisms.

LAUNDRY

If your client lives alone and is unable to wash linens, towels, and personal clothing, the work plan may call for the home care aide to perform these tasks. Clean clothing not only helps the client to feel more comfortable but also can be a morale booster.

How to Clean the Kitchen

TASK	MATERIALS NEEDED	BE SURE TO
Washing dishes	• Detergent or soap • Hot water	• Scrape dish to remove food. • Wash in hot, soapy water. • Rinse in hot water. • Air-dry. • Wash glassware first, utensils, then cups, saucers, plates, pots, and pans.
Using the automatic dishwasher	• Dishwasher detergent (type and amount according to directions only)	• Have client's family member demonstrate loading and starting, if unsure. • Empty glasses, cups, and dishes. • Load glasses, cups, and dishes. • Place eating and drinking surfaces toward spray of water (usually downward). • Do not overload.
Cleaning the refrigerator	• Soapy water • Baking soda solution (3 tablespoons to 1 quart [1000 mL] warm water) • Sponge or rags	• Dispose of food that is more than 3 days old or food that shows signs of spoiling (e.g., odor, color change). • Remove food, one shelf at a time. • Remove and wash shelves and trays with warm soapy water. • Wipe inside walls with baking soda solution. • Replace shelves and trays. • Replace food. • Place an open box or small perforated container of baking soda on shelf to absorb food odors and leave refrigerator odor free (optional).

How to Clean the Kitchen—cont'd

TASK	MATERIALS NEEDED	BE SURE TO
Cleaning kitchen counters	• Hot, soapy water and detergent or baking soda solution • Cloth or sponge	• Wipe countertops after each meal. • Use baking soda on a damp cloth to remove countertop stains. • Wipe food preparation surfaces with hot soapy water. • Rinse and dry thoroughly.
Cleaning the kitchen sink (stainless steel or porcelain)	• Hot, soapy water	• Clean daily after meal preparation.
Points to Remember:	• Some items should not be washed in an automatic dishwasher; they include electrical appliances, delicate glassware, fine china, sharp knives, silver (sterling) flatware, some types of pots and pans, and wooden bowls. • These items will need to be hand washed. • Use medium heat to keep food from boiling over or splattering. • Do not open the refrigerator door more often than necessary; warm air causes the motor to work harder to keep the desired temperature. • Use warm, soapy water and a cloth or sponge to wipe up cooking spills or splattered grease immediately from stove, oven, broiler, or microwave oven.	

Discuss with the client or client's family member preferences concerning use of detergents, softeners, or other laundry products.

Keeping laundry clean removes a source of potentially harmful organisms. When the client is recovering from an infection, frequent laundering of any item coming in contact with the client is necessary to prevent the spread of infection to others. Wear gloves when handling linens contaminated with body fluids. Place the linens in leak-proof containers. Treat and wash them as quickly as possible. Box 9-3 gives instructions for treating linens stained with body fluids.

See the "How to" box below for laundering instructions.

How to Do the Laundry

TASK	MATERIALS NEEDED	BE SURE TO

Sort items to be washed	• Laundry basket	• Read the care label on clothing.
		• Place items in piles according to care needed.
		  1. Sturdy white
		  2. Dark
		  3. Colored
		  4. Heavily soiled
		  5. Delicate (hand wash or dry clean)
		• Inspect items to be washed for spots, stains, or repairs needed.
		• Set aside and pretreat spots; repair as needed.
		• Empty pockets.
		• Turn dark socks inside out.
		• Button buttons.
		• Zip zippers.
		• Tie sashes and belts.
		• Hook hooks.
		• Treat linens soiled with body fluids (see Box 9-3).

How to Do the Laundry—cont'd

TASK	MATERIALS NEEDED	BE SURE TO
Select correct detergent	• Detergent • Fabric softener (if used) • Bleach, if needed for stains and odors • Borax, if needed for stains and odors	• Consult the client/family regarding preference. • Read the directions on the package.
Select correct water temperature	*Use* • Hot water 120°-140° F (40°-60° C) for heavily soiled clothes, diapers, whites, and light colored cotton • Warm water 100°-110° F (38°-43° C) for moderately or lightly soiled wash and wear and permanent press fabrics • Cold water 80°-100° F (27°-38° C) for bright colors, fragile fabrics, and lightly soiled items	• Select cold water for rinse cycle. • Select the proper setting for wash, rinse, and spin cycles. • Read the instructions usually found on the underside of the washer lid. • Receive instructions from your client or client's family regarding use of washing machine. • If still unsure, contact your supervisor for directions.
Load the machine Wash and dry load	• Washing machine • Dryer	• Put water in machine, and then add detergent. • Mix small and large items in the load for better washing action. • Do not overload; this damages items and is not efficient. • Machine-dry clothes. • Separate lightweight and heavy items to dry more evenly. • Remove permanent press items as soon as dryer stops to reduce wrinkling. • Remove clothes, fold, and store in appropriate place.

Points to Remember:
- Always wear gloves when handling linens stained with body fluids.
- Read the care label before selecting a laundering method.
- Treat stains appropriately (see Box 9-3).
- Some items attract lint, and others give off lint; separate them to avoid more work later in removing lint.
- Wash heavily soiled items in a separate load.
- More detergent does not always ensure a clean load of laundry; read the directions on the detergent package.
- **NEVER MIX CHLORINE BLEACH WITH AMMONIA BECAUSE IT CREATES A DEADLY GAS.**
- Do not overload washing machine or dryer; laundry needs enough water around the items to remove soil and enough air to dry items properly.
- Use cold water for washing when appropriate and especially for rinse cycle; it saves energy and prevents permanent press fabrics from wrinkling.
- Discuss with your client or client's family how home laundry is usually washed; some homes may not have a washing machine.
- Remember, your supervisor will advise you about your responsibilities if this situation occurs.

BOX 9-3   Cleaning Linens Soiled with Body Fluids

SAFETY AND BIOHAZARD CHECK

ALWAYS WEAR GLOVES WHEN HANDLING LINENS SOILED WITH BODY FLUIDS. STAIN REMOVAL MAY INVOLVE USE OF DANGEROUS CHEMICALS. FOLLOW THE LABEL INSTRUCTIONS CAREFULLY.

Ammonia is poisonous. Do not inhale fumes. Ammonia will cause burns or irritation if it comes in contact with the skin or eyes. Chlorine bleach is poisonous and will cause burns or irritation if it comes in contact with the skin or eyes.

General rules: These directions apply to white or colorfast linens. Before treating stains, flush the fabric with cold water to remove body fluids or solids on linens. Work quickly, before the stain becomes set in the fabric.

REMOVING URINE STAINS

1. Soak in a solution of 1 quart (1000 mL) warm water, ½ teaspoon liquid (hand) dishwashing detergent, and 1 tablespoon ammonia for 30 minutes.
2. Rinse with cold water.
3. Soak in a solution of 1 quart warm water and 1 tablespoon white vinegar for 1 hour.
4. Rinse with water.
5. Wash in the machine using detergent and chlorine bleach according to product directions. Dry as usual.

REMOVING FECAL STAINS

1. Soak in a solution of 1 quart (1000 mL) warm water, ½ teaspoon liquid (hand) dishwashing detergent, and 1 tablespoon ammonia for 30 minutes.
2. Rinse with cold water.
3. Wash in the machine using detergent and chlorine bleach according to product directions. Dry as usual.

REMOVING BLOOD STAINS

1. Soak in a solution of 1 quart (1000 mL) warm water, ½ teaspoon liquid (hand) dishwashing detergent, and 1 tablespoon ammonia for 15 minutes.
2. If fabric is strong enough, gently rub the stain. Continue as long as the stain responds to treatment.
3. Soak for another 15 minutes in the solution used in Step 1.
4. Soak in a solution of 1 quart warm water and 1 tablespoon enzyme product for 30 minutes.
5. Wash in the machine using detergent and chlorine bleach. Dry as usual.

CONTROLLING HOUSEHOLD PESTS

Household pests can be a source of infection, illness, and sometimes death. They can carry disease or cause illness to humans in a variety of ways, including bites and contamination of foods. Pests such as flies, mosquitoes, ants, roaches, mice, and rats enter the home in a variety of ways. After entering, they look for food and a place to grow and multiply.

There are two main rules for controlling pests: exclusion and sanitation.

Exclusion means keeping pests from entering the home. Keep screens repaired and in place to prevent flies and mosquitoes from entering. Seal up cracks and holes in walls or outside doors to keep out ants, mice, or roaches. If you see cracks, holes, or screens that need repair, notify your supervisor. Repairs will need to be made by someone skilled in the proper procedure.

Sanitation means performing proper techniques discussed in this chapter to remove sources of food and shelter needed for pests to grow and multiply. The following are some tips to maintain a home free of household pests:

- Refrigerate leftover cooked food immediately.
- Store all food properly, either in the refrigerator or in containers with tight lids, as appropriate.
- Wipe up crumbs and spills immediately.
- Remove garbage promptly, and place it in a container with a tight lid.
- Keep kitchen counters clean.
- Clean under the refrigerator and stove.
- Vacuum between cushions of the chair or couch where your client may drop crumbs from food or snacks.
- Dust and vacuum corners and behind and under furniture to keep pests from nesting.
- Throw out vase water and wilted flowers to prevent insects from growing and breeding in stagnant water.
- Check grains, flour, and seeds for signs of insects before storing in closed containers.
- Wash fruits and vegetables before eating.
- Remove sources of moisture.

BOX 9-4   Suggestions of Household Tasks

FOR YOUNG CHILDREN (5 YEARS OF AGE AND OLDER)

- Make own bed
- Put clothing back in the closet or drawer
- Put toys away
- Set the table
- Clean the table
- Pick up clutter
- Help with dishes
- Fold laundry
- Empty small wastebaskets

FOR OLDER CHILDREN AND ADOLESCENTS (INCLUDING ABOVE)

- Make beds
- Help younger children make beds
- Separate recyclables, and carry out trash
- Vacuum and dust
- Do laundry and dishes
- Clean bathrooms
- Clean woodwork and windows
- Clean and sweep the kitchen floor
- Carry in wood, and lay the fire
- Straighten closets
- Mend clothes
- Make small repairs

FOR ALL

- Straighten and put things away
- Put away own clothes
- Hang up own things
- Clean the tub or shower after use
- Restock supplies (e.g., toilet tissue, paper towels, facial tissue, soap)
- Clean up after yourself

Fig 9-4 Even the youngest family member can help.

Notify your supervisor if the home shows signs of pests. Do not use any chemicals to try to control household pests.

TEACHING OTHERS

Sometimes the home care aide will be asked to teach certain household tasks to the client or a family member. Perhaps the client has always performed all of the household duties, and, now, because of illness or disability, others must learn how to help. The home care aide can teach others to perform these tasks (Box 9-4).

When clients become disabled, they often must learn new ways to perform familiar tasks. The occupational therapist will teach the client new skills. Cleaning supplies and equipment may be adapted for your client's specific needs.

Families may need to learn to be organized and work together in home management. There are many chores children can do to help out around the home (Figure 9-4). When teaching clients or family members, use the following guidelines.

- Individualize the teaching for each family member.
- Get the person's full attention.
- Be sure the person wants to learn.
- Do not talk too fast.
- Do not teach too much at one time.
- Show and explain how to do each task, one step at a time, and then have the person perform the task; repeat the teaching if necessary.
- Be patient; it takes time to learn to do new things.
- Give praise for attempts and success.

CHAPTER SUMMARY

- A clean home environment contributes to the client's health and safety.
- The home care aide is responsible for maintaining a clean, safe, healthy environment by
  - Performing household duties.
  - Helping the client to perform household tasks.
  - Teaching disorganized families to care for their environment.
- Household responsibilities are listed in the work plan and may include: cleaning the client's area, bathroom, and kitchen.
- A work plan helps the home care aide to use time wisely and efficiently.
- Cleaning equipment and supplies require proper handling and storage to prevent accidents and injury.

STUDY QUESTIONS

1. Why is a clean home environment important for clients' health and safety?
2. List three ways the home care aide maintains a clean, healthy home environment. Describe three usual tasks.
3. Make a list of supplies and equipment needed to clean
   a. The client's area or bedroom
   b. The client's bathroom
4. What action would you take if
   a. You are asked to do spring housecleaning?
   b. The washing machine is broken?
   c. You do not know how to operate the dishwasher?
5. List five guidelines to remember when teaching others to perform household tasks.

10

Meeting the Client's Nutritional Needs

OBJECTIVES

After you read this chapter, you will be able to:

1. Discuss the importance of nutrition in maintaining health and preventing illness.
2. List three factors that influence individual and family food habits.
3. List five foods that belong in each of the following categories: proteins, carbohydrates, and fats.
4. Discuss the role of vitamins and minerals in the diet and major food sources of these substances.
5. Describe the importance of water, fluids, and dietary fiber.
6. Identify the five food groups of the MyPlate Food Guide and three foods found in each group.
7. Describe food shopping for clients, including: preparing a list, selecting products, and purchasing products.
8. Discuss food preparation, including food safety.
9. Recognize the need to follow agency policy regarding the client's money, expense receipts, travel, and transporting clients.
10. Feed clients who cannot feed themselves.
11. Describe the techniques for assisting clients who have difficulty eating.
12. Identify six therapeutic diets, and list foods to be included or avoided.

KEY TERMS

Anorexia Loss of appetite
Bacteria Microorganisms that cause disease
Deficiency A lack of one or more essential nutrients in the diet
Dehydrated/Dehydration Excessive water loss from body tissues resulting from insufficient fluid intake

Malnutrition Any disorder of nutrition
Nutrition The process by which food is taken in and used by the body
Unit prices A method of pricing food

Your body needs sufficient food and water to grow, develop, and function properly. Of course, the amount of food each person needs depends on age, sex, size, health, and activity level. For example, a healthy, physically active teenager needs to eat more food than an older adult who does not get as much exercise. Nutrition is the process in which food is taken in and used by the body.

FUNCTION OF FOOD

Food contains the nutrients (i.e., vitamins, minerals, dietary fiber, and water) a body needs to function 24 hours a day, every day. The human body uses the nutrients found in food for the following:

1. *Heat and energy production.* Brendan is a soccer player. He needs lots of energy to run up and down the field to chase and move the ball. He gets very hot and sweaty during soccer games.
2. *Growth and development.* Lisa is 6 months pregnant. She needs food for her own body to use and for her growing baby, too.
3. *Health and well-being.* Everyone needs the proper amount and type of nutrients. When essential nutrients are missing from the diet, malnutrition, weight loss, and deficiency disease may result. Leo has diabetes. To maintain a healthy body, he follows the diet ordered by his doctor.
4. *Healing and repair of body tissue.* Our bodies mend and repair injured and diseased tissue. Martha broke her leg in a fall. The doctor says it will take 6 to 8 weeks for it to heal. She needs the kinds of food that will help her leg to heal.

MEASURING FOOD ENERGY

Food energy is measured by means of a unit called a *calorie.* Our daily diet should include sufficient amounts of calories from nutritious foods. If the food that is eaten is less than the energy that is used by the body, weight loss will occur. If the food intake is more than the energy used by the body, weight gain will occur.

SOCIAL, CULTURAL, AND RELIGIOUS ASPECTS OF FOOD

For most people, food and eating mean much more than nutrition. Eating with others (family and/or friends) is a social activity, whether it be a burger and shake from the fast-food drive-in or a formal candlelight dinner. Eating with others is more enjoyable than eating alone. Many social events revolve around food (e.g., picnics, fiestas, banquets). Eating out can be fun, convenient, and entertaining.

Certain types of foods convey a sense of well-being. Many foods from one's childhood (sometimes called "comfort foods") provide comfort during illness and periods of stress. Everyone has heard of the curative powers of chicken soup. Most people have some special foods that just make them feel good. These vary with the person's ethnic background, and some of these "comfort" foods may not be available to immigrants in a new environment. Most of us grew up eating the kinds of food our families have eaten for generations.

Food customs are also closely linked to religious holidays or cultural celebrations. For example, roast lamb at Easter, matzos on Passover, and Mazeo for Kwanzaa are foods that have special meaning for observers of these holidays.

Some religions have rules about the kinds and amounts of food to be eaten, including food used for certain religious events and celebrations. Religious dietary laws indicate the regulations to follow, such as fasting, care of cooking and eating utensils, and other rules regarding food preparation. Table 10-1 outlines dietary requirements according to religious belief.

TABLE 10-1	Religion and Dietary Practices
RELIGION	**DIETARY RESTRICTION**
Baptist	Some groups may avoid coffee, tea, and alcohol.
Christian Scientist	Alcohol, tea, and coffee are not allowed.
Church of the Latter Day Saints (Mormon)	Alcohol and hot drinks, such as tea and coffee, are not allowed. Meat is not forbidden, but members are encouraged to eat meat infrequently.
Greek Orthodox	Wednesday, Friday, and Lent are days of fasting. Meat and dairy products are avoided during days of fast.
Islamic (Muslim/Moslem)	Alcohol, pork, and its by-products, gelatin, and vanilla extract cannot be eaten.
Judaism (Orthodox faith)	Foods must be kosher (prepared according to Jewish law); meat of kosher animals, kosher fowl, and kosher fish can be eaten. Pork and shellfish cannot be eaten. Milk, milk products, and eggs from kosher animals are acceptable; milk and milk products cannot be eaten with or immediately after eating meat; milk and milk products can be eaten 6 hours after eating meat; milk and milk products can be a part of the same meal with meat if they are served separately and before the meat. Kosher food cannot be prepared in pots/pans used to prepare non-kosher food. Kosher homes have separate sets of pots/pans, dishes, utensils for meat versus dairy. They cannot even be washed together. Breads, cakes, cookies, noodles, and alcoholic beverages are not consumed during Passover.
Roman Catholic	Fasting for 1 hour before receiving Holy Communion; no meat on Ash Wednesday, Good Friday, and Fridays during Lent.
Seventh Day Adventist (Adventist)	Coffee, tea, and alcohol are to be avoided; beverages with caffeine (colas) are not allowed. Some groups forbid pork and pork products; others forbid meat.

FOOD PREFERENCES

Some foods may be appetizing to you, yet the same foods are disgusting to someone else. A big, juicy steak may make your mouth water, but this food would offer no appeal to a vegetarian. Certain foods are not eaten for many reasons, including religious and cultural beliefs, personal taste, likes and dislikes, dietary restrictions, illness, pain, and allergies. Generally, mealtime has many different meanings. It is a time to eat, but, in some cultures, it is the gathering of a community together to eat, relax, and communicate. For others, mealtime means "grab something to eat, gobble it down, and run out the door." For some, it means eating alone (e.g., a hot meal delivered by a volunteer from Meals On Wheels, a bowl of cereal, cold rice). Many people who live alone just do not bother to prepare food; mealtime is often a frozen dinner heated in the microwave.

COMPONENTS OF FOOD

Food may be classified according to its basic composition: carbohydrates, proteins, and fats.

CARBOHYDRATES

Carbohydrates are composed of the chemicals carbon, hydrogen, and oxygen. They are the body's major source of energy. Carbohydrates:

1. Supply fiber, which contributes to good digestion and elimination.
2. Help the body to use proteins and fats effectively.
3. Supply other nutrients, such as vitamins and vegetable proteins.
   They are found in several forms in fruits, vegetables, and grains:
- Sugars—simple and complex sugars (e.g., table sugars, honey, fruit, jelly)
- Starches—the plant's food supply stored in roots, stems, and seeds (e.g., bread, pasta, grits, rice, potatoes, cereal)
- Fiber—part of the plant that acts as bulk to help the digestive system function (e.g., bran, nuts, seeds, popcorn, raw fruits and vegetables)

Digestion of carbohydrates starts in the mouth. They are broken down more rapidly than proteins or fats and are a quick source of energy. They produce 4 calories of energy per gram.

PROTEINS

Proteins are composed of compounds called *amino acids,* which contain carbon, hydrogen, oxygen, and nitrogen. Twenty amino acids have been discovered, of which 11 are manufactured by the body. The remaining nine, called *essential amino acids,* must come from the food we eat.

High-quality protein contains all nine essential amino acids, for example: milk, meat, fish, poultry, yogurt, cheese, eggs, and legumes (dried beans and peas). Lower-quality protein does not contain all of the essential amino acids and must be eaten with high-quality proteins to increase their effectiveness. Examples are: cereals, taco shells, bread, vegetables, spaghetti, and matzos.

Proteins are digested in the stomach and small intestine. While they are not a source of quick energy, protein intake is essential for energy production. They are also essential for growth, repair, and healing of body tissues. They produce 4 calories of energy per gram.

FATS

Fats are composed of fatty acids that contain carbon, hydrogen, and oxygen. They provide a highly concentrated source of energy—more than twice the amount of carbohydrates or proteins. Fats carry the fat-soluble vitamins: A, D, E, and K. They are essential for healthy skin and nervous systems; hold vital organs in place; and act as protection against injury. Fats provide flavor to food and give a satisfaction of fullness when eaten. They produce 9 calories of energy per gram.

Fatty acids are produced by the body or must come from the foods we eat (essential fatty acids). There are two categories of essential fatty acids:
1. Saturated fats contain all the hydrogen possible and are solid at room temperature (e.g., butter, lard, chocolate, lunch meat). (NOTE: Cholesterol is a chemical in the blood, digestive juices, and tissues. It is found in saturated fats.)
2. Unsaturated fats contain less hydrogen and become liquid at room temperature. Examples are: fish, vegetable oils, nuts.

Digestion of fats begins in the small intestine; fats are broken down by the action of bile and other digestive juices.

NOTE: Transfatty acids (*trans* fats) are made when hydrogen is added to vegetable oil. This creates a product with a longer shelf life and stability at room temperature. These products can be found in vegetable shortening, cookies, crackers, snack foods, and margarine. *Trans* fats, like saturated fats and cholesterol, increase the risk for coronary heart disease.

REMEMBER: Food may contain one component, or all of them. Legumes (dried peas or beans) contain protein and carbohydrates. Cheese may contain proteins, fats, and

TABLE 10-2	Fat-Soluble Vitamins	
VITAMIN	**PURPOSE**	**FOOD SOURCE**
Vitamin A	• Promotes growth • Prevents dry skin • Promotes good vision • Helps the body resist infection	Milk, liver, yellow and green leafy vegetables (carrots, sweet potatoes, spinach, greens), broccoli, and fruits (apricots and cantaloupe)
Vitamin D	• Keeps bones strong and healthy • Helps the body absorb and use calcium and phosphorus	Milk with vitamin D, fish oils, tuna fish, and salmon
Vitamin E	• Protects cells from harmful substances • Helps prevent cell destruction	Vegetable oils, green leafy vegetables, and asparagus
Vitamin K	• Clots blood	Green leafy vegetables, peas, green beans, and liver

carbohydrates. Olive oil contains only fat. The make-up of food is found on its contents label (see Figure 10-6).

VITAMINS

Vitamins are substances that are needed to maintain our health. Most of them cannot be produced by our bodies. Instead, they are provided by the foods we eat. Although carbohydrates, proteins, and fats contain calories, vitamins do not.

Groups of Vitamins

There are two groups of vitamins: vitamins that are dissolved in fats and vitamins that are dissolved in water.

Fat-Soluble Vitamins. Vitamins A, D, E, and K are dissolved in fatty foods and travel with these fats to reach the cells of the body. Fat-soluble vitamins are also stored in fatty tissues and in the liver. They are not easily eliminated from the body. Unused amounts of these vitamins can build up and cause harmful effects.

As the home care aide, you may be responsible for selecting nutritious foods and preparing meals for your client. Table 10-2 lists the major functions and food sources of vitamins A, D, E, and K. By using the information in this table, you will be able to select and prepare foods that supply natural forms of these important vitamins.

Water-Soluble Vitamins. Vitamins B and C are dissolved by water in the cells of our bodies. Water-soluble vitamins cannot be stored by the body. Excess amounts of these vitamins are eliminated from the body through urine and feces. When foods high in the B vitamins and vitamin C are cooked, some of the vitamins are lost in the cooking water and through the heating process.

Because these vitamins are not stored in our bodies, it is important to provide your client with foods rich in the B and C vitamins each day. Table 10-3 describes the functions of the water-soluble vitamins and lists good food sources.

Taking Vitamins

The best way to "take" vitamins is through a varied, well-balanced diet rich in natural sources of fat-soluble and water-soluble vitamins. Sometimes, because of poor appetite or other problems caused by illness, your client may not be receiving the desired

TABLE 10-3 | Water-Soluble Vitamins

VITAMIN	PURPOSE	FOOD SOURCE
Thiamin	• Promotes healthy nerves • Helps the body use carbohydrates, proteins, and fats	Pork products, whole grains and enriched grains, breads and cereals, and organ meats
Riboflavin	• Keeps skin and mucous membranes healthy • Helps the body use carbohydrates, proteins, and fats	Milk and milk products, enriched breads and cereals, meats, and eggs
Niacin	• Keeps the skin and gastrointestinal tract healthy • Helps the body use carbohydrates, proteins, and fats	Enriched breads and cereals, tuna and other fish, beef, chicken, and turkey
Folic acid	• Necessary for formation of red blood cells and growth and reproduction of cells • Promotes function of the gastrointestinal system	Beans, green leafy vegetables, citrus fruits, beets, wheat germ, and meats
Vitamin B_{12}	• Keeps the nervous system healthy • Helps the body use proteins	Organ meats, oysters, clams, eggs, beef, and pork
Vitamin C	• Helps to heal wounds • Promotes healthy teeth, gums, bones, and skin	Citrus fruits, broccoli, and strawberries

amount of vitamins in food. When this happens, the physician may advise adding vitamin supplements to the client's diet.

Taking large doses of vitamins without medical supervision can produce harmful results and may interfere with the effectiveness of other medications being taken. The natural way of taking vitamins, through the food we eat, is the best way.

MINERALS

Minerals are chemicals that come from water and the ground. Minerals become a part of the plant foods we eat because plants are nourished by soil, commercially prepared fertilizers, and water. Animal products are also good sources of minerals, because animals eat plants and consume water, too. Both plants and animal sources help us satisfy our needs for minerals.

Minerals are required in the daily diet for strong bones and teeth, nerve and muscle function, water balance, and other essential body functions. The best way to get adequate amounts of minerals is by eating a balanced diet of proteins, carbohydrates, and fats. Taking mineral supplements without medical supervision is dangerous because of possible harmful reactions.

Table 10-4 lists the key minerals and their food sources.

WATER

The human body is composed of about 60% water. Water is essential to life because it helps carry proteins, carbohydrates, fats, vitamins, and minerals to each cell. It also helps carry waste products to various organs to be excreted from the body. Water helps keep the body at a constant temperature.

TABLE 10-4   Minerals

MINERAL	PURPOSE	FOOD SOURCE
Calcium	• Helps to strengthen bones and teeth • Helps in blood clotting • Helps muscles to function	Milk, cheese, canned fish, yogurt, and tofu
Phosphorus	• Helps to strengthen bones and teeth	Milk, cheese, eggs, and meat
Iron	• Carries oxygen in the blood	Red meat, egg yolks, spinach, broccoli, and seafood
Iodine	• Helps thyroid gland function	Iodized salt, seafood, and shellfish
Sodium	• Transmits nerve impulses • Maintains body fluid balance	Table salt and processed foods
Potassium	• Promotes healthy function of nerves and heart	Bananas, orange juice, other fruits and vegetables, and milk

The Body's Need for Water

Adults can survive without eating food about 8 weeks because they use the nutrients that have been stored in the body, but the body cannot store water. Therefore, we can survive only a few days without drinking water.

Fluid Balance

A normal adult must consume 4 to 6 cups (1000 to 1500 milliliters) of fluids a day to maintain health. Besides drinking water, liquids such as milk, coffee, tea, juice, and soup provide water. Other foods, including fruits and vegetables, supply additional water. The body also produces water when digestive juices are made to help break down food. The total amount of fluids taken into the body each day is almost 8 to 12 cups (2500 milliliters) from all sources. Because fluids cannot be stored, they are eliminated from the body in the form of urine, feces, perspiration, and the air we exhale (Figure 10-1 and Box 10-1).

The phrase *What goes in, must come out* is very true about water. For proper balance, the fluids we take in (intake) must be removed (output). If sufficient fluids are not taken in, the person becomes dehydrated, and serious problems can occur if not treated immediately. If the output is much smaller than the intake, fluid has accumulated in body tissues (Figure 10-2). Information on procedures used to measure fluid intake and output (I&O) is found in Chapter 15.

DIETARY FIBER

Commonly called *roughage*, dietary fiber produces the bulk needed for proper elimination of solid waste products from the bowel. Dietary fibers are substances found in foods, such as wheat bran, citrus fruits, oat products, beans, and vegetables. They are parts of plant structures that absorb water. By holding water, dietary fiber helps to enlarge and soften feces. Therefore, elimination of feces becomes easier. A diet high in dietary fiber and adequate amounts of water helps prevent constipation.

Excellent sources of dietary fiber include kidney and lima beans, citrus fruits, cereals with wheat and oat brans, popped popcorn, dried figs, prunes and dates, corn, and baked potatoes with skins.

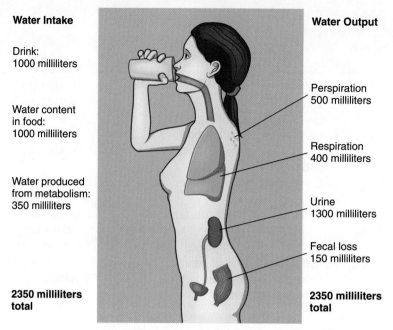

Fig 10-1 Water balance.

Water Intake

Drink:
1000 milliliters

Water content
in food:
1000 milliliters

Water produced
from metabolism:
350 milliliters

**2350 milliliters
total**

Water Output

Perspiration
500 milliliters

Respiration
400 milliliters

Urine
1300 milliliters

Fecal loss
150 milliliters

**2350 milliliters
total**

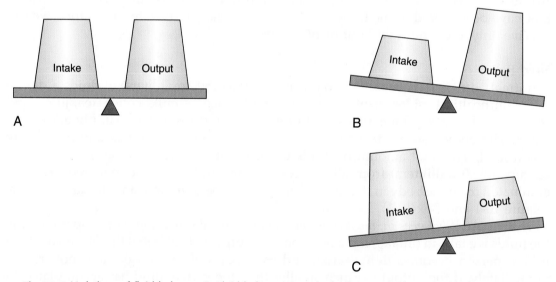

Fig 10-2 Variations of fluid balance. **A,** Fluid balance. **B,** Dehydration. **C,** Fluid accumulates in the body.

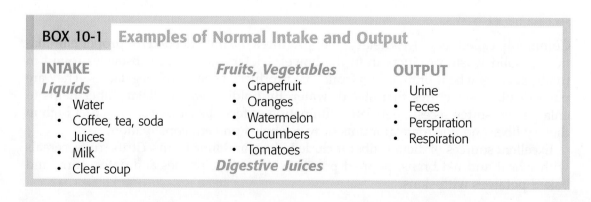

BOX 10-1 **Examples of Normal Intake and Output**

INTAKE

Liquids
- Water
- Coffee, tea, soda
- Juices
- Milk
- Clear soup

Fruits, Vegetables
- Grapefruit
- Oranges
- Watermelon
- Cucumbers
- Tomatoes

Digestive Juices

OUTPUT
- Urine
- Feces
- Perspiration
- Respiration

MYPLATE FOOD GUIDE

The U.S. Department of Agriculture has issued Dietary Guidelines for Americans. Developed by nutrition experts, the guidelines and icon, MyPlate Food Guide (Figure 10-3) are designed to help people to make better, more informed, healthy food choices. The icon is a dinner plate, divided into four sections, and a glass of milk. It shows the groups of food that should make up a healthy meal. These five groups are: grains, vegetables, fruits, protein foods, and dairy. Boxes 10-2 to 10-6 describe the foods included in each group.

Fig 10-3 The MyPlate Food Guide. (Courtesy of U.S. Department of Agriculture, Washington, DC.)

BOX 10-2   Grains

DESCRIPTION

Foods made from cereal grains (e.g., wheat, rice, oats, barley, corn meal). Types:
<u>Whole grain</u> contains the entire grain kernel (e.g., whole wheat, brown rice, oatmeal).
<u>Refined grain</u> is processed to remove the grain kernel (e.g., white flour, white rice).

POINTS TO REMEMBER

- There are many sources of grains: cereal, bread, crackers, pasta, tortillas, cookies, cake, and pretzels.
- Choose foods that contain whole grains rather than "enriched" products.
- Look for the word *whole* before the grain name on the list of ingredients. See Box 10-10 for other smart food choices.
- Make at least half your grains whole grains.

DO YOU KNOW?

- Grains are excellent sources of carbohydrates and some B vitamins.
- Whole grains are good sources of dietary fiber. Watch out for labels that read, "made from whole grains." This may be misleading. Look for the fiber content on the Nutrition Facts label (see Figure 10-7).

BOX 10-3 Vegetables

DESCRIPTION

Fresh, canned, frozen, and 100% vegetable juices. May be raw or cooked.
<u>Dark green vegetables</u>—spinach, broccoli, collard greens, bok choy, kale, and
   other dark leafy greens
<u>Red and orange vegetables</u>—carrots, sweet potatoes, beets, tomatoes, acorn and butternut
   squash
<u>Dry beans and peas</u>—kidney beans, chick peas, pinto beans, black-eyed peas
<u>Starchy vegetables</u>—corn, white potatoes, green peas
<u>Other vegetables</u>—cabbage, celery, onions, cauliflower, and so on

POINTS TO REMEMBER

- Eat more dark green, orange, and red vegetables and dry beans and peas.
- Vegetables are excellent sources of vitamins, dietary fiber, and vegetable protein
  (dry beans and peas).
- Vary the type of vegetables each day to add interest and texture to the meals.

DO YOU KNOW?

- Frozen vegetables have the same vitamin content as fresh ones. Cook both properly to
  keep the vitamin content at maximum levels.
- For the freshest vegetables, try to buy locally grown produce.

BOX 10-4 Fruits

DESCRIPTION

Fresh, canned, frozen, dried, and 100% fruit juices. May be raw or cooked. There
are many different kinds, including:
<u>Citrus</u>—orange, grapefruit, lemon, lime
<u>Berries</u>—blueberries, strawberries, raspberries
<u>Melons</u>—watermelon, cantaloupe, honeydew
<u>Others</u>—apple, peach, pear, banana, mango, papaya

POINTS TO REMEMBER

- Vary the kinds of fruit. There are so many to choose.
- Avoid fruit drinks. They have limited amounts of actual fruit juices and are usually high in
  sugar content.
- Select fresh fruit in season when possible.
- Canned fruit packed in water has fewer calories than fruit packed in syrup.

DO YOU KNOW?

- Prunes, raisins, and other dried fruits are concentrated fruits. They are higher in sugar
  content and calories than fresh fruit.
- Fruits are excellent sources of dietary fiber and vitamins.

The amount of food to be eaten from each group depends on the following factors.
There is no one standard to be used for everyone.
- Age
- Sex
- Amount of physical activity
- Height
- Weight

BOX 10-5 Protein Foods

DESCRIPTION

Includes: foods made from meat, poultry, fish, beans and peas, eggs, nuts, and seeds.

POINTS TO REMEMBER

- Many of these foods contain fat and cholesterol. Read labels, and select lean or low-fat products.
- Avoid frying meat, poultry, or fish.
- Drain or skim off any fat accumulated in cooking (e.g., when browning meat for tacos or chili).
- Choose unsalted seeds and nuts to limit sodium intake.

DO YOU KNOW?

- Processed meats (hot dogs, sausage, bacon, and cold cuts) have high amounts of sodium (salt). Check labels. Try to use more poultry and fish.
- Meat and beans are good sources of high-quality protein, B vitamins, and minerals.
- Tofu (soybean curd) is an excellent source of vegetarian protein.

BOX 10-6 Dairy

DESCRIPTION

Includes milk and products made from milk: yogurt, cottage cheese, string cheese, cheddar cheese, milk-based desserts (pudding, ice cream), and soy beverages.
   Note: Cream, cream cheese, and butter are examples of oil.

POINTS TO REMEMBER

- Milk builds and maintains bones throughout life.
- Low-fat or fat-free products should be selected.
- Lactose-free products are available for those who cannot consume milk.

DO YOU KNOW?

- Milk and milk products contain calcium, protein, and vitamin D.
- Pregnant and nursing women need extra milk products for themselves and their infants.

For example, an older woman is usually less active and therefore needs less food from each group than a growing, active adolescent girl. However, both of them need foods from each group to maintain health. MyPlate is designed to meet the unique needs of each person. Help in planning daily meals is available on the ChooseMyPlate.gov Internet website. To receive an individualized Daily Food Plan, when prompted, enter the person's age, sex, height, weight, and amount of daily physical activity.

The following list shows the amounts needed daily from each food group for a healthy adult on a 2000 calorie diet.

Grains	6 ounces
Vegetables	2½ cups
Fruits	2 cups
Dairy	3 cups
Protein foods	5½ ounces

NOTE: For children, teenagers, pregnant women, nursing mothers, older adults, and others with special nutritional needs, the amount of food from each group will vary. Additional information is available from the home care agency's dietitian or from the ChooseMyPlate.gov Internet website.

OILS (FATS) AND EMPTY CALORIES

Oils

Oils are fats in liquid form. Some examples are: canola oil, sunflower oil, peanut oil, olive oil, and cream. They may be used in cooking foods or flavoring foods, as in salad dressing.

Solid fats include butter, meat and poultry fat, oleo, and shortening. Fats may also be "hidden," as in nuts, seeds, egg yolks, and avocados.

The MyPlate Food Guide does not indicate the amount of oil needed because sufficient oil/fat from foods is usually obtained from the foods we eat each day. In fact, the typical American meal of french fries, milk shake, and burger is loaded with calories from oils and fats.

For healthier eating, remember to select fats from those found in fish, nuts, and vegetable oil. Oils from plant sources do not contain cholesterol. Animal fats do contain cholesterol, so limit solid fats such as butter, shortening, and foods that contain these products. Check the Nutrition Facts label, and choose low-fat foods.

Empty Calories

Calories from foods containing solid fats and/or added sugars are called "empty calories." Foods such as cookies, cakes, donuts, pizza, energy drinks, and hot dogs are high in calories but low in nutritional value. So, limit the amount of these types of food. Eat them occasionally, not as part of your regular daily food plan.

BALANCING FOOD AND PHYSICAL ACTIVITY

Daily physical activity is an important part of maintaining a healthy lifestyle. It should be enjoyable and not a chore. Some people join an exercise class at the local gym or ride a stationary bike at home. Others get exercise by walking the dog, caring for a vegetable or flower garden, maintaining a home, or mowing the lawn with a push mower. Whatever the method, physical activity should become a part of each day—the more physical activity, the greater the health benefits.

PLANNING THE MENU USING THE MYPLATE FOOD GUIDE

So far, you know the food sources of proteins, carbohydrates, fats, vitamins, minerals, dietary fiber, oils, and the value of water and other fluids in the diet. You know the food groups of the MyPlate Food Guide. The next step is to put this information into practical use.

No matter how many ounces or cups of food are recommended, there are general guidelines to follow. These include:
- Make ½ your plate from the vegetable and fruit groups
  Vary the types of vegetables (e.g., dark green, red, orange)
- Make ¼ your plate from the grains group
  At least half should be whole grains
- Make ¼ your plate from the protein foods group
  Use a variety of lean meats, and include 8 ounces of seafood per week
- Include food from the dairy group
  Use fat-free or low-fat (1%) milk instead of whole milk
- Limit the amount of "empty calories"

BOX 10-7 Serving Sizes

WHAT IS:

One Ounce

1 slice of bread
½ cup cooked pasta or rice
1 cup ready-to-eat cereal
1 egg
1 slice of processed cheese
¼ cup baked beans or refried beans

One Cup

2 cups raw leafy greens
1 small apple

8 large strawberries
2 slices processed cheese
½ cup raisins
1 half-pint container of milk

Other Serving Sizes

3 ounces lean meat or fish = a deck of cards
½ cup nuts = 2 ping pong balls
1 tablespoon salad dressing = a thumb tip
1 pancake = a compact CD
1 cup ready-to-eat cereal = a large handful
2 ounces peanut butter = 2 tablespoons

- Enjoy your food—just eat less
- Drink water instead of sugary drinks
- Avoid oversized portions of food

When planning your client's menus, consider the following:
- **Food preferences:** Know the likes and dislikes of the person.
- **Quantity:** Know the amount of food the client should eat. Follow suggested amounts per serving in Box 10-7.
- **Meal patterns:** Know when the main meal and lighter meals and snacks are usually eaten.
- **Variety:** Select different foods within each food group every day for a variety in flavors, textures, colors, and shapes.
- **Moderation:** Use fats, oils, sweets, and salt sparingly.
- **Balance:** Choose foods from each of the groups according to the requirements of the MyPlate Food Guide.
- **Fluids:** Meet the needs for adequate fluid intake: a minimum of 4 to 6 cups (1000 to 1500 milliliters) per day.
- **Therapeutic diet:** Follow the client's dietary plan.

BEFORE PLANNING THE MENU, DISCUSS FOOD LIKES AND DISLIKES WITH YOUR CLIENT. THIS IS IMPORTANT TO KNOW SO THAT YOU WILL INCLUDE FOODS THAT THE CLIENT LIKES TO EAT. THE MOST SUCCESSFUL MENU IS ONE THAT THE CLIENT ENJOYS EATING AND PROVIDES THE NECESSARY NUTRIENTS. YOU CAN PLAN A GOOD, NUTRITIONALLY BALANCED MEAL, BUT IF THE CLIENT DOES NOT EAT IT, YOUR WORK HAS BEEN IN VAIN. Some clients prefer to eat the main meal in the evening. Others are used to having this meal at noon. Perhaps some prefer a lighter breakfast with snacks in mid-morning and mid-afternoon. Plan according to these preferences, too (Figure 10-4).

Choosing foods from all the groups provides that balance of nutrients so necessary for good nutrition. Varying the foods within each group allows for different tastes, textures, and colors. Variety helps to make each meal more interesting, attractive, and less boring to the client.

Many of your clients will have well-established food habits. For example, Father Kowalski has eaten the same food for breakfast for the past 25 years—two cups of coffee and a donut. This food habit will be very difficult to change, perhaps impossible. Your challenge is to add foods for the remaining meals, including snacks, to make up for the lack of a well-balanced breakfast.

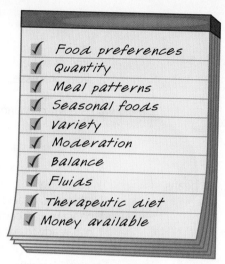

Fig 10-4 Planning the menu involves many factors.

Planning the menu to include adequate amounts of fluid is essential for good health. Some clients prefer to drink fluids with the meal, but others will tell you that they become too full and cannot finish their food if fluids are served during the meal. Be sure to provide water, milk, fruit juices, and other fluids during the day to meet the daily fluid requirement of 4 to 6 cups (1000 to 1500 milliliters).

SHOPPING FOR FOOD

The home care aide may do the food shopping, if the client cannot and there is no one else to assume this responsibility. **ASSISTING YOUR CLIENT TO SHOP MAY BE PART OF THE CARE PLAN. YOU MAY GO TO THE MARKET ALONE OR YOU MIGHT BE TAKING THE CLIENT TO THE MARKET. WHATEVER THE CASE, BE SURE THAT YOU UNDERSTAND AND FOLLOW THE POLICY OF YOUR AGENCY REGARDING HANDLING CLIENTS' MONEY AND TRANSPORTING CLIENTS IN CARS. THIS IS VERY IMPORTANT BECAUSE YOU AND THE AGENCY COULD BE HELD LEGALLY RESPONSIBLE IF THERE ARE ANY LOSSES, INJURIES, OR ACCIDENTS INVOLVING YOU AND THE CLIENT. BE SURE THAT YOU FOLLOW THE RULES AND REGULATIONS OF THE AGENCY.**

Think of food shopping as a challenge. Your goal will be to get the most for your client's money by
- Purchasing the best-quality, most healthful foods
- Staying within the food budget

PREPARE A SHOPPING LIST

Preparation for shopping begins with menu planning and preparing a shopping list. Each time you use up an item, write it on a list. This way there is a continuing record of what is needed. Keep the list in the same place, and encourage your client to use it when possible. On marketing day, rewrite the list to include the following:
- Items needed and replaced frequently, such as milk, soap, toilet tissue
- Sale items listed in newspaper advertisements and supermarket circulars
- Items needed because of dietary needs or restrictions, such as sugar substitute and low-sodium or low-fat foods

Try to write the list according to the layout of the store, so you will not waste time and energy running all over the market. The time allotted for shopping may be limited,

Expiration Date

Sell Date

Freshness Date

Fig 10-5 Food labels.

Rotini
Ingredients: Semolina (wheat); durum flour (wheat); niacin; iron (ferrous sulfate); thiamin mononitrate; riboflavin; folic acid. **ALLERGEN INFORMATION: CONTAINS WHEAT INGREDIENTS AND IS MANUFACTURED IN A FACILITY THAT USES EGGS**

Bitesize Wheat Cereal
Ingredients: Whole wheat, sugar, sorbitol, gelatin, Vitamins and Minerals: iron, niacinamide, zinc oxide, pyridoxine hydrachloride, (vitamin B$_6$), riboflavin (vitamin B$_2$), thiamin hydrochloride (vitamin B$_1$) folic acid and vitamin B$_{12}$. To maintain quality, BHT has been added to the packaging.

Pink Grapefruit Juice Cocktail
Ingredients: Pink grapefruit juice from concentrate, filtered water, high fructose corn syrup, pectin, citric acid, natural grapefruit flavor, vitamin C (ascorbic acid), canthaxanthin (color).

Fig 10-6 Contents labels.

so do the job quickly and thoroughly. Use the list so you will not forget anything your client needs. Coupons can help to save money; keep these with the marketing list.

READ LABELS

Read the label to help you choose foods that can be used to make up a healthful diet. For example, too much saturated fat and cholesterol can increase the level of cholesterol in the blood (a risk for heart disease). Large amounts of sodium can increase the risk for high blood pressure. A food label (Figure 10-5) may give several types of information, including the following:

- **Open dates.** This helps to determine the freshness of the food. There are three commonly used dates (see Figure 10-5).
  1. **Sell by. ...** This is the last recommended date of sale. Most products will keep about 3 days beyond the date stamped.
  2. **Best if used by. ...** This is the last date that the manufacturer will guarantee full freshness and quality.
  3. **Expiration date. ...** This is the last date the product can be safely used. The date appears after the statement, "Do not use after (date)."
- **Contents.** This label is found on processed foods and lists the ingredients in the product (Figure 10-6). The contents are listed in descending order. That is, the first ingredient listed is present in the largest amount. For example, an orange juice container label only lists one ingredient, orange juice, whereas the label for orange drink lists water, high-fructose corn syrup, citric acid, and orange juice.
- **Nutrition Facts.** This label contains nutrition information and is required on almost all packaged foods. This information can be used to help in planning a healthy diet. Figure 10-7 shows a Nutrition Facts label and how to read it. Terms used on food labels are defined in Box 10-8.
- **Food package symbol.** A food package may also display a symbol—a quick way for shoppers to identify the food as contributing to a healthy lifestyle. "Heart Healthy" and "100% Whole Grain" symbols are two examples.

Serving size ——

Calories from serving ——

Nutrients in each serving ——

Fat

Carbohy-drates

Proteins

Vitamins

Minerals

—— Calories from fat

Percent of daily value listed for vitamins and minerals to meet daily requirements

Nutrition Facts
Serving Size 1 packet (35g)
Servings Per Container 10

Amount Per Serving

Calories 130   Calories from Fat 15

% Daily Value*

Total Fat 1.5g	2%
Saturated Fat 0.5g	3%
Polyunsaturated Fat 0.5g	
Monounsaturated Fat 0.5g	
Cholesterol 0mg	0%
Sodium 105mg	4%
Total Carbohydrate 26g	9%
Dietary Fiber 3g	11%
Soluble Fiber 1g	
Sugars 11g	
Protein 4g	
Vitamin A	15%
Vitamin C	0%
Calcium	15%
Iron	30%
Thiamin	20%
Riboflavin	10%
Niacin	15%
Vitamin B6	20%
Folate	20%

* Percent Daily Values are based on a 2,000 calorie diet. Your daily values may be higher or lower depending on your calorie needs:

		Calories:	2,000	2,500
Total Fat	Less than		65g	80g
Sat Fat	Less than		20g	25g
Cholesterol	Less than		300mg	300mg
Sodium	Less than		2,400mg	2,400mg
Total Carbohydrate			300g	375g
Dietary Fiber			25g	30g

More nutrients may be listed on some labels

g = grams (about 28g = 1 ounce)
mg = milligram (1000mg = 1 gram)

Fig 10-7 A Nutrition Facts label.

- **Size of product.** This label tells the total amount of the product you are purchasing, such as 5 pounds of potatoes, 500 napkins, or 1 dozen eggs.

COMPARE PRICES

There are several ways to compare prices. Most supermarkets display unit prices on the shelf above or below the products for sale. The unit price will vary. Items may be priced according to
- **Weight,** as coffee by the pound, or sugar by the kilogram
- **Volume,** as milk by the quart or soda by the liter
- **Count,** as tea bags by the hundred or toilet tissue by the sheet

Check prices by comparing cost, unit for unit, according to what amount has been posted on the supermarket shelf. Also, check the ingredients in the product. When buying frozen meals, compare the serving size and the contents.

BOX 10-8   Food Label Terms

- **Light or lite:** One-third fewer calories or 50% less fat per serving than the regular product
- **Low fat:** Three grams of fat or less per serving
- **Low cholesterol:** Less than 20 milligrams of cholesterol and 2 grams or less of saturated fat per serving
- **Low calorie:** Less than 40 calories per serving
- **Low sodium:** Less than 140 milligrams of sodium per serving
- **Fat free/sugar free:** Less than 0.5 gram of fat or sugar per serving
- **Reduced:** 25% less of the specified nutrient or calories than the usual product
- **High fiber:** Five or more grams of fiber per serving
- **Good source:** Serving contains 10% to 19% of Daily Value for a particular nutrient or vitamin per serving
- **High in:** Serving contains 20% or more of Daily Value for a particular nutrient
- **Healthy (individual food item):** Low fat, low saturated fat, less than 480 milligrams sodium, less than 95 milligrams cholesterol, and at least 10% of the Daily Value of vitamins A, C, iron, protein, calcium, and fiber
- **Lean (meat, poultry, seafood):** Ten grams of fat or less, 4.5 grams of saturated fat, and less than 95 milligrams of cholesterol per 3-ounce serving
- **Calorie free:** Less than 5 calories per serving

Buying in quantity can be very economical, but this is not always practical for clients who live alone. They may not be able to use or store large quantities of food.

Buy food in its "original" form. Usually, the more a food is processed, the greater the cost. Do most of your shopping in the "outside aisles" of the supermarket for fresh and frozen foods.

SHOP FOR FRESHNESS

Try to buy foods that are "in season," such as apples in the fall and berries in the spring and summer. Today, we are able to buy produce grown in other countries—foods that are "in season" in another part of the world. When these products are "on special" at the market, they are usually fresh and a good buy.

Farmers' markets and "green grocers" offer freshly picked produce right from the grower. This is an opportunity to obtain the freshest fruits and vegetables available.

When shopping at the supermarket, always check the dates on food packages before making a purchase. Also check the appearance of the food. Does it look and smell fresh? Frozen foods should be solid, and refrigerated foods should be cold. Purchase refrigerated and frozen foods last to prevent warming and thawing.

When you shop, include some food from each of the groups found in the MyPlate Food Guide.

RETURNING TO THE CLIENT'S HOME

BE CERTAIN THAT YOU HAVE THE MARKET RECEIPT, THE CORRECT CHANGE, AND THE MARKETING LIST. YOU WILL GIVE THESE TO YOUR CLIENT AS A RECORD OF YOUR PURCHASES AND EXPENDITURES. KEEP RECORDS IN THE SAME PLACE, AND ALWAYS FOLLOW YOUR AGENCY'S PROCEDURES REGARDING THE CLIENT'S MONEY AND RECEIPTS.

The following information for storing and preparing food is important to prevent and/or reduce the risk of foodborne illnesses. Be aware that foods such as milk,

---

BOX 10-9 Food Storage Guidelines

FREEZER: TEMPERATURE 0° F

- Use moisture-proof wrap; label and date all packages.
- Keep a list of freezer contents; any foods stored beyond the appropriate time (quality and safety may be questionable) should be discarded.
- Do not store foods longer than 1 month beyond recommended time.

REFRIGERATOR: TEMPERATURE 34° TO 40° F AT ALL TIMES

- Wrap perishable foods to prevent mingling of tastes and odors.
- Wrap raw meat loosely; store on a plate so that juices do not drip onto other foods.
- Refrigerate leftovers immediately; wrap tightly to prevent drying; use within 2 to 3 days.
- Keep eggs cold; store inside the refrigerator, not inside the door.

PANTRY

- Use cool, dry storage areas; avoid damp and hot locations.
- Date packages not already dated.
- Keep foods in moisture-proof containers (except for fresh produce).
- If pests are a problem, store dry goods (e.g., cereal, pasta) in glass or heavy plastic storage containers.

---

cheese, and juice that are labeled "natural" and not pasteurized are at high risk for foodborne illnesses. So, these foods should be avoided.

FOOD STORAGE

Proper storage is essential to maintain the quality and the safety of food. Meat, poultry, and fish must be refrigerated or frozen until used. Thaw in the refrigerator or microwave, never at room temperature. Recommended storage times are different for each product. Quality cannot be maintained if foods are improperly stored. For example, if the bag inside a cereal box is not closed tightly, the product becomes limp and soggy, and the quality is poor. Try to use items before the expiration date. Some recommendations about storage are listed in Box 10-9.

PREPARING FOOD

Your goal in preparing food is to promote the client's nutrition according to the care plan. Certainly, you want to prepare food that the client is able to eat and that will be enjoyable. Color, flavor, and variety make a meal appealing to see, smell, and taste. Use cooking methods that will preserve color and taste, as well as vitamins and minerals. Do not add unnecessary and unwanted ingredients, such as large quantities of salt, sugar, and fats. Try to offer variety in the meals; no one wants to eat the same thing every day. If the choice of available foods is limited, try to vary the methods of preparation. Potatoes can be baked, mashed, boiled, or fried. They can be served hot, cold, and in stews and soups. The use of the same food each day does not have to be boring. Box 10-10 offers some suggestions for choosing healthy foods.

FOOD SAFETY

During the past few years, the number of deaths caused by harmful bacteria in meat and poultry has been steadily rising. Because of this, the U.S. Department of

BOX 10-10   Smart Food Choices

GRAINS

- Choose whole grain breads and flour.
- Use cereals where sugar is listed as a third ingredient or lower on the label.
- Do not add salt to cooking water for pasta and rice.
- Avoid creamed sauces on pastas and large amounts of butter or margarine on bread.

VEGETABLES AND FRUITS

- Eat fruits without sugar or whipped toppings.
- The best choice is whole fruit; then choose fruit juices over fruit drinks or soda.
- Steam or microwave fresh vegetables; season with herbs, pepper, or lemon juice.
- To boost fiber, leave the skin on potatoes, tomatoes, apples, pears, and peaches.

DAIRY

- Use skim (fat-free) or 1% milk.
- Replace cream in recipes with evaporated milk.
- Nonfat yogurt is a good substitute for sour cream.
- Limit high-fat cheeses (cheddar, American, Swiss, and cream).
- Use small amounts of sharp cheese as flavoring.
- Select fat free cottage cheese.

PROTEIN FOODS

- Serve 3-ounce portions (the size of a deck of cards).
- Use cooking methods that let the fat drain away—grilling, broiling, roasting, and baking; trim fat from meats, and remove skin from poultry before cooking.
- Select lean cuts of meat.
- Limit breaded and fried chicken and seafood.
- Use ground turkey instead of ground beef.
- Limit
  Organ meats (liver)—high in cholesterol
  Smoked fish—high in sodium
  Lunch meats, cold cuts, hot dogs, and sausage—high in sodium and fat

OILS, FATS, AND SWEETS

- Limit intake.
- Always use oils by the level teaspoon.
- Use nonstick cooking sprays.
- Select fat-free and reduced-calorie salad dressings.
- Try herb vinegars and lemon juice on salads instead of salad dressing.
- Use jams and jellies (if allowed) instead of butter.
- Avoid foods containing trans fats.

FROZEN AND CANNED FOODS

- Read labels, and select products with less than 400 calories, and low in sodium and fat.
- When serving a frozen dinner, add a green salad, fresh fruit, and skim milk for a complete meal.
- Frozen yogurt and ice milk are lower in fat than premium ice creams.
- Avoid canned soups that are high in fat and sodium.
  The agency staff dietitian will be able to help you with special dietary needs for your clients.

Agriculture developed rules regarding the safe handling and cooking of meat and poultry.

Labels on uncooked meat and poultry outline four steps for safety of meat and poultry.

1. Store it properly (as discussed earlier in the chapter).
2. Avoid cross-contamination by keeping raw meats and poultry separate from other foods. Wash all work surfaces (including cutting boards), utensils, and hands after touching raw meat or poultry.
3. Cook food thoroughly. Meat and poultry should be fully cooked. Hamburgers should not be pink on the inside.
4. Keep hot foods hot and cold foods cold until serving. Refrigerate leftovers immediately or discard.
5. Wash raw fruits and vegetables before cooking or serving.

ALWAYS WASH YOUR HANDS THOROUGHLY WITH WARM WATER AND SOAP BEFORE YOU BEGIN MEAL PREPARATION. IF YOU ARE INTERRUPTED (E.G., TO GIVE CLIENT CARE, ANSWER THE TELEPHONE, BLOW YOUR NOSE), WASH YOUR HANDS AGAIN BEFORE RESUMING YOUR FOOD DUTIES (SEE SECTION ON HANDWASHING IN CHAPTER 11).

SERVING THE FOOD

Before serving the meal, help your client to use the toilet, commode, or bedpan and to wash his or her hands. Make sure the bedpan or urinal is stored properly after use. Assist with oral hygiene (Chapter 14) if appropriate.

The food should be attractively arranged on the plate. Try not to serve foods that are all one color, such as white fish, white potatoes, and white cauliflower. This is not appealing to the eye. Carrots or green beans instead of cauliflower would liven up the appearance of the dish. Try your best to make things look good. Set the table with the proper utensils. If your client uses adaptive eating utensils, such as a plate guard or built-up silverware (Figure 10-8), place these properly and within easy use. Cut the food, and assist the client as required. Encourage the client to be as independent as possible.

If your client stays in bed, take the food to him or her on a tray. You can substitute a baking sheet for a tray or cut a cardboard box to make a tray (Figure 10-9). Set the tray as you would set the table. Do not forget napkins. Use several napkins, paper

Fig 10-8 Adaptive eating utensils and a plate guard.

Fig 10-9 A cookie sheet can be substituted for a tray.

PROCEDURE 10-1   Feeding the Client

MATERIALS NEEDED

- Utensils: knife, fork, spoon
- Dishes, bowls, cup, glass
- Napkins (2)
- Towel or bib
- Straws
- Adaptive supplies
  Plate guard
  Special utensils
  Universal cup holder
  Bed tray

PROCEDURE

1. Explain what you are going to do.
2. Wash your hands.
3. Obtain materials listed above.
4. Prepare client for mealtime.
   - Offer to assist with toileting.
   - Offer to assist client to wash hands.
   - Position client to sit up
     In bed
     In a chair
   - Place table or bed tray over client's lap so he or she can see and reach the food.
5. Drape napkin across client's chest and under the chin.
6. Serve food on tray, if needed.
7. Sit near the client.
8. Explain what is being served.
9. Cut food, butter bread, pour and prepare liquids as needed.
10. Ask the client what he or she would like to eat first.
11. Encourage client to do as much self-feeding as possible.
12. Feed client one bite at a time. Use a spoon, and fill only half full according to ability to chew and swallow.
13. Alternate solids and liquids. Use a straw for drinking.
14. Talk pleasantly with the client, and encourage him or her to eat. Offer praise.
15. When client is finished, wipe client's mouth and then remove tray (if used).
16. Wash client's hands and face. Remove napkin or bib.
17. Offer oral hygiene.
18. Make sure client is safe and comfortable.
19. Note amount eaten, and record the percent of food consumed (100% = all; 50% = half) in care record.
20. Wash your hands.
21. Wash dishes and utensils used for meal.
22. Clean and straighten kitchen.

towels, or a dish towel to protect the client's clothing. It is not easy to eat in bed and be neat.

FEEDING THE CLIENT

If your client is unable to feed himself or herself, assist with feeding. See Procedure 10-1, Feeding the Client.

SPECIAL SITUATIONS

Many clients have problems eating because of missing teeth. Illness can also result in poor appetite or trouble swallowing. Some clients are so tired that they just do not have the energy to eat. These situations provide opportunities for the home care aide to adjust the menu or method of food preparation so that the client is more likely to eat. A client with many missing teeth will probably not be able to eat a raw apple. By adjusting the menu to substitute applesauce, one of the requirements of the food group of the MyPlate Food Guide will be met.

The client who is blind may or may not require adjustments to the menu or method of food preparation, but this person will need to know where foods are placed on the plate to select what to eat. If your client has weakness on one side of the face, feed the strong side.

> ### BOX 10-11   The Client With a Poor Appetite
>
> - Make meals attractive and colorful; serve on dinnerware that client is used to.
> - Offer small meals and snacks frequently.
> - Select foods and snacks high in nutrients and calories.
> - Prepare snacks in advance, and have them readily available.
> - Avoid foods high in fat, which can cause a feeling of fullness.
> - Give high-calorie liquids in place of plain water or diet soda.
> - Serve foods at the desired temperature; they may need to be cool or warm rather than cold or hot.
> - Give liquids 30 to 60 minutes before a meal rather than with a meal, which fills the stomach quickly.
> - Provide companionship while the client is eating if he or she is alone.
> - Do not force foods; if a food is not appealing today, try it again another day.
> - Serve the same foods each day if the client wants to eat them.
> - Record and report unusual difficulties in eating to your supervisor.

POOR APPETITE

Mrs. Stevens has had chemotherapy for cancer. She says, "Food doesn't taste the same. Just looking at a big plate of food makes me sick."

The term used to describe a loss of appetite is anorexia. There are many reasons for this complaint. The illness itself, medical treatments such as cancer therapies, worry, anxiety, or fear can result in lack of interest in eating. Box 10-11 gives some advice for preparing and serving foods for the client with a poor appetite.

DIFFICULTY CHEWING AND SWALLOWING

Anna Petrova's client, Brigid (82 years of age), has no teeth. Brigid's daughter insists that she wear the full set of dentures, but when her daughter leaves the apartment, Brigid takes out the dentures and refuses to wear them.

Difficulty chewing can be caused by many factors, as in the case of Brigid. Poorly fitting dentures, missing teeth, or a sore mouth can make chewing very difficult. In addition, chewing takes a lot of energy. Clients whose illnesses result in low energy levels may find chewing to be exhausting.

The act of swallowing is a complex process that requires coordination of the nerves and muscles of the throat. Saliva helps lubricate food so that swallowing takes place without effort. When clients do not produce enough saliva or have illnesses that affect nerves and muscles of the throat, swallowing becomes difficult. The speech-language therapist may teach your client techniques to help improve swallowing. Your encouragement to use these techniques is important. Box 10-12 gives information about ways to plan and prepare meals for the client who has difficulty chewing or swallowing.

CLIENTS WITH LOW ENERGY LEVELS

Russ Larson's client, Louis Roupp, has great difficulty breathing. "I have such a hard time breathing that I haven't any strength to do anything else."

BOX 10-12 The Client With Difficulty Chewing and Swallowing

CHEWING

- Select ground meats: beef, turkey, lamb, and ham.
- Include high-calorie, high-protein drinks.
- Prepare foods such as eggs, fish, and cheese for sources of high protein.
- Use a food processor or blender to soften or puree food.
- Include soups or puddings.
- Cut food into small pieces.
- High-fiber foods (e.g., vegetables, bran cereals) must be soft.
- Be patient with the client; do not rush.

SWALLOWING

- Have the client sit upright, slightly forward, with the chin tilted down, if conditions permit.
- Have the client lower the chin during the swallowing process.
- Select foods with similar textures for ease in chewing and swallowing; thick, soft foods are easiest to swallow.
- Thicken liquids to ease the swallowing process.
  Add commercially available thickening agents to hot liquids.
  Add gelatin to cold liquids.
- Have the client remain in the sitting position for 20 to 30 minutes after the meal.
- Record and report unusual difficulties in eating to your supervisor.

BOX 10-13 The Client With Low Energy Levels

- Allow plenty of time to eat.
- Encourage a rest period for about $\frac{1}{2}$ hour before and after eating.
- Serve small meals at least six times a day.
- Select foods high in nutrient value.
- Select foods that do not require a lot of chewing.
- Use a blender to puree food.
- Provide a straw to eliminate the need to lift a cup or glass.
- Cut food into small pieces.
- Butter the bread; pour liquids.
- Assist with feeding as needed.
- Prepare nutritious drinks, such as milk shakes.
- Use liquid dietary supplements, if ordered by the doctor.
- Prepare foods in advance that can be served without delay.
- Use the microwave, if available, to reduce time spent cooking or reheating foods.
- Use cups, glasses, and eating utensils that are light and easy to handle; place each within easy reach.
- Record and report unusual difficulties in eating to your supervisor.

For clients whose illnesses cause severe fatigue to occur, energy must be conserved so that activities of daily living, like eating, can be performed with as little effort as possible. Drinking, chewing, and swallowing require a lot of energy. Lifting a fork or cup, reaching for the salt shaker—these actions take energy to perform. Usually, the morning hours are best for clients with low energy because energy reserves are at their highest point. Therefore, breakfast may become the best meal of the day.

Because Mr. Roupp has low energy, Russ follows the guidelines in Box 10-13 when he assists Mr. Roupp with meals.

THE BLIND CLIENT

Mohammed has been blind since birth. He can feed himself, but he says, "I like to eat all my vegetables first, then the rest of the food."

Mealtime can be a pleasant experience for your blind client if you take the following steps.

- Explain where foods are on the plate; describe the plate as a clock—"The broccoli is at 3 o'clock, the baked flounder is at 6 o'clock, and the mashed potatoes are at 9 o'clock."
- Keep utensils, napkin, cup, glass, saltshaker, and so on, in the same location on the table or tray.
- Avoid the urge to "help" the client unless he or she requests your assistance.

SPECIAL DIETS TO MEET THE CLIENT'S NEEDS

Treatment of the client's illness may include changes in the diet. This is called *nutritional therapy*. In combination with other types of treatment—such as medications, physical therapy, and speech therapy, nutritional therapy contributes to the client's recovering process.

The type of diet ordered by the doctor depends on the nutritional needs of the client. Perhaps there are problems with the way the food is digested or absorbed. Or the body requires increased amounts of certain nutrients so that the healing of tissues can take place. Nutritional therapy is an important part of the client's overall plan of care.

MODIFYING THE DIET

The MyPlate Food Guide forms the foundation for modifying the diet to meet the client's needs. In fact, the diet ordered by the doctor should be as similar as possible to the client's regular diet. Changes may need to be made in the frequency of meals, the quantity of certain types of foods, and/or the texture or digestibility of the foods consumed. The dietitian meets with the client and family to discuss the client's food preferences and explain the dietary changes needed. The dietitian will also answer questions concerning food selection, preparation, and serving. When teaching the client and family about the modifications needed, the dietitian considers food preferences, existing diet, cultural and religious requirements, budget, and kitchen facilities available.

YOUR ROLE IN NUTRITIONAL THERAPY

Nutritional therapy is an important part of the care plan. Your responsibility is to prepare meals according to the diet plan. Because you will visit the client more frequently than other staff members, you can observe and record information about how the diet is being tolerated. Accurate record keeping of the food eaten and fluids consumed is very important. The dietitian may need to visit again to review the diet modifications. Table 10-5 provides information about therapeutic diets frequently used for clients. Remember, the food groups of the MyPlate Food Guide form the foundation for each of the diets listed. The kinds of foods selected or the method of food preparation will vary according to the specific diet.

No matter what type of diet your client receives, the keys to healthy eating are *balance, variety,* and *moderation.* The following tips can help you to provide good nutrition for your client.

- Serve a variety of nutrient-rich foods.
- Use the MyPlate Food Guide as a reference in meal planning.

TABLE 10-5	Therapeutic Diets Using MyPlate Food Guide	
NAME	PURPOSE	FOODS
Regular	Provides all nutrients.	*Include:* All food groups. *Avoid:* None.
Soft	Provides foods that are easy to chew, swallow, and digest.	*Include:* All food groups that have been strained, chopped, and/or pureed. *Avoid:* High-fiber foods, seeds.
Bland	Promotes easy digestion and avoids irritation to digestive system.	*Include:* All food groups. *Avoid:* Highly seasoned foods, pepper, coffee, alcohol, high-fiber foods, seeds.
High calorie	Increases caloric intake.	*Include:* All food groups. Add nourishing snacks with high nutrient and caloric value, such as milk shakes. *Avoid:* None.
Low calorie	Decreases caloric intake.	*Include:* All food groups. Choose high-nutrient, low-fat foods: skim milk, yogurt, fresh fruits and vegetables, lean meats. *Avoid:* Foods high in fat, sodas, fried foods, beer, gravies.
Sodium restricted	Limits sodium intake.	*Include:* All food groups. Choose fresh fruits and vegetables, but limit cheese, milk, bakery bread. *Avoid:* Table and cooking salts, lunch meat, bacon, canned vegetables and soups, salted butter and margarine, commercially prepared frozen dinners.
Diabetic	Regulates the amount of carbohydrates in the diet.	*Include:* All food groups. Use lists of recommended foods (available from the agency's dietitian). *Avoid:* Table sugar, honey, sweetened carbonated sodas, alcoholic beverages, pastries, cookies, cakes, pies.
Low fat	Limits the amount of fat in the diet.	*Include:* All food groups. Skim milk, lean meat, fish and poultry, low-fat cottage cheese, fruits, and vegetables. *Avoid:* Fried foods, cooking oil, cheese, butter, margarine, ice cream, salad dressings, eggs, gravies, bacon, lunch meat, and avocados.
Low cholesterol	Reduces the amount of cholesterol in the blood.	*Include:* All food groups. Skim milk, lean meat, fish, poultry, fruits, and vegetables. *Avoid:* Foods and fats that come from animals, such as liver, bacon and bacon fat, egg yolks, butter, cheese, mayonnaise, sour cream, and ice cream.

- Serve whole grains, fruits, and vegetables according to diet requirements.
- Offer moderate portions of food.
- Avoid too much sugar and sodium.
- Encourage adequate fluid intake.
- Avoid too much fat, saturated fat, and cholesterol.

CHAPTER SUMMARY

- Good nutrition is an important part of maintaining health.
- Many factors influence food selection: likes and dislikes, culture, religion, physical condition, and income.
- Foods are classified as carbohydrates, proteins, and fats.
- Carbohydrates include sugars, starches, and fiber.
- Milk, meat, eggs, and legumes are good sources of protein.
- Fats are found in butter, oils, nuts, and chocolate.
- Vitamins and minerals must be consumed daily for good health.
- Fluids are essential for life; the normal adult must drink 4 to 6 cups (1000 to 1500 milliliters) of fluids each day.
- Fiber helps to promote proper bowel function.
- The MyPlate Food Guide is a resource for meal planning.
- The home care aide may be responsible for the client's food shopping.
- Prepare foods according to recommendations included in this chapter; proper food handling and storage are essential to maintaining the quality and safety of food.
- Follow agency policy regarding the client's money, expense receipts, travel, and transportation of clients.
- Assist the client to eat according to the care plan and the client's individual needs.
- Nutritional therapy is an important part of the care plan; prepare meals according to this plan.

STUDY QUESTIONS

1. How does good nutrition help to maintain health and prevent illness?
2. List three factors that influence individual and family food habits.
3. From the foods listed below, identify which are good sources of carbohydrate, protein, or fat.

orange juice	butter	milk
oatmeal	carrots	olive oil
turkey	hamburger	flounder
bacon	bread	potato chips
bagel	cream cheese	yogurt
ice cream	strawberries	tuna fish

4. Prepare a chart listing the vitamins and minerals. Include their functions and three food sources of each.
5. Explain why water, other fluids, and dietary fiber are needed in the diet each day.
6. Describe how each of the following is stored.
   a. Fresh ground beef
   b. Dry boxed cereal
   c. Leftover turkey
   d. Eggs
7. Review your agency's written policies regarding
   a. Handling clients' money
   b. Traveling and transporting clients
8. Describe the step-by-step procedure for feeding clients.
9. Describe what you would do for clients who have difficulty chewing and swallowing.
10. Identify foods to be included or avoided for the following therapeutic diets.
    a. Sodium restricted
    b. Diabetic
    c. Bland
    d. Low cholesterol

11

Preventing Infection/Medical Asepsis

OBJECTIVES

After you read this chapter, you will be able to:

1. Discuss microorganisms, pathogens, and nonpathogens.
2. Describe the cycle of infection.
3. Identify four ways infection can be spread.
4. Discuss the terms *medical asepsis, surgical asepsis,* and *standard (universal) precautions*.
5. Demonstrate correct practice of standard (universal) precautions in a client's home.
6. Demonstrate correct handwashing technique.
7. Apply nonsterile gloves, and remove contaminated gloves.
8. Describe the importance of following CDC and OSHA regulations about bloodborne pathogens.
9. Understand methods of disinfection in the home.
10. Demonstrate correct use of the mask and moisture-resistant gown or apron.

KEY TERMS

Aerobic Able to live in the presence of oxygen

AIDS Abbreviation for *acquired immunodeficiency syndrome,* an infectious disease caused by a virus and spread through contact with blood, body fluids, and/or unprotected sexual intercourse

Anaerobic Able to live without air or oxygen

Biohazard A biologic agent, such as harmful bacteria and viruses, or condition, such as chemical fumes, that threatens human life or health; potential danger, risk, or harm from exposure to such organisms or agents

Bloodborne pathogens Pathogenic microorganisms that are present in human blood and can cause disease in humans

Carrier A person or animal that spreads disease to others but does not become ill

Catheters Hollow, flexible tubes made of soft plastic or rubber that can be inserted into the body to withdraw or to insert fluids

Contaminated Dirty and/or exposed to harmful organisms, making the object unsafe for use as intended

Exposure incident A specific eye, mouth, other mucous membrane, nonintact skin, or parenteral contact with blood or other potentially infectious material that results from the performance of an employee's duties

Hepatitis B, hepatitis C Infectious diseases of the liver caused by a virus and spread through contact with blood, body fluids, and/or unprotected sexual intercourse

KEY TERMS—cont'd

HIV Abbreviation for *human immunodeficiency virus;* the virus that causes AIDS

Infection Occurs when harmful organisms enter the body and grow, causing illness or disease

Intravenous (IV) infusions Administration of nutrients or medications through a vein or veins

Invasive Entering the body

Medical asepsis Use of techniques and practices to prevent the spread of pathogenic organisms

Nonpathogenic Usually not capable of causing or producing a disease

Parenteral Piercing mucous membranes or skin through needlesticks, human bites, cuts, and/ or scrapes

Pathogenic Capable of causing or producing a disease

Personal protective equipment (PPE) Specialized clothing or equipment worn by an employee for protection against a biohazard

Reservoir A place where a pathogen is stored, can live, and grow

Sputum Material coughed up from the lungs and spit out through the mouth

Standard (universal) precautions An approach to infection control, designed to prevent the spread of bloodborne and other pathogens

Transmitted Passed from one person or place to another

Vomitus Material expelled from the stomach when vomiting

The Waters twins came home from kindergarten coughing and sneezing. They had no appetite, complained about runny, sore noses, and felt hot and sick. Their mother took their temperature, called the doctor, and followed instructions for treating their symptoms.

The twins were home from school for several days. Grandma Waters took care of the children while their parents went to work.

About a week later, Grandpa Waters began to cough, sneeze, and have a runny nose. "It's all your fault," he told his wife. "You brought those darned germs home, and now I feel awful."

Infection occurs when harmful organisms enter the body and grow, causing illness or disease. Microorganisms are small living plants or animals that can be seen only through a microscope. Even though we cannot see them, they are everywhere—on our skin, under the nails, on clothing, in food, in water, and in the air we breathe. Animals and insects also carry microorganisms (Figure 11-1).

MICROORGANISMS

Many microorganisms are nonpathogenic, meaning that they do not usually produce an infection. Some nonpathogens are helpful and are used in the production of certain foods, such as bread, cheese, yogurt, beer, and wine. Other nonpathogens live in and on the human body and cause no harm. Some of these are also helpful. For example, the *Escherichia coli* is a bacteria that normally lives in the bowel. This organism assists with bowel function and the manufacture of vitamin K in the body. (But *E. coli* can cause serious infection if it invades other parts of the body, such as the urinary bladder, upper digestive tract, or surgical wounds.)

There is, however, another group of microorganisms, known as pathogens, or pathogenic organisms, that are harmful and capable of producing illness known as *infectious disease.*

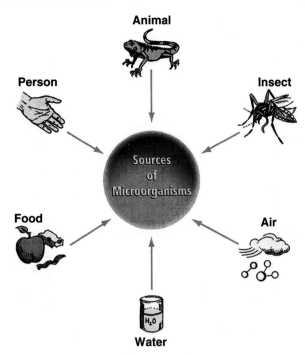

Fig 11-1 Microorganisms come from many sources.

GROWTH OF MICROORGANISMS

As living substances, microorganisms must have the following to live and grow:
- **Host:** A person, animal, or food on which to live.
- **Warmth:** Microorganisms grow best at body temperature; extreme heat will destroy microorganisms, and cold will slow their growth but will not prevent it; food stored in the refrigerator too long eventually becomes "spoiled" due to the action of growing microorganisms.
- **Darkness:** Microorganisms thrive in dark places, but light can destroy them.
- **Oxygen:** Is necessary to living organisms and needed by aerobic organisms; other microorganisms thrive where there is little or no oxygen; these are called anaerobic organisms.
- **Moisture:** Microorganisms grow in moist areas.
- **Food:** As living things, microorganisms need food to multiply; this food may be leftover green beans in the back of the refrigerator or the tissues of the human body.

Pathogenic microorganisms flourish where it is warm, dark, and moist with oxygen and a food supply. Can you think of any places in the body that act as a suitable home for pathogens? How about the mouth, throat, and nose? These and other body tissues meet all the requirements needed by pathogens to set up housekeeping and to cause an infection.

THE CYCLE OF INFECTION

For a pathogenic microorganism to cause an infection, a definite cycle or chain of infection occurs (Figure 11-2). This cycle includes six parts.

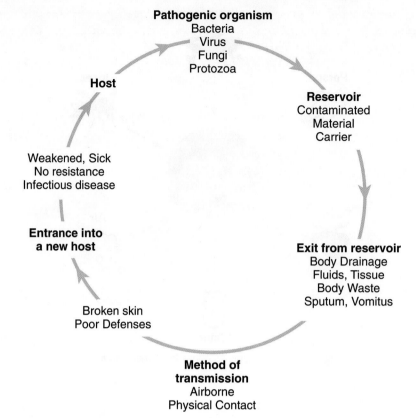

Fig 11-2 Cycle of infection.

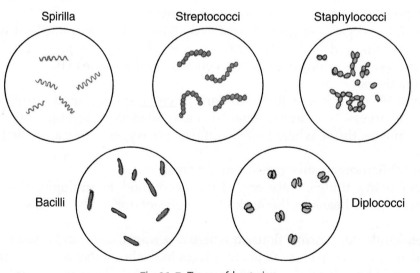

Fig 11-3 Types of bacteria.

1. THE PATHOGENIC ORGANISM

The most common groups of pathogenic microorganisms include the following.

- **Bacteria:** One-celled microscopic plants that multiply very quickly (Figure 11-3). There are many types of bacteria. Bacteria commonly found in the client's environment are
  - **Streptococcus:** May cause wound, heart, respiratory, and other infections.
  - **Staphylococcus:** May cause wound and soft-tissue infections.

The term *strep infection* is used when the streptococcal organism is the cause of the disease. Likewise, the term *staph infection* refers to a disease resulting from an invasion of one of the staphylococcal organisms.

- **Viruses:** The smallest known living disease-producing organisms. They cause many illnesses, ranging from the common cold and influenza to AIDS, hepatitis B, and hepatitis C.
- **Fungi:** Tiny plants that live on other plants or animals and can cause disease. Fungi (singular form of the word is *fungus*) are very plentiful in the environment; they can be seen growing on old bread or oranges: We might describe that food as being *moldy*. Among the diseases caused by fungi are athlete's foot and vaginal yeast infections.
- **Protozoa:** One-celled microscopic organisms that usually live in water and can cause disease. Infectious diseases caused by protozoa include malaria and a type of pneumonia associated with AIDS.

2. RESERVOIR OF INFECTION

The place where the pathogen is stored, lives, and grows is called a reservoir. Examples of reservoirs are persons with infectious diseases, soiled tissues and linens, client supplies, and equipment such as thermometers, bedpans, and commodes. Another reservoir may be a carrier, a person or animal that does not become ill but spreads the disease to others.

3. EXIT FROM THE RESERVOIR OF INFECTION

The pathogen must escape from the original host to cause disease in another host. Pathogens can be found in body fluids, such as blood, urine, semen, saliva, sputum, and vomitus, and in mucous membranes, tissues, and organs of the body. Secretions from the eyes, ears, nose, vagina, or penis may also contain pathogens. Of course, draining sores and infected wounds are excellent sources of pathogens.

4. METHOD OF TRANSMISSION

Organisms are transmitted by means of many routes: through direct or indirect contact, in the air, by animals and insects, and by food and water.

Direct Contact

Microorganisms are transmitted through direct contact with the person who is infected, including sexual contact. It is said that the 10 greatest carriers of disease are the fingers (Figure 11-4 and Box 11-1). Touching body secretions and handling body fluids without

Fig 11-4 The 10 greatest carriers of disease.

BOX 11-1   Do You Know?

- Your 10 FINGERS are the 10 greatest carriers of disease.
- Long, artificial nails act as excellent hiding places for bacteria to live and grow.
- If you wear long, artificial nails, your clients may be at greater risk for infection.
- Chipped, polished nails can also harbor germs that cause illnesses.
- YOUR BEST BET IS TO KEEP NAILS NATURAL, UNPOLISHED, AND SHORT.
- WASH YOUR HANDS FREQUENTLY AND THOROUGHLY (PROCEDURE 11-1, HANDWASHING)—IT IS THE BEST DEFENSE AGAINST SPREADING DISEASE.

protecting your hands are ways to carry pathogens from the infected person to yourself.

Examples: Syphilis and gonorrhea

Indirect Contact

Organisms can be transmitted through contact with items used by the infected person. Using another person's washcloth, towel, razor, toothbrush, and comb can result in microorganisms being transferred from the infected person to yourself without any direct personal contact. Drinking from the client's cup or glass or handling used tissues are ways organisms travel from one person to another.

Example: The common cold

Air

Some pathogens travel through the air in tiny droplets of water or dust. When we breathe in this air, organisms enter our respiratory systems. If we sneeze without covering the nose and mouth with a tissue, millions of organisms enter the air. Breathing in this air can cause pathogens to enter the body.

Example: Tuberculosis

Animals and Insects

The transmission of disease can occur through animals and insects. They carry organisms from place to place. Flies, mosquitoes, rats, mice, and ticks are examples of common carriers of disease.

Examples: Malaria and Lyme disease

Food and Water

Eating contaminated food or undercooked meat or poultry, eating unrefrigerated leftovers, and drinking unsafe water are ways in which organisms travel from the source to a human. Information about proper preparation and storage of food is found in Chapter 10.

Example: Hepatitis A

5. ENTRANCE INTO A NEW HOST

The pathogen must find a way to enter the body of the new host. Remember that the first line of defense is the skin. When skin is broken from a cut or a surgical wound, by injection, or from a bedsore, there is the opportunity for infection. Drainage tubes and catheters are often the route by which pathogens invade the body. Intravenous (IV) infusions provide a direct line through the skin and into the blood and may be used by pathogenic microorganisms as a "superhighway" for entrance into the host.

BOX 11-2   Signs and Symptoms of Infection

1. Redness of tissue
2. Swelling of area
3. Pain in area
4. Warmth in area (warm to touch)
5. Fever, chills, and headache
6. Nausea, vomiting, diarrhea
7. Coughing
8. Skin rash
9. Pus or foul-smelling drainage from a wound or body opening
10. Fatigue
   If your client develops any of these symptoms, notify your supervisor.

6. HOST

Microorganisms are all around us, but most of us do not have an infection because we have resistance to many microorganisms. BUT WHEN PATHOGENS INCREASE IN NUMBERS AND STRENGTH AND BODY DEFENSES CANNOT DESTROY THEM, AN INFECTION MAY OCCUR. SOME SIGNS AND SYMPTOMS OF INFECTION ARE LISTED IN BOX 11-2. BE ALERT FOR THESE SYMPTOMS IN YOUR CLIENT, AND REPORT THEM TO YOUR SUPERVISOR IMMEDIATELY.

Some people are more susceptible to infection than others. Factors that place persons at risk for infection include the following:
- Age—either the very old or the very young
- Great stress
- Chronic or acute illness
- Some medications
- Inadequate nutrition
- Poor living conditions
- Poor personal hygiene

If the host acts as a good place for pathogens to live and multiply, the cycle of infection will be complete and ready to start all over again.

BREAKING THE CYCLE OF INFECTION

Protecting the client from becoming a new host is an important role for every home care aide. The cycle of infection must be broken to prevent the transmission of a pathogen from one host to another. The organism can be removed, destroyed, or blocked in its progress through the cycle. Keep clean things "clean," and dispose of contaminated materials promptly. Follow all practices of good housekeeping and other measures (listed in this chapter) to prevent the spread of disease.

PREVENTING THE SPREAD OF DISEASE

PRACTICING GOOD PERSONAL HYGIENE IS IMPORTANT IN COMBATING THE SPREAD OF DISEASE. MAINTAINING YOUR OWN HEALTH IS ESSENTIAL SO YOU DO NOT BECOME A HOST FOR DISEASE-PRODUCING ORGANISMS. Using proper techniques of housekeeping, including food preparation and

---

BOX 11-3 **Ten Common-Sense Rules to Prevent Transmission of Disease**

1. Wash your hands after using the bathroom.
2. Wash your hands before and after handling or preparing food and before and after eating.
3. Cover your nose and mouth when coughing, sneezing, and blowing. (Cough or sneeze into your sleeve, if necessary.)
4. Wash your hands after coughing, sneezing, or blowing your nose.
5. Do not use another person's soiled drinking or eating utensils.
6. Do not use another person's personal items, such as toothbrush, razor, washcloth, or towels.
7. Practice good personal hygiene, and maintain good grooming habits.
8. Wash raw fruits and vegetables before eating or serving.
9. Prepare and store food properly.
10. Use good housekeeping practices to eliminate household pests and maintain a clean environment.

---

storage, also helps to prevent the spread of disease. Information about these techniques is found in Chapters 9 and 10.

Box 11-3 lists 10 common-sense rules to follow in preventing the transmission of disease.

MEDICAL ASEPSIS

The practice of **medical asepsis** is the use of techniques and practices to prevent the spread of pathogenic organisms from one person or place to another person or place. Medical asepsis is also known as *clean technique*.

HANDWASHING IS A KEY COMPONENT IN THE PRACTICE OF MEDICAL ASEPSIS. EXPERTS ON INFECTION CONTROL OFTEN SAY THAT HANDWASHING IS ONE OF THE MOST EFFECTIVE WAYS OF PREVENTING THE SPREAD OF INFECTION. Establish a place in the client's home where you can keep all of your supplies for handwashing. This may be next to the kitchen sink and/or on top of the toilet tank in the bathroom. Bar soap should not be used. Ask your client to get liquid soap, or bring your own to be kept at your "special handwashing place." These materials are for your use only.

The inside of the sink and the faucets are considered to be contaminated. Do not touch these areas when handwashing. After you have washed your hands, turn off the water using a dry paper towel. Procedure 11-1 gives the steps needed for proper handwashing. Other medical aseptic practices are listed in Table 11-1.

If running water is not available, your supervisor will advise you about what to use to clean your hands. Hand rubs using alcohol-based gels or detergent-containing towelettes may be used. Be sure to wash your hands with soap and water as soon as possible. Alcohol-based gels are flammable. Keep them away from heat and flame.

SURGICAL ASEPSIS

With surgical asepsis, sterile equipment and supplies are used. The term *sterile* means "free from all microorganisms, pathogens, and nonpathogens." Sterile technique is a specialized skill used during surgical procedures, injections, and other **invasive** procedures. Sterile technique is not usually the responsibility of the home care aide.

PROCEDURE 11-1 Handwashing

Materials Needed
- Liquid soap in a pump container
- Paper towels: Remove from the roll and separate four individual towels
- Warm running water
- Wastebasket
- Hand lotion, if desired

Procedure
1. Collect all materials at the sink (Figure 11-5).
2. Remove your wristwatch or push it up onto your forearm about 4 to 5 inches. Remove rings.
3. Stand back from the sink so that your clothing does not become wet.
4. Turn on the faucet. Adjust the water to a comfortable temperature.
5. Completely wet hands and wrists under the running water. Always keep your fingers and hands below your elbows to prevent dirty water from contaminating your arms (Figure 11-6).
6. Apply soap to your hands.
7. Lather hands well by rubbing the palms together (Figure 11-7). Spread lather over the entire area of the hands and wrists. Get soap under your nails and between your fingers.
8. Use a rotating and rubbing motion (friction) for 30 seconds.
   a. Vigorously rub one hand against the other and around wrist. Repeat with the other hand and wrist (Figure 11-8).
   b. Wash between fingers by interlacing them (Figure 11-9).
   c. Rub your fingernails against the palms of your hands to clean this area.
9. Wash at least 2 inches above your wrists.

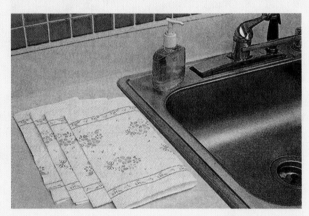
Fig 11-5 Collect materials at sink (Step 1).

Fig 11-7 Lather hands well (Step 7).

Fig 11-6 Keep fingers and hands below elbows (Step 5).

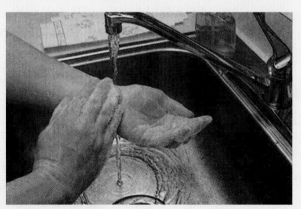
Fig 11-8 Use rotating rubbing motion to create friction. (Step 8).

PROCEDURE 11-1   Handwashing—cont'd

Fig 11-9 Wash between fingers (Step 8).

Fig 11-10 Rinse hands and wrists (Step 10).

10. Rinse well under the running water, one hand at a time. Rinse from 2 inches above the wrist. Keep hands and fingers below the elbows so water flows from the fingertips directly into the sink (Figure 11-10).
11. Dry your hands and wrists with paper towels.
12. Drop the used paper towels into the wastebasket.
13. Turn off the faucets using another dry paper towel (Figure 11-11).
14. Discard towel.
15. Apply hand lotion, if desired.

Fig 11-11 Use dry paper towel when turning off faucets (Step 13).

STANDARD (UNIVERSAL) PRECAUTIONS

Standard (universal) precautions is a method of infection control by which all human blood and body fluids are treated as though they are infected with pathogens. In other words, every client is treated as if he or she has a potentially infectious disease. Handwashing is a vital part of the practice of standard (universal) precautions, along with the proper use of gloves. Gloves are always worn when there is risk of direct contact with body fluids or moist body surfaces. They are used to protect

- You from infectious disease
- The client from you (sometimes health care workers bring infection to clients)
  HANDWASHING IS ALWAYS DONE BEFORE AND AFTER USING GLOVES.
Other rules for handwashing are listed in Box 11-4. Explain the reasons for using gloves to both the client and family. When applying and removing gloves, follow Procedure 11-2, Applying Gloves and Removing Contaminated Gloves.

PROTECTING AGAINST BLOODBORNE DISEASES

Health care workers can be exposed to blood and other infectious body fluids while caring for patients and clients. If proper precautions are not taken, **bloodborne**

TABLE 11-1	Breaking the Cycle of Infection Through Medical Asepsis

STEP IN CYCLE	HOME CARE AIDE ACTIVITY
1. Pathogenic organism	Keep the environment clean. Practice disinfection.
2. Reservoir of infection	Eliminate reservoir, when possible. Use gloves to handle contaminated material (e.g., tissues, sanitary napkins). Double bag and discard into covered trash container to keep animals out of trash. Empty bedpan, urinal, and commode promptly. Disinfect properly. Remove and treat soiled linens promptly. Keep client clean; bathe when necessary. Clean refrigerator; discard leftovers.
3. Exit from reservoir of infection	Block exit. Do not cough or sneeze on client or permit anyone to sneeze or cough on you. Teach client to cough into tissue and to discard in plastic bag. Do not go to work if you have an open, draining sore anywhere on your body. Notify supervisor if you have an infection. Seek advice about caring for clients when you have an infection. Wear gloves when handling body fluids. Wear other PPE as needed. Place soiled linens in plastic bags. Wear gloves when doing laundry contaminated with body fluids.
4. Method of transmission	WASH HANDS. Clients should have their own personal care items (e.g., linens, razor, toothbrush). There should be no sharing. Do not let client care items touch the floor; discard or disinfect any items that touch the floor. Do not let soiled linens touch your uniform. Keep drainage bags and tubes off the floor. Do not shake linens when changing the bed. Do not put linens on the floor. Cover nose and mouth when sneezing. Cough or sneeze into your sleeve if necessary. Discourage people with infections, especially colds and flu, from visiting the client. Keep window and door screens in place to prevent entrance of insects. Drink safe water only. Prepare and store food properly. Keep clean and contaminated items apart.
5. Entrance into a new host	Protect client's skin. Keep clean, dry, and prevent breakdown. Wear gloves if there is a risk of exposure to blood or other body fluids. Do not handle "sharps"—have client discard into a puncture-proof container (e.g., coffee can or plastic milk jug) according to agency and/or local community policy.
6. Host	Maintain and encourage healthy practices: good nutrition, sufficient rest. Avoid people with infections.

pathogens may be transmitted from the client to the health care worker and lead to disease, perhaps even death. The health care worker in turn can spread the disease to his or her family and/or friends.

HUMAN IMMUNODEFICIENCY, HEPATITIS B, AND HEPATITIS C VIRUSES

Human immunodeficiency virus (HIV), hepatitis B virus (HBV), and hepatitis C virus (HCV) are pathogens carried by the blood. HIV can eventually lead to AIDS and death.

> ## BOX 11-4   Rules for Handwashing
>
> Wash your hands
> - When you arrive in the client's home.
> - Before and after you give "hands-on" care or have personal contact with a client or his or her personal care items.
> - During care if you are interrupted for any reason.
> - Between tasks or procedures.
> - After using the toilet.
> - When you cough, sneeze, or blow your nose.
> - Before and after meals.
> - Before and after handling food.
> - If your hands become contaminated with body fluids.
> - Before you leave the client's home.
> - Before and after using gloves.
>
> For a 30-second handwash, sing the song "Happy Birthday" twice.
> Keep nails short, and remove jewelry from fingers.
> Rings and long fingernails may harbor pathogenic organisms.

Hepatitis B and C both attack the liver and can lead to chronic liver disease and death. At the present time, there are no cures for these diseases.

HIV is a more fragile virus than HBV. *Fragile* means that HIV is easily destroyed when it is outside the body in blood or other body fluids. HBV, however, is very strong. It resists normal hygiene practices used to destroy organisms. In fact, this virus can live for more than 1 week in dried saliva or blood on clothing or surfaces. HCV was identified in 1989. It is the most common chronic bloodborne infection in the United States; about 4.1 million people in the United States are infected.

Every year, hundreds of thousands of people in the United States become infected with HBV and HCV. Many become carriers of these bloodborne diseases. The number of HIV-infected people has increased rapidly. About one million Americans have HIV, which damages the immune system and leads to AIDS.

Federal Regulations

Because of the rapid increase in the numbers of persons with HIV, HBV, and HCV, the federal government has issued regulations to safeguard health care workers who come in contact with body fluids. Doctors, nurses, dentists, emergency medical workers, and home care workers are examples of health care personnel who may be at risk.

The U.S. Government's Centers for Disease Control and Prevention (CDC) and Occupational Safety and Health Administration (OSHA) require health care workers to protect themselves against exposure to bloodborne diseases.

Sometimes a health care worker accidentally comes in direct contact with the client's blood or other potentially infectious material. This is called an exposure incident. Bloodborne pathogens can enter the health care worker's body through several routes: the eye, mouth, other mucous membranes, tiny breaks in the skin, especially the hands or around the fingernails, or parenteral contact. OSHA REQUIRES THAT THE EXPOSURE INCIDENT BE REPORTED IMMEDIATELY TO THE EMPLOYER. THIS ALLOWS TREATMENT TO BEGIN WITHOUT DELAY. IT ALSO HELPS TO PREVENT THE SPREAD OF DISEASE TO OTHERS. During your training program, you will learn how to protect yourself from the possibility of being exposed to harmful organisms.

PROCEDURE 11-2 Applying Gloves and Removing Contaminated Gloves

APPLYING GLOVES

Materials Needed
- Pair of gloves (available from agency)

Procedure
1. Wash your hands.
2. Dry hands thoroughly.
3. Inspect gloves for tears or perforations.
4. Put gloves on when ready to begin client care.

REMOVING CONTAMINATED GLOVES
Procedure
With both hands still gloved,
1. Use right hand to grasp the glove on the left hand. Grasp the outer surface of the glove only, just below the wrist cuff (Figure 11-12).
2. Pull the left glove downward until it is off and turned inside out (Figure 11-13).
3. Continue holding the left glove in your right hand. Gather up the glove in your right hand (Figure 11-14).

4. Insert two fingers of your left hand inside the cuff of the right glove. Do not touch the outside of the glove with your bare hand (Figure 11-15).
5. Pull the right glove down and inside out and completely over the left glove (Figure 11-16).
6. Deposit both gloves into the proper container.
7. Wash your hands.

Fig 11-14 Gather up the left glove in your right hand (Step 3).

Fig 11-12 Use right hand to grasp outer surface of left-hand glove just below the wrist cuff (Step 1).

Fig 11-15 Insert two fingers of your left hand inside the cuff of the right glove (Step 4).

Fig 11-13 Pull left glove downward until it is off and turned inside out (Step 2).

Fig 11-16 Pull right glove down and over the left glove (Step 5).

Health Care Employer's Responsibilities

The federal OSHA regulations require that health care employers

- Provide hepatitis B immunizations for at-risk employees at no cost to the employee.
- Establish, in writing, tasks and procedures to be used when employees are working with clients.
- Establish procedures to eliminate or reduce employee exposure to bloodborne diseases.
- Provide employee training about biohazard exposure, precautions, and procedures when working with clients.
- Establish procedures for employees who have had an exposure incident to possible bloodborne pathogens.
- Require employees to use personal protective equipment (PPE) that the agency provides.

Home Care Aide's Responsibilities

The federal OSHA regulations also affect you, the home care aide. They are designed to help to eliminate or reduce your exposure to HIV, HBV, and HCV. Rules and regulations are effective only if they are carried out properly. Therefore, for your own protection, it is essential that you

1. Treat all blood, body fluids, and waste as if they are infectious (Box 11-5).
2. Use correct techniques for handwashing, handling body secretions, and disposing of wastes.
3. Use appropriate PPE (Box 11-6).
4. Obtain a hepatitis B vaccination, provided by your employer.
5. Attend training sessions provided by your employer.
6. Report, immediately, to your employer any exposure incident.
7. Notify your agency when you are ill and unable to work so that you do not transmit your illness to your client and client's family.
    Box 11-7 gives additional information about ways to protect yourself.

STERILIZATION AND DISINFECTION

Sterilization is the process used to destroy all living microorganisms, both nonpathogenic and pathogenic. *Disinfection* is the process that retards or inhibits the growth of pathogens. Sterilization and disinfection are methods used to prevent the spread of microorganisms and to reduce the spread of disease. Although disinfection destroys most pathogens, it usually does not destroy all of them.

Equipment, materials, linens, towels, clothing—anything used by the client or health care worker can be sterilized or disinfected. In health care institutions, specially trained workers use complicated equipment to keep all departments supplied with sterile materials, but in the client's home, this equipment is not usually available. It is very difficult to destroy all pathogens without using special sterilization equipment. Fortunately, many items now can be purchased for home care use in sterile packages that are discarded after use.

DISINFECTION IN THE HOME

You will not usually be responsible for sterilizing equipment or other materials in the home, but you will be responsible for disinfecting equipment used by the client and performing housekeeping tasks to disinfect various areas in the home. See Chapter 9 for more information.

BOX 11-5   Basic Rules for Standard (Universal) Precautions

- Wear disposable gloves when there is a chance of being in contact with client's blood, semen, vaginal secretions, or other body fluids.
- Wear gloves when the skin of your hands is broken or irritated.
- Wash hands before applying gloves and immediately after removing gloves.
- Wash hands immediately after being contaminated with blood or other body fluids.
- Clean up blood or body fluid spills immediately with bleach and water solution (1:10); remember to prepare solution daily.
- Do not handle used "sharps" such as needles.
- Ask client to place used "sharps" in puncture-resistant container or Biohazard Needle Box container provided by your agency or community (Figure 11-17).
- Wear personal protective equipment as required by your agency.
- Avoid splashing when disposing of contents of bedpan, urinal, or commode; if splashing occurs, clean area immediately.
- Wear gloves when disposing of soiled sanitary napkins or tampons.
- Do not eat, drink, apply cosmetics, or handle contact lenses in areas where exposure to blood or other potentially infectious materials is possible.

Fig 11-17 Wastebasket with biohazard symbol.

BOX 11-6   Personal Protective Equipment (PPE) for Bloodborne Diseases

Disposable gloves: Use when there is risk of direct contact with body fluids or moist body surfaces or when the skin of your hands is broken or irritated.

Plastic aprons or moisture-resistant gowns: Use when there is risk of body fluids splashing onto clothing and/or skin.

Mask: Use when there is risk of spraying or splashing of body substances into the nose and mouth.

Protective eyewear: Use when there is risk of body substances spraying or splashing into the eyes.

WET AND DRY HEAT

The usual methods of disinfection are by wet or dry heat (boiling water and baking) and by chemicals. The method used depends on the type of item to be disinfected. For example, glassware is disinfected using wet heat, whereas dressings are disinfected using dry heat. Urinals are chemically disinfected. If in doubt about the correct method of disinfecting items in your client's home, contact your supervisor. Procedure 11-3, Disinfecting Using Wet Heat, and Procedure 11-4, Disinfecting Using Dry Heat, describe wet and dry disinfection.

BOX 11-7   Basic Rules to Protect Yourself in the Client's Home

- Remember that your fingers are the 10 best carriers of disease.
- Wear gloves if you have cuts on your hands, chapped hands, or other breaks in the skin.
- Wear gloves when cleaning up blood and body fluids.
- Wear gloves when touching mucous membranes.
- Wear gloves when using disinfecting solutions.
- Wash your hands before and after using gloves.
- Wash your hands before and after giving personal care to your client, even if gloves are worn.
- Treat all blood, body fluids, and waste as if they are infectious.
- Discard cracked or torn utility gloves.
- Wear protective clothing, as required (e.g., gloves, mask, goggles, face shield).
- Use proper techniques to avoid spattering of body fluids and waste.
- Dispose of body fluids and waste according to agency policy.
- Do not handle client's used needle and syringe; ask client to dispose of them in puncture-resistant container.
- Do not recap, bend, or break a needle after use.
- Wear utility gloves when removing trash.
- Wash hands even after removing utility gloves.
- Contact your supervisor when in doubt about proper procedures.

PROCEDURE 11-3   Disinfecting Using Wet Heat

Materials Needed
- Items to be disinfected, cleaned, and dried
- Clean pot, large enough to hold items and lid
- Clean lid for pot
- Cold water
- Clock or timer
- Stove, hot plate, or other source of heat
- Pot holder

Procedure
1. Wash your hands.
2. Place items in pot so that all surfaces will be in contact with water.
3. Cover items with water. Provide some space at top of pot for steam to escape.
4. Place lid on top of pot.
5. Place covered pot on stove or other source of heat. Be sure bottom of pot is in full contact with heat source.
6. Turn pot handle(s) to the side(s).
7. Turn on heat and bring water to a boil. Do not open lid any time during this process (Steps 7 to 10). Steam begins to escape from sides of pot.
8. Boil for 20 minutes.
9. Turn off heat.
10. Allow water and contents to cool.
11. Remove cover with potholder.
12. Remove disinfected item. Place on clean towel to air-dry. Store properly.
13. Wash, dry, and return disinfecting supplies to appropriate location.
14. Wash your hands.

CHEMICAL DISINFECTION

The most common, least expensive chemical solution used in the home is soap or detergent and hot water. Friction caused by scrubbing surfaces with a brush or the rotating action of the automatic dishwasher or clothes washer loosens microorganisms from the surfaces. Heat from the hot water solution helps to destroy pathogens.

Other solutions can be made by diluting chemicals with water. FOR EXAMPLE, OSHA STANDARDS REQUIRE A BLEACH SOLUTION MADE WITH WATER BE

PROCEDURE 11-4 Disinfecting Using Dry Heat

Materials Needed
- Items to be disinfected: Cloth-wrapped dressings or other items
- Flat pan of metal (pie tin) or ovenware
- Oven
- Timer or clock
- Pot holder

Procedure
1. Wash your hands.
2. Place cloth-wrapped dressings in flat pan.
3. Place flat pan in the oven.
4. Turn on oven to 350° F (180° C).
5. Bake for 1 hour. Do not open oven while items are baking.
6. Turn off oven, and allow items to cool.
7. Remove flat pan using pot holder.
8. Unwrap cloth carefully without touching dressings.
9. Return items to appropriate location.
10. Wash your hands.

PROCEDURE 11-5 Making Bleach Solution

Materials Needed
- Household bleach
- Water
- Plastic container with cap
- Label
- Pen or pencil (for writing label)
- Measuring cup
- Rubber utility gloves (for cleaning)

Procedure
1. Wash your hands.
2. Put on rubber utility gloves.
3. Measure 5 cups of water (1200 milliliters), and pour into container.
4. Measure ½ cup (120 milliliters) of household bleach, and pour into container.
5. Place cap on container, and shake to mix solution.
6. Prepare label, "Bleach Solution 1:10," add date and time, and put label on container (Figure 11-18).
7. Store in closed cabinet out of reach of children and away from foods. Return materials to appropriate location.
8. Remove and rinse gloves. Hang to dry.
9. Wash your hands.

Fig 11-18 Prepare label and put on container (Step 6).

USED TO TREAT BLOOD AND BODY FLUIDS BECAUSE IT DESTROYS BLOOD-BORNE PATHOGENS. THEREFORE, IT IS IMPORTANT THAT YOU KNOW THE CORRECT METHOD OF PREPARING THIS SOLUTION. MAKE ONLY ENOUGH SOLUTION TO BE USED DURING A 24-HOUR PERIOD; THE SOLUTION LOSES ITS STRENGTH AFTER THAT TIME. (SEE PROCEDURE 11-5, MAKING BLEACH SOLUTION).

Cleaning the client's bedpan, urinal, toilet, or commode with a vinegar-and-water solution will disinfect these items and prevent offensive odors (Procedure 11-6, Making Vinegar Solution).

PROCEDURE 11-6   Making Vinegar Solution

Materials Needed
- White vinegar
- Water
- Plastic container with cap
- Label
- Pen or pencil (for writing label)
- Measuring cup

Procedure
1. Wash your hands.
2. Measure 3 cups (720 milliliters) of water, and pour into container.

3. Measure 1 cup (240 milliliters) of white vinegar, and pour into container.
4. Place cap on container, and shake to mix solution.
5. Prepare label, "Vinegar Solution 1:3," add date and time, and put on container.
6. Store in closed cabinet out of reach of children and away from food. Return materials to appropriate location.
7. Wash your hands.

TABLE 11-2   Household Disinfecting Solutions

SOLUTION	USED FOR
Detergent and hot water	Towels, bed linens, clothing, dishes, drinking glasses/cups, eating utensils, pots, and pans
Bleach and water	Bathroom and kitchen surfaces, blood, body fluids, feces, vomitus stained clothing, and toilet
Vinegar and water	Urinal, bedpan, toilet, commode, surfaces in shower, tub, and kitchen
Commercial disinfectants	Toilet, bathtub, shower, sink, and other surfaces in bathroom; floors, sink, and other surfaces in kitchen

Commercially prepared disinfectants are also available. Before using these products, remember to **READ THE LABELS** for instructions on proper use and precautions.

Table 11-2 gives information about household disinfecting solutions and their uses. Procedure 11-7, Disinfecting with Household Solutions, gives steps to follow when disinfecting with household solutions.

OTHER PRECAUTIONS

There may be times when the client's illness requires other precautions to be taken, in addition to the procedures already discussed. When the client has a highly contagious disease, isolation is necessary to decrease the chance of spreading the disease to caregivers and others. Perhaps a member of the family has an illness that could be spread to the client whose immune system is not working well; protecting the client from the chance of infection is another reason for using isolation procedures.

The care plan will indicate what procedures are necessary to protect you and your client. Your supervisor will give special instructions concerning these procedures, including the use and disposal of PPE such as masks and gowns.

PROCEDURE 11-7 | Disinfecting With Household Solutions

Materials Needed
- Items to be disinfected
- Plastic pan
- Container with solution (bleach 1:10, vinegar 1:3, or commercial solution)
- Detergent and warm water
- Paper towels
- Utility gloves
- Timer

Procedure
1. Wash your hands.
2. Put on utility gloves.
3. Wash items with detergent.
4. Rinse items with warm water.
5. Pour solution into plastic pan.
6. Submerge washed items in solution for 10 minutes.
7. Remove items.
8. Rinse well with hot water.
9. Lay items on paper towel to dry, or hang on towel rack or shower rail to dry.
10. Clean area, and return materials to appropriate location.
11. Remove and rinse gloves. Hang to dry.
12. Wash your hands.

PERSONAL PROTECTIVE EQUIPMENT

The most common equipment used in the home are disposable gloves, masks, and moisture-resistant aprons or gowns.

Disposable gloves are used as protection against pathogens from the client entering the home care aide. Examples of activities that require the use of gloves include changing linens or clothing soiled with body fluids, giving personal care where there is risk of coming in contact with the client's blood, caring for the client's mouth, shaving a client, and performing certain housekeeping tasks. GLOVES ARE ALWAYS WORN WHEN THERE IS CONTACT OR RISK OF CONTACT WITH BODY FLUIDS. IF YOU HAVE CUTS, CHAPPED HANDS, OR OTHER SKIN PROBLEMS, NOTIFY YOUR EMPLOYER. GLOVES MUST BE WORN.

Before putting on gloves, remove all jewelry and keep your nails short. Rings and long fingernails can tear gloves. Discard disposable gloves immediately after use. Use a new pair of disposable gloves each time. If gloves are required to give your client care, the agency will provide them for your use.

Masks are used to cover the nose and mouth of the wearer. When the client's illness is spread by airborne pathogens, wearing a mask acts as a barrier to prevent organisms from entering the caregiver's respiratory system. Masks and protective eyewear are used when there is a chance of splashing or spraying body fluids into the mouth, nose, or eyes. A mask should be worn for no longer than 20 to 30 minutes. After that time, the mask usually becomes damp or wet due to breathing. It is no longer an effective barrier and is considered to be contaminated. See Procedure 11-8, Applying a Mask and Removing a Contaminated Mask.

Moisture-resistant gowns or aprons are used when there is a chance of soiling clothing with blood, other body fluids, or wastes while giving client care. Gowns used in the home are usually disposable and are discarded into the trash container in the client's room. See Procedure 11-9, Applying a Gown and Removing a Contaminated Gown, and Box 11-8 for the sequence for removing contaminated PPE.

If other PPE is required to care for your client, such as goggles or a face shield, your agency will provide this equipment. Any question you have about using this PPE should be answered by your supervisor, not the client or family.

PROCEDURE 11-8 | Applying a Mask and Removing a Contaminated Mask

APPLYING A MASK

Materials Needed
- Disposable mask (from agency)

Procedure
1. Wash your hands.
2. Pick up mask by top strings (or upper elastic band).
3. Position mask over nose and mouth (Figure 11-19) with top strings over ears. Tie strings behind head (or position elastic band over ears and high up on head). Tie lower strings (or position lower elastic band low on back of head, under ears).

REMOVING A CONTAMINATED MASK

Procedure
1. Wash your hands.
2. Untie lower strings of mask (or pull lower elastic band up to top of head).
3. Untie upper strings, and remove mask while still holding strings (or lift both elastic bands over head and remove mask) (Figure 11-20).
4. Discard mask in proper container.
5. Wash your hands.

Fig 11-19 When applying a mask, position it over the nose and mouth (Step 3).

Fig 11-20 Untie upper strings and remove mask while still holding strings (Step 3).

BOX 11-8 | Sequence for Removing Contaminated Personal Protective Equipment

1. Remove contaminated gloves and discard.
   Hands are the most contaminated.
2. Remove mask and discard.
3. Remove gown and discard.
4. Wash your hands.

PROCEDURE 11-9   Applying a Gown and Removing a Contaminated Gown

APPLYING A GOWN

Materials Needed
- Disposable, moisture-resistant gown (from agency)

Procedure
1. Wash your hands.
2. Insert arms into sleeves of gown with opening in the back.
3. Tie the neck strings (or close Velcro strips).
4. Close the back opening by overlapping one side of gown over the other.
5. Tie at waist (or close Velcro strips).
6. Give client care.

REMOVING A CONTAMINATED GOWN

Procedure
1. Untie waist strings.
2. Untie neck strings.
3. Pull gown down from the shoulder with neck ties (Figure 11-21).
4. Leaning forward, turn the gown inside out while removing it. Do not touch the outside of the gown. This surface is contaminated (Figure 11-22).
5. Keeping one hand inside the sleeve of the gown, use it to pull off the other sleeve. Do the same on the other side.
6. Roll the gown into a ball. Keep contaminated area inside (Figure 11-23).
7. Discard into proper container (Figure 11-24).
8. Wash your hands.

Fig 11-22 When removing gown, lean forward and turn it inside out (Step 4).

Fig 11-23 Roll gown into a ball, keeping contaminated area inside (Step 6).

Fig 11-21 Pull gown from shoulder with neck ties (Step 3).

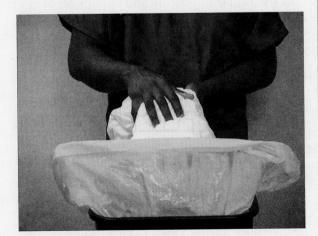

Fig 11-24 Discard gown (Step 7).

PROCEDURE 11-10   Double Bagging

MATERIALS NEEDED

- Two plastic bags—one "clean" and one "dirty"
- Isolation gown
- Gloves
- Helper (family member)

Procedure

1. Position helper with "clean" bag outside door of client's room. If you are alone, place clean, open bag in doorway, and go ahead with procedure.
2. Wash your hands.
3. Apply gown and gloves.
4. Enter room. Take "dirty" bag in.
5. Place contaminated materials in "dirty" bag. Seal.
6. Ask person with "clean" bag to open it so you can insert second bag. Have helper seal "clean" bag. If alone, place "dirty" bag in "clean" bag, but do not seal until hands are clean.
7. Remove gloves and gown. Discard in proper container.
8. Wash your hands.
9. Seal "clean" bag, if alone. Dispose of double-bagged material appropriately.

REMOVING CONTAMINATED MATERIAL

Contaminated material is removed from the client's room through a process known as *double bagging*. Trash or linens are placed in a plastic bag inside the room. This is known as the "dirty" bag. Another person, outside the client's room, holds open another plastic bag (the "clean" bag) ready to receive the contaminated material. See Procedure 11-10, Double Bagging.

CHAPTER SUMMARY

- The home care aide has an important role to play in preventing infection.
- Pathogenic microorganisms produce disease as they travel through the cycle of infection.
- Medical asepsis and standard (universal) precautions are used in the home to prevent the spread of disease.
- Proper handwashing technique is one of the most effective ways to prevent infection.
- Standard (universal) precautions MUST be used whenever there is risk of contact with blood or body fluids.
- It is always important to follow CDC, OSHA, and your agency's regulations concerning bloodborne pathogens.

STUDY QUESTIONS

1. List four requirements for microorganisms to live and grow.
2. Describe the cycle of infection, and give two methods for blocking each part.
3. Define the following terms:
   a. Medical asepsis
   b. Surgical asepsis
   c. Standard (universal) precautions
   d. Bloodborne pathogens
4. List five rules to follow when using standard (universal) precautions.
5. Describe how to prepare a bleach solution for use in the home.

12

Body Mechanics

OBJECTIVES

After you read this chapter, you will be able to:

1. Demonstrate good body mechanics when standing, sitting, lifting, and moving objects.
2. List three effects of immobility.
3. Describe the procedures for moving, positioning, and transferring clients.
4. Define the term *assistive devices,* and give three examples.
5. List six rules to follow when assisting the client to walk.
6. Discuss 10 safety factors to consider when assisting clients to use walkers, canes, wheelchairs, and mechanical lifts.
7. Explain what you would do if the client begins to fall.
8. Practice infection control when positioning, moving, and lifting clients.

KEY TERMS

Ambulate To move the body with or without assistance; to walk

Bed cradle A device used to keep the top bedding from resting on the client's legs and feet

Body mechanics Proper use of muscles to move and lift objects and to maintain correct posture

Bony prominence Part of the bone that is near the skin's surface

Contracture Shortening of a muscle whereby a joint becomes permanently immovable

Fatigue Loss of strength and endurance

Footboard A positioning device used to keep the client's feet in an upright position

Footdrop Inability to keep the foot in a normal walking position

Lifting or turning sheet Folded sheet placed under the client from shoulders to thighs

Muscle atrophy Wasting of muscle

Muscle tone Readiness of the muscle to work

Pneumonia Inflammation of the lung

Pressure ulcer Sore on the skin caused by prolonged pressure on the part; also called *bedsore* or *decubitus ulcer*

Shearing Pressure against the surface of the skin and skin layers as the client is being moved; one surface rubs against another surface

Transfer Moving the client from one place to another

Today is home care aide Rosina Chavez's first visit to her client, Jorge, a 250-pound young adult who is partially paralyzed. The care plan requires that she give him a bed bath, get him out of bed using a mechanical lift, and prepare and assist him to eat a noontime meal. When she introduces herself to him, his first remarks are, "You're too thin. You'll never be able to take care of me. You'll hurt yourself just trying to move me in bed." Rosina explains that she's been taught how to perform the tasks necessary to care for him. "It's not my size that counts but how I use my muscles that makes the difference." Jorge smiles and says, "Perhaps you're right. Let's see what happens." Jorge was pleased and surprised that Rosina performed her tasks efficiently and safely.

The proper use of muscles to move and lift objects and maintain correct posture is called body mechanics. It is a way of using your body so that the work is performed by several groups of muscles with the strongest ones being used.

USING GOOD BODY MECHANICS

The way you use your body to walk, sit, stand, lift, push, pull, or move objects is very important, not only at work but everywhere and every day. The body is like a finely tuned machine. When used properly, it performs very well. When misused, it performs poorly and eventually breaks down.

BENEFITS TO THE HOME CARE AIDE

Practicing good body mechanics offers the following benefits.
• Correct muscle groups are used for the task being performed.
• Muscle fatigue, strain, and body injury are reduced.
• Personal safety is maintained.
• Tasks are performed efficiently.

BENEFITS TO THE CLIENT

When the home care aide uses correct body mechanics, the client benefits in the following ways:
• Anxiety and fears about moving are reduced.
• Position changes are made smoothly and without injury to the client.
• Concerns about falling are reduced.
• Confidence in the home care aide's ability to perform tasks correctly is increased.

STEPS TO GOOD BODY MECHANICS

USING CORRECT POSTURE

The first step toward good body mechanics is correct posture. It helps to promote proper balance, conserve energy, prevent muscle strain, and maintain the natural curves of the spine (Figure 12-1). Tips for good posture include the following:

When Standing (Figure 12-2)
• Head erect
• Shoulders back and at ease

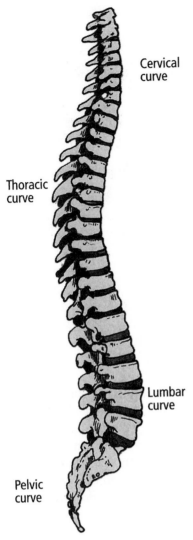

Fig 12-1 Natural curves of the spine.

Fig 12-2 Correct posture when standing.

Fig 12-3 Correct posture when sitting.

- Chest up and forward
- Arms at sides
- Abdomen flat
- Buttocks tucked in
- Feet parallel to each other; one foot slightly forward
- When standing for a long time, put one foot on a stool and change position every 20 minutes

When Sitting (Figure 12-3)
- Head erect
- Shoulders back and at ease
- Chest up and forward
- Hips bent at right angles
- Weight supported by thighs
- Sit back in chair
- Rest both feet on floor

> ### BOX 12-1   The Muscular System: A Review
>
> - Muscles are attached to bones by tendons.
> - Joints permit movement according to the type of joint: ball and socket, hinge, or pivot.
> - The muscular system maintains the body's correct posture.
> - Back and abdominal muscles help to provide correct posture.
> - The large, strong muscles of the arms, legs, abdomen, and buttocks are used for lifting and moving objects.
> - Back muscles are weak ones.
> - Muscles are strengthened by use; proper exercise helps keep muscles in good working condition.

MAINTAINING GOOD MUSCLE TONE

Muscles work best when they are in good condition or tone. See Box 12-1 for a review of the muscular system. Muscle tone means the readiness of the muscle to work. Poor muscle tone occurs when muscles are not used frequently. They become weak, tire easily, and cause fatigue. Good muscle tone means that the muscle is strong and ready to work. Muscles that are in good condition do not tire easily. Therefore, fatigue is reduced.

Muscle tone can be improved by a program of regular exercise. Before starting such a program, always consult your physician. The program should begin gradually and be performed under the direction of a qualified person. Stretching large muscle groups, such as the arms and legs, is important before starting each exercise session because it prepares the muscles to work and helps prevent strains. One of the best exercises is walking briskly for 20 minutes at least three or four times a week. Exercising regularly should increase muscle tone and strength, reduce stress and fatigue, and strengthen the heart muscle, too.

MAINTAINING BALANCE

When standing, lifting, or moving, it is important to keep your body in proper balance. Remember: When standing, keep your feet apart with one foot slightly forward. This will provide a wider base of support and better balance (Figure 12-4).

PROTECTING YOUR BACK

Back injuries usually occur because of a combination of many factors. Examples include: incorrect use of body mechanics; poor posture; maintaining one body position for too long; and lack of rest and relaxation to reduce the stresses of life. Developing poor habits at work and at home can contribute to back problems.

Being overweight places additional strain on the lower back. It is estimated that being overweight by 20 pounds equals 200 pounds of extra stress on the lower back. Therefore, it is important for the home care aide to maintain a healthy weight to avoid extra strain on the lower back.

Home care aides, who have previously injured their backs or require additional support for the back, may benefit from using a back belt when lifting or moving objects or clients (Figure 12-5). It is important to have the belt specially fitted by a skilled professional. Consult your physician for further information.

MOST PEOPLE HAVE A MAXIMUM AMOUNT OF WEIGHT THAT THEY CAN LIFT SAFELY. KNOW YOUR BODY. KNOW YOUR LIMITS. IF UNSURE ABOUT WHETHER YOU WILL BE ABLE TO LIFT THE WEIGHT, STOP AND GET HELP.

Fig 12-4 Good balance means keeping the feet apart with one foot slightly forward.

Fig 12-5 A back belt. (Courtesy JT Posey Company, Arcadia, CA.)

DO NOT ATTEMPT TO BEGIN TO LIFT THE WEIGHT; YOU MAY INJURE YOURSELF OR YOUR CLIENT.

Some clients may be able to assist when you are moving them in bed or when you are getting them out of bed. It is important to explain the steps they can take to help you and to avoid strain on themselves or on you.

The following tips will help protect your back and practice good body mechanics. Make it a habit of following these guidelines each day whether at work or at home.

Basic Rules for Protecting Your Back and Practicing Good Body Mechanics
1. Wear appropriate clothing
   * Nonskid, comfortable shoes: low-heeled or wedge.
   * Back belt, if needed.
2. Plan the move, and prepare the client
   * Go through the entire move mentally, before starting.
   * Know where you are taking the client (e.g., chair, commode).
   * Tell the client what you are planning to do.
   * Instruct the client about how he or she can assist you; make sure the client understands—get feedback before proceeding.
   * Use assistive devices, if available.
   * Get help, if necessary; instruct your helper about the correct technique to use; remember, you are the leader; count 1-2-3 and MOVE TOGETHER.
3. Move objects safely
   * Get help when lifting heavy objects.
   * Push, slide, or roll objects, when appropriate.
   * Get as close to the object as possible.
   * Keep your feet apart for a wider base of support.
   * Get on the same level of the load; squat, or get on one knee.
   * Stagger your feet, and point them in the direction of the move.
   * Keep your back straight.
   NEVER BEND OVER FROM THE WAIST.
   * Grasp the object firmly, and breathe in.
   * Tighten abdominal muscles and lift slowly, by straightening the legs.
   * Exhale as you perform the move.
   * Avoid sudden jerking movements; lift smoothly.
   * Turn your body as a unit, using your legs and feet.

DO NOT TWIST YOUR UPPER BODY.

- Adjust work heights to avoid reaching, twisting, or bending.
- Never lift a load that is overhead; use a footstool to get as close to the load as possible; test weight of the load before lifting.
- Set the object down slowly, bending your knees and keeping your back straight.

THE CLIENT IN BED

EFFECTS OF IMMOBILITY

Clients who spend long periods of time in bed may experience the effects of immobility.

- Muscle atrophy and/or contractures
- Pressure ulcers
- Slowed circulation that may lead to blood clots
- Constipation
- Reduced lung expansion, which could lead to pneumonia
- Emotional effects of illness, as discussed in Chapter 7
- Generalized discomfort

Properly positioning and moving clients in bed help reduce the effects of immobility by

- Encouraging effective moving and overall body function
- Reducing excessive pressure on certain areas
- Improving circulation and lung expansion
- Promoting comfort and rest

CHANGING POSITIONS IN BED

Many clients are able to move about in bed and should be encouraged to do so. However, if moving is difficult or impossible, the home care aide is expected to provide the necessary assistance. Explain what you are going to do and, if appropriate, how the client can help. For example, if the bed has side rails, you might ask the client to use them to help you make the move.

For those who are unable to help with the move, a useful device for moving and turning clients is the lifting or turning sheet. A regular drawsheet or a flat sheet that has been folded into fourths may be used. The turning sheet should be placed under the client and extend from the shoulders to the thighs. When you are ready to move the client, roll the edges of the turning sheet so you can hold it firmly as you move the client into a new position. The turning sheet provides ease in movement for both the client and the aide.

THE CARE PLAN FOR A CLIENT WHO IS UNABLE TO MOVE WILL INCLUDE A SCHEDULE FOR TURNING THE CLIENT EVERY 1 TO 2 HOURS. A CLIENT'S POSITION MUST BE CHANGED AT LEAST EVERY 2 HOURS TO PREVENT COMPLICATIONS THAT ARISE FROM IMMOBILITY. Each time you turn your client, observe the skin for any changes. Immediately report redness, paleness, or white discoloration of the skin, particularly over bony prominences, as these signs may indicate a beginning pressure ulcer.

RAISING THE CLIENT'S HEAD AND SHOULDERS

Sometimes it is necessary to raise the client's head and shoulders to readjust pillows, bed linens, or clothing. Instruct the client to assist you (if appropriate), and follow Procedure 12-1, Raising Client's Head and Shoulders.

PROCEDURE 12-1 | Raising Client's Head and Shoulders

1. Explain what you are going to do.
2. Wash your hands.
3. Provide privacy (close door, shut drapes, pull shades).
4. Raise bed to convenient working height.*
5. Lock wheels on bed, or push bed against wall if there are no brakes.
6. Lower rail on side of bed where you are working.*
7. Lower head of bed, and remove pillows. Fold back top sheet.
8. Stand facing bed, with feet about 12 inches apart.
9. Ask client to place near arm under your near arm and shoulder. Client's hand should reach to your shoulder (Figure 12-6, A).
10. Place your near arm under client's arm and shoulder. Your hand should reach to client's shoulder.
11. Slip your farthest arm under client's neck and shoulders (Figure 12-6, B).
12. On a count of "3," shift your weight from foot nearest to head of the bed to your other foot. At the same time, rock client to a semisitting position (Figure 12-6, C).
13. Support client with arm locked under shoulder; use other arm to remove or readjust pillows.
14. Assist client to lie back on bed using locked arms and supporting neck and shoulders as before.
15. Make sure client is safe and comfortable. Replace top sheet.
16. Place bed in lowest position. (Raise side rail, if indicated.)*
17. Wash your hands.

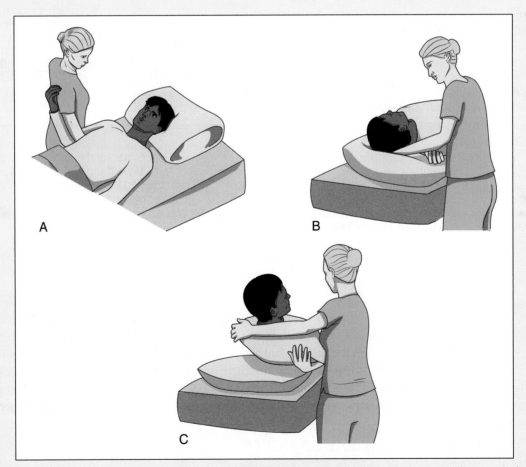

A

B

C

Fig 12-6 **A,** Ask the client to place his or her arm under your arm and shoulder (Step 9). **B,** Slip your farthest arm under the client's neck and shoulders (Step 11). **C,** Rock the client to a semisitting position (Step 12).

*Your client may not have an adjustable hospital bed; those steps marked with an asterisk (*) will not apply.

PROCEDURE 12-2   Moving Client to the Side of the Bed

1. Explain what you are going to do.
2. Wash your hands.
3. Provide privacy (close door, shut drapes, pull shades).
4. Raise bed to convenient working height.*
5. Lock wheels on bed, or push bed against wall if there are no brakes.
6. Lower rail on side where you are working.*
7. Fold back top sheet.
8. Stand facing bed, with feet about 12 inches apart, one foot in front of the other. As you perform each move, shift your weight from your front foot to your rear foot.
9. Slip one arm under client reaching across to the opposite shoulder. Place other arm under middle of client's back.
10. On a count of "3," rock back and shift upper segment of client's body to edge of bed (Figure 12-7, A).
11. Place arms under client's waist and buttocks. Move client's waist and buttocks to edge of bed in same manner (Figure 12-7, B).
12. Place arms under client's thighs and lower legs. Move client's thighs and lower legs to edge of bed in same manner (Figure 12-7, C).
13. Make sure client is in good body alignment. Replace top sheet.
14. Place bed in lowest position. (Raise side rail, if indicated.)*
15. Wash your hands.

A

B

C

Fig 12-7 **A,** Shift upper part of the client's body to edge of the bed (Step 10). **B,** Move the client's waist and buttocks to edge of the bed (Step 11). **C,** Move the client's thighs and lower legs to edge of the bed (Step 12).

*Your client may not have an adjustable hospital bed; those steps marked with an asterisk (*) will not apply.

MOVING THE CLIENT TO THE SIDE OF THE BED

For you to perform certain procedures safely and properly, clients are positioned near the side of the bed. This is often one of the first few steps in a procedure, such as making an occupied bed, giving a bed bath, and placing clients in side-lying positions. (See Procedure 12-2, Moving Client to the Side of the Bed.) Some clients may not be moved in segments, as described in Procedure 12-2, because of back injuries or other problems. Check with your supervisor for the proper procedure to use with these clients.

MOVING THE CLIENT UP IN BED

There are many reasons that a client will need to be moved up in bed. One of the most important is to help your client maintain proper body alignment. A client who is correctly positioned in bed will be more at ease and comfortable. In addition, moving a client up in the bed is the first step in many positioning and personal care procedures. Refer to Figures 12-8 and 12-9 and Procedure 12-3, Moving Client Up in Bed When Client Can Help, and Procedure 12-4, Moving Client Up in Bed When Client Cannot Help, for the correct methods of moving a client up in bed.

PROCEDURE 12-3 Moving Client Up in Bed When Client Can Help

1. Explain what you are going to do.
2. Wash your hands.
3. Provide privacy (close door, shut drapes, pull shades).
4. Raise bed to convenient working height.*
5. Lock wheels on bed, or push bed against wall if there are no brakes.
6. Lower rail on side where you are working.*
7. Fold back top sheet. Lower client's head; remove pillows.
8. Prop one pillow against headboard. This will protect the client from hitting his or her head when moving up.
9. Stand facing head of bed, with knees bent, and feet 12 inches apart.
10. Slip one arm under client's shoulders and other arm under client's thighs (Figure 12-8, *A*).
11. Instruct client to bend his or her knees, and firmly place feet against mattress. On a signal from you, client will push with feet and hands to assist with move up in bed (Figure 12-8, *B*).
12. Help client move toward head of bed by shifting your body weight from your rear leg to your front leg.
13. Several small upward moves may be used rather than one large move to reach head of bed.
14. Make sure client is in good body alignment. Replace top sheet and pillows.
15. Place bed in lowest position. (Raise side rail, if indicated.)*
16. Wash your hands.

A

B

Fig 12-8 **A,** Slip one arm under the client's shoulders and the other arm under the client's thighs (Step 10). **B,** Client pushes with feet and hands (Step 11).

*Your client may not have an adjustable hospital bed; those steps marked with an asterisk (*) will not apply.

POSITIONING THE CLIENT IN BED

POSITIONS FREQUENTLY USED

Proper positioning will provide comfort and relieve pressure on joints and bony prominences. Several positions are usually used.

Supine position is also known as the *dorsal recumbent position* (Figure 12-10). The client lies on his or her back, with the bed flat. A small pillow is placed under the head and shoulders. Arms and hands are on the side, with the palms facing down. As an option, arms and hands may be elevated on pillows, and a small pillow or folded towel may be placed under the small of the back as needed. Sometimes, small pillows may be placed under the lower leg to raise the heels off the bed. Positioning devices, such as splints, hand rolls, or a footboard, may be used. Supine position is used for sleeping and resting (Procedure 12-5, Positioning Client in Supine [Back-Lying] Position).

Fowler's position is a sitting position. The head of the bed is elevated to a semisitting position, with the client's hips at the bend in the bed. A pillow is placed behind the

PROCEDURE 12-4   Moving Client Up in Bed When Client Cannot Help

1. Explain what you are going to do.
2. Wash your hands.
3. Provide privacy (close door, shut drapes, pull shades).
4. Raise bed to convenient working height.*
5. Lock wheels on bed, or push bed against wall if there are no brakes.
6. Lower rail on side where you are working.*
7. Fold back top sheet. Lower client's head; remove pillows.
8. Prop one pillow against headboard. This will protect the client from hitting his or her head when moving up.
9. Be sure turning sheet is in position under client's body.
10. One person
    a. Keep side rails up.*
    b. Stand at head of bed, with feet about 12 inches apart, one foot in front of the other, facing foot of bed.
    c. Roll top of turning sheet toward client's head.
    d. Firmly grasp top of turning sheet in both hands.
    e. Use good body mechanics—bend knees and hips, keep back straight.
    f. On a count of "3," shift your weight from front leg to rear leg, and pull the turning sheet and client up toward head of bed (Figure 12-9, A).

g. Several small moves may be necessary and are easier to do than one large upward move.
11. Two persons
    a. Lower both side rails.*
    b. Each person stands at side of bed with feet 12 inches apart, one foot in front of the other, facing head of bed.
    c. Roll sides of turning sheet close to client's body.
    d. Firmly grasp edges of turning sheet with both hands.
    e. Use good body mechanics—bend knees and hips, keep back straight.
    f. On a count of "3," both persons shift their weight from rear leg to front leg, lifting turning sheet and moving client toward head of bed (Figure 12-9, B).
    g. Several small moves may be necessary and are easier to do than one large upward move.
12. Check lower sheets for wrinkles; smooth, if necessary.
13. Make sure client is in good body alignment. Replace top sheet and pillows.
14. Place bed in lowest position. (Raise side rail, if indicated.)*
15. Wash your hands.

A

B

Fig 12-9 **A,** Shift your weight from the front to rear leg, and pull the turning sheet and client toward head of the bed (Step 10f). **B,** Both persons shift weight while lifting the turning sheet and moving the client (Step 11f).

*Your client may not have an adjustable hospital bed; those steps marked with an asterisk (*) will not apply.

head and neck. Support the client's arms with pillows (Figure 12-11). Positioning devices may be used as described earlier. Fowler's position is used when clients are eating, taking medications, reading, and watching television. This position also provides comfort and easier breathing for clients who have cardiac and respiratory conditions. If a hospital bed is not available, you will need to improvise a backrest for this

PROCEDURE 12-5   Positioning Client in the Supine (Back-Lying) Position

1. Explain what you are going to do.
2. Wash your hands.
3. Provide privacy (close door, shut drapes, pull shades).
4. Raise bed to convenient working height.*
5. Lock wheels on bed, or push bed against wall if there are no brakes.
6. Lower rail on side where you are working.*
7. Fold back top sheet. Position client on back.
8. Adjust pillows properly.
   a. Small pillow under head and shoulders
   b. Support arms and hands with pillows
   c. Small pillow or folded towel under small of back, if your supervisor tells you to do so
9. Position other devices, such as footboard, trochanter rolls, bed cradle, as indicated in care plan.
10. Make sure client is in proper body alignment. Replace top sheet.
11. Place bed in lowest position. (Raise side rail, if indicated.)*
12. Wash your hands.
13. Record what you have done. Watch for and report any unusual symptoms to your supervisor.

Fig 12-10 Supine position.

*Your client may not have an adjustable hospital bed; those steps marked with an asterisk (*) will not apply.

PROCEDURE 12-6   Positioning Client in the Fowler's (Semisitting) Position

1. Explain what you are going to do.
2. Wash your hands.
3. Provide privacy (close door, shut drapes, pull shades).
4. Raise bed to convenient working height.*
5. Lock wheels on bed, or push bed against wall if there are no brakes.
6. Lower rail on side where you are working.*
7. Fold back top sheet. Position client on back.
8. Raise head of bed to 45-degree angle. If bed is not adjustable, use other devices to position client (see Figure 12-12).
9. Adjust pillows properly.
   a. Small pillow under head and shoulders
   b. Support arms and hands with pillows
10. Position other devices such as footboard, trochanter rolls, bed cradle, as indicated in the care plan.
11. Make sure client is in good body alignment. Replace top sheet.
12. Place bed in lowest position. (Raise side rail, if indicated.)*
13. Wash your hands.
14. Record what you have done. Watch for and report any unusual symptoms to your supervisor.

Fig 12-11 Fowler's position.

*Your client may not have an adjustable hospital bed; those steps marked with an asterisk (*) will not apply.

position. Sofa pillows, a pillow armrest, or a wedge pillow can be used (Figure 12-12). (See Procedure 12-6, Positioning Client in the Fowler's Position.)

Lateral position is a side-lying position. The lower leg bears the weight, while the upper leg is positioned so that it does not rest on the one underneath. Pillows are placed under the client's head, between the legs, under the uppermost arm, and along the back (Figure 12-13). The lower arm must be positioned properly to allow for movement and circulation. Watch the lower arm for signs of impaired circulation, such as cool,

Fig 12-12 Types of backrests. **A,** Wedge pillow. **B,** Pillow armrest. **C,** Sofa pillows.

PROCEDURE 12-7   Positioning Client in the Lateral (Side-Lying) Position

1. Explain what you are going to do.
2. Wash your hands.
3. Provide privacy (close door, shut drapes, pull shades).
4. Raise bed to convenient working height.*
5. Lock wheels on bed, or push bed against wall if there are no brakes.
6. Lower rail on side where your are working.*
7. Lower client's head; remove pillows. Fold back top sheet.
8. Ask client to move to side of bed nearest you. Assist client as needed, (see Procedure 12-2).
9. Raise side rail.*
10. Go to other side of bed. Lower side rail.*
11. Place one hand around client's farthest shoulder and your other hand around farthest hip. Roll client toward you, turning on side facing toward center of bed. Bend upper leg. Both arms are slightly bent.
12. Adjust pillows properly.
    a. Small pillow under head and neck
    b. Support upper arm and leg on pillows

    c. A folded towel or pillow may be placed along the back to maintain the side-lying position; this is optional
13. Position other devices as indicated in the care plan.
14. Make sure client is in good body alignment. Replace top sheet.
15. Place bed in lowest position. (Raise side rail, if indicated.)*
16. Wash your hands.
17. Record what you have done. Watch for and report any unusual symptoms to your supervisor.

Fig 12-13 Lateral (side-lying) position.

*Your client may not have an adjustable hospital bed; those steps marked with an asterisk (*) will not apply.

discolored skin, and blue fingernails. If the client complains of numbness, tingling, and pain in the lower arm and hand, change the position immediately. Record observations. If the symptoms are not relieved within 3 to 5 minutes, call your supervisor. (See Procedure 12-7, Positioning Client in the Lateral Position.)

Sims' position is also a side-lying position, but the client lies partially on the abdomen (Figure 12-14). This position is used for taking rectal temperatures, administering enemas, and other types of treatments. However, some clients are comfortable in this position, and it can be used to relieve pressure on the bony prominences of the back.

PROCEDURE 12-8   Positioning Client in the Sims' Position

1. Explain what you are going to do.
2. Wash your hands.
3. Provide privacy (close door, shut drapes, pull shades).
4. Raise bed to convenient working height.*
5. Lock wheels on bed, or push bed against wall if there are no brakes.
6. Lower rail on side where you are working.*
7. Lower client's head; remove pillows. Fold back top sheet.
8. Ask client to move to side of bed nearest you. Assist client as needed (see Procedure 12-2).
9. Raise side rail.*
10. Go to other side of bed. Lower side rail.*
11. Place one hand around client's farthest shoulder and your other hand around farthest hip. Roll client toward you, turning on side facing toward center of bed. Position upper leg so it does not rest on lower leg. Lower arm is behind client.

12. Adjust pillows properly.
    a. Small pillow under head and neck
    b. Support upper arm and leg on pillows
13. Position other devices as indicated in the care plan.
14. Make sure client is in good body alignment. Replace top sheet.
15. Place bed in lowest position. (Raise side rail, if indicated.)*
16. Wash your hands.
17. Record what you have done. Watch for and report any unusual symptoms to your supervisor.

Fig 12-14 Sims' position.

*Your client may not have an adjustable hospital bed; those steps marked with an asterisk (*) will not apply.

The upper leg is bent and rests on a pillow. The lower arm is behind the client. Pillows are positioned under the head and upper arm. The client's head is turned toward the upper arm. Observe for proper circulation in the lower arm and hand. (See Procedure 12-8, Positioning Client in the Sims' Position.)

Prone position places the client on his or her abdomen with the head turned to the side (Figure 12-15). The feet may be elevated on a pillow or can hang over the end of the mattress to prevent pressure on the toes and ankle discomfort (Figure 12-16). The arms are bent, and a pillow is placed under the head. A small pillow or folded towel can be placed under the waist, if needed for comfort. The prone position is not for everyone, in fact, some people find it very uncomfortable and complain about feeling "stuck" and unable to move in this position. Make sure the client is able to breathe and that the pillows do not interfere with respiration, speech, and vision. This position is not usually used unless specified in the care plan. (See Procedure 12-9, Positioning Client in the Prone [Abdominal] Position.)

See Table 12-1 for information about what to observe, record, and report when positioning clients.

POSITIONING DEVICES

Devices are used to maintain proper positioning and good body alignment.
* Pillows: Placed under the limbs and joints to prevent pressure, keep skin surfaces separate, promote comfort, increase circulation, provide support, and maintain correct alignment.
* Trochanter roll: Rolled towel, pillow, or blanket placed next to the hip to keep the leg from turning outward (Figure 12-17, *A*).
* Footboard: Padded board attached to the mattress at the foot of the bed; this device keeps the client's feet in an upright position and helps to prevent footdrop (Figure 12-17, *B*).

PROCEDURE 12-9   Positioning Client in the Prone (Abdominal) Position

1. Explain what you are going to do.
2. Wash your hands.
3. Provide privacy (close door, shut drapes, pull shades).
4. Raise bed to convenient working height.*
5. Lock wheels on bed, or push bed against wall if there are no brakes.
6. Lower rail on side where you are working.*
7. Lower client's head; remove pillows. Fold back top sheet.
8. Ask client to move to side of bed nearest you. Assist client as needed.
9. Raise side rail.*
10. Go to other side of bed. Lower side rail.*
11. Place one hand around client's farthest shoulder and other hand around client's farthest hip. Roll client toward you, turning on side and then onto the abdomen. Turn client's head to the side for comfort and ease in breathing. Arms are flexed on each side of head.
12. Adjust pillows properly.
    a. Small pillow under head and neck
    b. Optional small pillow under abdomen
    c. Pillow under lower legs to relieve pressure on toes; client may be positioned so that toes hang over mattress

13. Make sure client is in good body alignment. Replace top sheet.
14. Place bed in lowest position. (Raise side rail, if indicated.)*
15. Wash your hands.
16. Record what you have done. Watch for and report any unusual symptoms to your supervisor.

Fig 12-15 Prone position.

Fig 12-16 Prone position with client's feet hanging over mattress.

*Your client may not have an adjustable hospital bed; those steps marked with an asterisk (*) will not apply.

- High-top sneakers: May be used instead of a footboard to maintain proper positioning of the feet. Remove the sneakers according to the schedule listed in the care plan. Inspect the skin; wash and dry the client's feet. Put on clean socks, and replace the sneakers.
- Bed cradle: Device used to keep the top bedding from resting on the client's feet and legs (Figure 12-17, C). Cradles are available from medical supply companies, or you may improvise with a large carton (Figure 12-17, D).
- Hand rolls: Padded rolls or rolled washcloths that are placed in the client's hand to maintain a desired position as listed in the care plan (Figure 12-17, E). Remove during bathing. Wash and dry the hand before replacing the hand roll.
- Splints: Devices of cloth, plastic, and metal used to keep joints in a desired position as listed in the care plan (Figure 12-17, F). Remove during bathing, wash and dry skin, and replace splint according to the care plan.

Be sure that you understand the proper use of each device. If you have any questions, check with your supervisor.

RULES TO FOLLOW

Use the following principles of good body mechanics when positioning clients.
1. Encourage the client to do as much as possible within physical limits.
2. Do not pull on the client's arms or legs. Roll the client by placing your hands behind the client's hips and shoulders or under the shoulders or hips.

TABLE 12-1	Observe, Record, Report: Positioning in Bed		
POSITIONING IN BED	OBSERVE	RECORD	REPORT

Lateral/Sims'	Signs of poor circulation in lower arm and hand
	   Cool
	   Discolored skin
	   Blue fingernails
		Signs observed	

	Signs of skin changes over bony prominences
	   Redness
	   Paleness
	   White discoloration
		Area affected
		(e.g., heel, elbow)
		Color and size
		(e.g., "red," "size of dime")
			To supervisor, immediately

	Client's complaints • Numbness in arm, hand • Tingling in arm, hand • Pain in arm, hand	Client's complaints	
		What you did: Changed client's position immediately, and then every 1 to 2 hours	To supervisor if symptoms are not relieved in 3 to 5 minutes
Prone	Difficulty breathing; pillow interferes with speech or vision	Signs observed	
	Client's complaints; unable to move or feels "stuck"	Client's complaints	
		What you did: Changed client's position to relieve symptoms Changed client's position every 1 to 2 hours	To supervisor if symptoms or difficulty breathing continues after position is changed

3. As you move the client, shift your weight from one leg to the other. This assists in the moving process and allows you to use effective body mechanics.
4. Use a lifting or turning sheet, or get a helper when necessary.
5. Whenever possible, completely lower the head of the bed, to prevent uphill movement.
6. Move the client carefully to avoid any shearing motion that could damage the skin and cause a pressure ulcer.

CHECK THE CLIENT'S SKIN EACH TIME YOU CHANGE THE POSITION, AT LEAST EVERY 2 HOURS. OBSERVE SKIN OVER BONY PROMINENCES AND IN AREAS WHERE THERE MAY BE PRESSURE ON SOFT TISSUE, SUCH AS EARS, BREASTS, AND BUTTOCKS.

HELPING THE CLIENT TO BE MOBILE

There are several methods to help clients to become mobile. Moving the client from one area to another is called a transfer. There are three main ways to transfer clients depending on their ability to perform the task.
1. *Standing transfer:* Client is able to bear weight on one or both legs.
2. *Sitting transfer:* Client is unable to support weight on both legs. A sliding board is used.

Fig 12-17 Positioning devices. **A,** Trochanter roll. **B,** Footboard. **C,** Bed cradle. **D,** Carton bed cradle. **E,** Hand rolls. **F,** Splints.

BOX 12-2   Preparing for Transfers

- Transfer across the shortest distance.
- Try to keep transfer heights the same.
- Obtain all necessary equipment (wheelchair, chair, assistive devices) BEFORE beginning the transfer. Make sure equipment is in working order.
- Make sure there is enough space for a safe transfer; remove obstacles.
- Position chair as close to client as possible.
- Lock brakes on hospital bed and wheelchair, or make sure bed and chair are stable.
- Remove throw rugs or other hazards.
- Offer client bedpan/urinal.
- Assist client to put on SAFE FOOTWEAR—no socks, no floppy or slick-bottomed bedroom slippers.
- Check position of catheters or other tubing to be protected in the move.
- Know your client's strength and endurance.
- Obtain helper, if necessary.
- Place transfer belt on client, if needed.
- Put on your back belt, if needed.

---

3. *Lifting transfer:* Client is unable to move or cannot be moved by one or more persons. A mechanical lift is used.

The transfer procedure is one that you will perform frequently. Getting the client out of bed to sit in a chair or wheelchair or to use the bedside commode are two common activities. Box 12-2 gives suggestions for preparing to safely transfer clients while using proper body mechanics. Follow these guidelines when performing the transfer procedures listed below.

PREPARING THE CLIENT TO GET OUT OF BED

Most clients look forward to getting out of bed for the first time. For many, it is the first big step toward regaining independence. It is also a sign of improvement—of "getting better." Your supervisor will usually visit and evaluate the client's environment to ensure that it is safe to get him or her out of bed. The care plan will indicate how frequently the client is to get out of bed, the activity when out of bed (e.g., sitting in a chair, walking), and the duration (e.g., 10 minutes, a half hour). Getting out of bed for the first time can produce some anxiety for the client. "Will I fall?" "Can I reach the chair?" Your calm reassurance can help reduce some concerns. Explaining what you will do and how the client can assist you is a way to focus on the positive, not the negative.

ALWAYS USE THE SAME SEQUENCE OF STEPS IN THE PROCEDURE EACH TIME YOU ASSIST THE CLIENT. BE CONSISTENT; DO NOT CONFUSE THE CLIENT BY CHANGING THE PROCEDURE. BEGIN THE PROCEDURE ONLY WHEN THE CLIENT UNDERSTANDS WHAT YOU WILL DO AND HOW HE OR SHE CAN HELP. The first step is to have the client sit on the side of the bed with both feet on the floor. (See Procedure 12-10, Assisting Client to Sit on the Side of the Bed.)

PROCEDURE 12-10	Assisting Client to Sit on the Side of the Bed

Materials Needed
- Robe
- Sturdy footwear
- Chair, if needed

Fig 12-18 Swing the client's legs over edge of the bed (Step 16).

Procedure
1. Explain what you are going to do.
2. Wash your hands.
3. Obtain materials listed above.
4. Provide privacy (close door, shut drapes, pull shades).
5. Raise bed to convenient working height.*
6. Lock wheels on bed, or push bed against wall if there are no brakes.
7. Lower rail on side where you are working.*
8. Fold back top bedding.
9. Get as close to side of bed as possible, legs touching side of bed, so that you are level with client.
10. Position feet apart, with one foot staggered. Bend your hips and knees.
11. Ask client to move to side of bed nearest you. Assist client as needed (see Procedure 12-2).
12. Put up side rail and raise head of bed.*
13. Place client in Fowler's position without pillows (see Procedure 12-5).*
14. Lower bed and put side rail down.*
15. Place one arm around the shoulder area and the other arm under client's knees.
16. On a count of "3," shift your weight to rear leg, and slowly swing client's legs over edge of bed while pulling shoulders to sitting position (Figure 12-18).

Continued

PROCEDURE 12-10   **Assisting Client to Sit on the Side of the Bed—cont'd**

17. Place bed in lowest position so client's feet are touching the floor.*
18. Remain facing client with both hands supporting shoulders until client is stable.
19. Assist client to put on robe and footwear. Apply transfer or gait belt, if needed for transfer (see Procedure 12-12).
20. Place back of chair next to bed, facing client. Have client hold back of chair to keep balance, if needed (Figure 12-19).
21. Remain with client.
22. Reverse procedure to return client to Fowler's position.
23. Wash your hands.
24. Record client's reaction to the procedure, amount of time spent sitting on side of bed, and any other observations.

Fig 12-19 Client sits on side of the bed (Step 20).

*Your client may not have an adjustable hospital bed; those steps marked with an asterisk (*) will not apply.

TABLE 12-2	Observe, Record, Report: Transfers	
OBSERVE	**RECORD**	**REPORT**
Pale, sweaty Rapid increase in pulse Difficulty breathing	Signs observed	
Client's complaints • Dizziness • Feels faint, weak • Pain, discomfort	Client's complaints	
	What you did: Returned client to bed; placed client in Fowler's or supine position	To supervisor for further directions

It is important that the circulatory system becomes accustomed to this position before the client begins to stand. It is not unusual for the client to experience some dizziness, which usually subsides in a few minutes. If the client remains dizzy, begins to sweat, or becomes weak or pale or there is a rapid increase in the pulse rate or change in the pulse rhythm, return him or her to a supine or Fowler's position in bed. Record your findings, and report to your supervisor for further directions.

See Table 12-2 for information about what to observe, record, and report when transferring clients from place to place.

TRANSFERRING THE CLIENT TO A CHAIR/WHEELCHAIR

Once the client has adjusted to sitting at the side of the bed, he or she is ready to transfer to a chair or wheelchair. The care plan should indicate the client's strong side. Be sure to place the chair or wheelchair parallel to this side so that the client can assist you with the transfer procedure (Box 12-3). (See Procedure 12-11, Transferring Client from Bed to Chair/Wheelchair: Standing Transfer, and Procedure 12-12, Transferring Client from Bed to Chair/Wheelchair: Standing Transfer Using Transfer Belt). Explain what you are going to do and how your client can help. Encourage him or her to do as much as possible to foster independence.

BOX 12-3 | **Safety Tips: Using the Wheelchair**

- Place chair next to client's stronger side before making the transfer.
- Put footrests out of the way before client gets in or out of the chair.
- Make sure BOTH wheel brakes are locked before client gets in or out of the chair.
- Replace footrests in proper position, and assist client, as needed, to put feet on footrests after being seated.
- Make sure client is in a comfortable and safe sitting position before releasing the wheel brakes.
- Release both wheel brakes before attempting to move the chair.
- Make sure client's clothing or lap blanket does not trail on the floor or become caught in the wheels.

PROCEDURE 12-11 | **Transferring Client From Bed to Chair/Wheelchair: Standing Transfer**

Materials Needed
- Chair or wheelchair
- Blanket, if needed
- Special chair cushion, if needed
- Robe
- Sturdy footwear

Procedure
1. Explain what you are going to do.
2. Wash your hands.
3. Obtain materials listed above.
4. Provide privacy (close door, shut drapes, pull shades).
5. Place chair parallel to bed and on client's strong side.
6. When using a wheelchair, lock brakes and move footrests out of the way (Figure 12-20).
7. Lower bed, lock wheels, and lower rail on side where you are working.*
8. Assist client, as needed, to sit on side of bed (see Procedure 12-9) and put on robe and footwear.
9. Stand directly in front of client, with your feet slightly apart. Bend hips and knees so that you are level with client.
10. Place your arms under client's arms and around client's back, locking fingers together or clasping one hand over the other wrist (Figure 12-21). Have client hug your back (not your neck).

Fig 12-20 Lock brakes, and move footrest out of the way (Step 6).

Fig 12-21 Place your arms under the client's arms. Clasp one hand over the other wrist (Step 10).

Continued

PROCEDURE 12-11   Transferring Client From Bed to Chair/Wheelchair: Standing Transfer—cont'd

11. Lock your knees against client's knees to provide additional support and to prevent the knees from buckling (Figure 12-22).
12. Bend your knees and ask client to rock with you as you count 1-2-3. Stand on a count of "3."
13. Count to 10 before continuing. This allows time for the body to adjust to the standing position.
14. Walk with client to chair, taking small steps, while guiding client's back to chair. Continue until chair's sitting surface touches back of client's legs.
15. Have client reach back and grasp the farthest arm of the chair, then the nearest arm.
16. Bend your hips and knees while guiding client into chair (Figure 12-23).
17. Make sure client is safe and comfortable.
    a. If in wheelchair, replace footrests and have client put feet on them.
    b. Place necessary items within client's reach.
18. Wash your hands.
19. Record client's reaction to the procedure, amount of time sitting in chair, and any other observations.

Fig 12-22 Lock your knees against the client's knees (Step 11).

Fig 12-23 Bend your knees, and guide client into the chair (Step 16).

*Your client may not have an adjustable hospital bed; those steps marked with an asterisk (*) will not apply.

PROCEDURE 12-12   Transferring Client From Bed to Chair/Wheelchair: Standing Transfer Using Transfer Belt

Materials Needed
- Chair or wheelchair
- Blanket, if needed
- Special chair cushion, if used
- Transfer belt
- Robe
- Sturdy footwear

Procedure
1. Explain what you are going to do and how the client can help you.
2. Wash your hands.
3. Obtain materials listed above.
4. Provide privacy (close door, shut drapes, pull shades).

5. Apply transfer belt (see Procedure 12-14).
6. Place chair parallel to bed and on client's strong side. If using a wheelchair, lock brakes and move footrests out of way. If bed has wheels, lock them.
7. Stand directly in front of client.
8. Make sure client's feet are firmly on the floor.
9. Have client place fists on bed next to thighs and lean forward.
10. Grasp transfer belt firmly at each side (Figure 12-24).
11. Lock your knees against client's knees to provide additional support and to prevent client's knees from buckling.

PROCEDURE 12-12   Transferring Client From Bed to Chair/Wheelchair: Standing Transfer Using Transfer Belt—cont'd

12. Ask client to push fists down on bed and stand on a count of "3."
13. Pull client into standing position as you straighten knees and legs.
14. Count to 10 before continuing, to allow client's body to adjust to standing position.
15. Instruct client to
    a. Take small steps while turning back to chair until legs touch the chair.
    b. Reach back and grasp the farthest arm of chair, then nearest arm.
    c. Lower buttocks into chair, leaning slightly forward while sitting down.
    d. Slide hips back into chair and sit erect.
16. Make sure client is safe and comfortable.
    a. If in wheelchair, replace footrests and have client put feet on them.
    b. Place necessary items within client's reach.
17. Wash your hands.
18. Record client's reaction to the procedure, amount of time sitting in chair, and any other observations.

Fig 12-24 Grasp the transfer belt firmly at each side (Step 10).

RETURNING THE CLIENT TO BED

Assist the client to return to bed according to the care plan (see Procedure 12-13, Returning Client to Bed).

USING ASSISTIVE DEVICES

Assistive devices are items used to help clients to perform activities of daily living more easily. In Chapter 10, devices such as plate guards and built-up utensils were described to help clients to eat. Likewise, there is equipment that can be obtained to assist and support the client to move more easily and safely. Assistive devices can be purchased or rented on recommendation of the physician or the agency's physical therapist. Many community agencies loan this equipment on a temporary basis.

TRANSFER (GAIT) BELT

A transfer, or gait, belt is a belt worn by the client and used by the home care aide to hold on to the client during a transfer. It is used to help support a weak or unsteady client to move or walk. Apply the belt before beginning the transfer or before assisting the client to walk (see Procedure 12-14, Applying a Transfer [Gait] Belt).

SLIDING BOARD

This board acts as a bridge between two surfaces. For clients who have difficulty standing or are unable to bear weight on their legs, the sliding board can be used to move

PROCEDURE 12-13   Returning Client to Bed

1. Explain what you are going to do and how the client can help you.
2. Wash your hands.
3. Provide privacy (close door, shut drapes, pull shades).
4. Prepare the bed; fold down top bedding.
5. Lower height of bed to lowest level.*
6. Place chair parallel to bed; client moves toward strong side.
7. If wheelchair is used, lock brakes and place footrests out of the way. If bed has wheels, lock them.
8. Direct client to
   a. Hold onto armrests.
   b. Slide to edge of chair.
   c. Push down on armrests, straighten legs, and stand up.
   d. Take small steps while turning back to bed until back of legs touch bed.
   e. Reach back and place hands on bed.
   f. Lower buttocks into bed and slide back in bed.
9. Assist client to remove robe and shoes; place in closet.
10. Make sure client is safe and comfortable.
11. Place bed in lowest position. (Raise side rails, if indicated.)*
12. Wash your hands.
13. Record what you have done and client's reaction.

*Your client may not have an adjustable hospital bed; those steps marked with an asterisk (*) will not apply.

PROCEDURE 12-14   Applying a Transfer (Gait) Belt

Materials Needed
• Transfer (gait) belt

Procedure
1. Explain what you are going to do.
2. Wash your hands.
3. Obtain transfer (gait) belt.
4. Assist client to a sitting position on side of bed.
5. Apply belt over clothing and around waist. Never apply over bare skin.
6. Place belt buckles off-center in the front or in back, for client's comfort (Figure 12-25).
7. Tighten belt, using buckles, until it is snug. Belt should not be uncomfortable, cause pain, or cause breathing difficulties.
8. Check that the female's breasts are not caught under the belt.
9. Prepare client for transfer.

Fig 12-25 Place belt buckles off-center (Step 6).

the client from one area to another. The client pushes himself or herself onto the board and scoots along the board to the other side. Keep hands on top of the board, not around the edges, to prevent injury to the fingers. Sliding boards are available from commercial home care supply companies. A leaf from the client's dining room table may also be used, but check first with the client's physician or physical therapist (Figure 12-26, *A*).

THE TRAPEZE

A trapeze is a pull-up device attached to the bed. It can be used to help the client to raise himself or herself from a flat position in bed to a sitting position. The client grasps

Fig 12-26 Assistive devices. **A,** Sliding board. **B,** Trapeze at the foot of the bed. **C,** Overhead trapeze.

BOX 12-4 Safe Operation of the Mechanical Lift

- Read and understand the manufacturer's instructions before using the lift, if you are unsure of the procedure.
- Follow these instructions when operating the lift.
- Keep the client's body as low as possible during the transfer (e.g., just clear of the bed, chair, commode).
- Lower client SLOWLY so the client is not injured by the swivel bar.
- Do not exceed the weight limitation as posted on the lift.
- Do not use a torn, cut, or frayed sling.
- Use the mechanical lift for transfers only, not for transporting the client from place to place.

---

the handles of the trapeze and pulls up. Using this device requires strength in the arm muscles. The home care aide assists the client, as needed, to assume the sitting position (Figures 12-26, *B* and *C*).

THE MECHANICAL LIFT

A mechanical lift is used when the client is unable to assist with transfers from bed and back to bed. It can be used to move the client to a chair, wheelchair, commode, shower chair, or automobile. Proper use of the lift conserves the energy of both the client and caregiver because the lift supports the entire weight of the client.

There are various types of lifts. In the home, the hydraulic lift is commonly used. The lift is usually rented from a local medical supply company. Before using the lift, make sure that you know the proper procedure according to the manufacturer's instruction manual. See Box 12-4 for suggestions on safe operation of the mechanical lift. If you are unsure of the correct procedure, notify your supervisor.

For safe operation, two persons are needed: one to operate the lift and the other to guide the client as he or she is being moved. (See Procedure 12-15 for general steps to follow.)

PROCEDURE 12-15   Using a Mechanical Lift

Materials Needed
- Mechanical lift with sling
- Sheet, folded into quarters (optional)
- Chair or wheelchair
- A helper (family member)

Procedure
1. Explain what you are going to do.
2. Wash your hands.
3. Obtain materials listed above.
4. Provide privacy (close door, shut drapes, pull shades).
5. Raise bed to convenient working height, and lower side rails.*
6. Lower head of bed to level comfortable for client, as low as possible.*
7. Center sling (with sheet on top) placing it underneath client by turning client from side to side (as if placing a drawsheet under client while making an occupied bed; see Procedure 13-3) (Figure 12-27, A).
8. Position sling according to manufacturer's instructions.
9. Place chair/wheelchair at head (or foot) of bed, about 1 foot away from side of bed.
10. Lock wheels on bed.
11. Raise lift, and position over client (Figure 12-27, B).
12. Roll base of lift as far under bed as possible, locating swivel bar over client.
13. Attach sling to swivel bar. Check placement of sling straps for safety (Figure 12-27, C).
14. Raise head of bed to sitting position.*
15. Place client's arms across chest. DO NOT have client touch swivel bar.
16. Pump lift high enough for client and sling to be free of the bed (Figure 12-27, D).

Fig 12-27 **A,** Place sling under the client (Step 7). **B,** Raise lift, and position over the client (Step 11). **C,** Attach sling to swivel bar (Step 13). **D,** Pump lift to raise the client from the bed (Step 16).

PROCEDURE 12-15   Using a Mechanical Lift—cont'd

17. Ask helper to support client's legs and guide client as you move lift and client away from bed (Figure 12-27, *E*).
18. Position lift so that client's back is toward chair.
19. Lower client into chair as helper guides client into chair. Follow manufacturer's instructions for lowering lift (Figure 12-27, F).
20. Lower swivel bar to unhook sling. Leave sling in place (Figure 12-27, G).
21. Put on client's footwear; position feet.
22. Cover client's lap and legs with blanket, as needed.
23. Make sure client is safe and comfortable.
24. Wash your hands.
25. Record what you have done. Report any unusual conditions to your supervisor.
26. Reverse procedure to return client to bed.

Fig 12-27 cont'd **E,** Helper supports the client's legs (Step 17). **F,** Lower client into the chair (Step 19). **G,** Lower swivel bar to unhook sling (Step 20).

*Your client may not have an adjustable hospital bed; those steps marked with an asterisk (*) will not apply.

It is important to observe your client during and after the transfer procedure. Signs of dizziness, fatigue, difficulty breathing, pain, or discomfort must be recorded and reported to your supervisor.

AMBULATION

The term ambulate means to move the body by walking with or without assistance. Once the client has tolerated sitting in a chair, the next step is to begin to walk. The physical therapist will instruct the client and caregiver about any special techniques required and will prepare a schedule for daily ambulation. Your role as the home care aide is to assist the client, as needed, making sure that the physical therapist's

TABLE 12-3	Observe, Record, Report: Ambulation	
OBSERVE	**RECORD**	**REPORT**
Pale, sweaty Difficulty breathing	Signs observed	
Client's complaints • Dizziness • Feels faint, weak • Pain, discomfort	Client's complaints	
	What you did: Assisted client Distance walked Time spent walking Returned to chair/bed About client's complaints and your observations	To supervisor for further directions

directions are followed. Sometimes the client may want to walk longer than the directions allow. Always follow the physical therapist's directions. Record your client's request, and notify your supervisor for further instructions.

When assisting your client to walk, follow these general rules.

- Assist the client to put on the gait belt, if needed.
- Assist the client to standing position, and then count to 10 before proceeding.
- Stand by the client's weaker side and slightly behind, with your feet apart.
- Grasp the gait belt in back with one hand while placing other hand in front of collarbone on the weaker side.
- Do not rush the client; allow plenty of time.
- Practice good body mechanics.
- If the client becomes tired, wait a few minutes before proceeding.
- Calmly encourage and reassure the client, as needed.
- Record the distance walked, amount of time spent walking, and how the client tolerated the activity.
- Record and report any difficulty, such as dizziness, weakness, pain, or breathing difficulties.
- See Table 12-3 for information about what to observe, record, and report when assisting clients to ambulate.

USING WALKING DEVICES

Walking devices, such as walkers, canes, and crutches, may be needed to help support clients when walking. The physician determines the type(s) of assistive device according to the client's needs and abilities. The physical therapist fits the device to the client's size. Then, the client is instructed about the proper use and care of the device. It is your responsibility to make sure that the client follows these directions. Never change the directions given by the physical therapist. If the client is having difficulty using the device correctly, contact your supervisor for advice.

WALKERS

Walkers are small metal stands that the client leans on when walking from place to place (Figure 12-28). They are used for clients who have difficulty with balance or are

Fig 12-28 A walker helps this client to keep his balance.

Fig 12-29 Common types of canes. **A,** Regular cane. **B,** Broad-based cane.

weak and need additional support. Of all the types of assistive walking devices, walkers offer the greatest amount of stability because they provide four points of support. Some walkers have wheels and are pushed around; some are moved by lifting; and others have seats attached so that the client may rest when necessary. The type of walker is ordered by the doctor and usually obtained from a medical supply company. The physical therapist will instruct the client and caregiver about the proper technique when using the walker. Listed below are some basic guidelines that the client should follow to use the walker correctly and safely.

The client is using the walker correctly and safely when

- He or she stands BEFORE grasping the walker; walkers are not meant to support the client's full weight when rising from a sitting position. However, the client may use it to pull up to a standing position if you hold it steady; remind the client that, when unattended, the walker must never be grasped to rise from a sitting position or to lower self to a sitting position.
- All four legs of the walker are on the floor in a level position BEFORE taking a step; this technique will provide a solid base of support.
- The walker without wheels is advanced by picking it up and moving it forward while standing still; this technique will help keep the body in proper position and balance.
- The walker, with wheels, is advanced by pushing it forward.
- One foot is moved and then the other into the walker, after the walker is in proper position.
- When getting into a chair from the walker, the client releases the walker, grasps the arms of the chair, and lowers self into the chair.

CANES

Canes are sticks that clients lean on for balance while walking. There are two types.
1. *Regular:* Has a curved handle and provides one point of support (Figure 12-29, *A*).
2. *Broad-based:* Has three or four prongs (tripod or quad cane) that provide a greater base of support than the regular cane (Figure 12-29, *B*).

Canes provide limited support to the client's weak side. Therefore, they should be used by those clients who are able to walk without much assistance. Like all assistive walking devices, canes must be properly fitted to the client. The physical therapist fits the cane and gives instructions about its proper use and care.

The client is using a cane correctly and safely when

- It is held in the stronger hand with the elbow slightly bent.
- It is held in the hand opposite the weak leg.
- The rubber cap is in place and replaced when worn.

CRUTCHES

Crutches are walking aids that are held in place by the arms. The client must have strong shoulders, arms, wrists, and hands. At least one leg must be strong enough to bear weight. Other requirements include the ability to stand erect, have good balance, and be able to wear sturdy walking shoes.

There are three types of crutches.

1. *Axillary crutches:* Made of wood or aluminum and fit under the axilla
2. *Nonaxillary crutches (Canadian crutches):* Fit half-way between the shoulder and elbow and held in place by a cuff that encircles the forearm
3. *Adjustable ("Adjusto") or telescopic crutches:* Can be adjusted to full length or elbow length or used as a cane

Before preparing to crutch walk, the doctor usually prescribes special exercises to strengthen the muscles of the upper body that will be used to bear weight. The physical therapist will instruct the client about how to do the exercises, when to practice, and for how long each day. When the client is strong enough, the therapist selects the type of crutch best suited to the client's physical condition. Measuring and fitting the crutch also are responsibilities of the therapist.

The client is using crutches correctly and safely when

- Weight is placed on upper arms, wrists, and hands—NOT under the arms; nerves in the axillary area can be damaged if the client bears weight on the top of the crutches.
- Instructions given by the therapist are followed accurately.
- The rubber crutch caps are in place and replaced when worn (Box 12-5).

A WORD OF CAUTION

There may be situations where your client or family member has developed poor habits of positioning, lifting, moving, or using assistive devices incorrectly. When

---

BOX 12-5   Safety Tips: Using Walkers, Canes, and Crutches

- Make sure that all bolts are tightened and tips have rubber safety protectors.
- Place walkers, canes, or crutches, when not in use, near the client but out of traffic pattern of the room.
- Assist client to put on walking shoes, not floppy slippers.
- Remove obstacles from the client's path.
- Reinforce instructions of the physical therapist.
- Do not rush the client; allow plenty of time to practice walking.
- Practice using assistive devices when the client's energy level is high.

Fig 12-30 Ease the client down to the floor by bending your knees. Keep your back straight.

you observe this, explain, in a tactful manner, the dangers to the client or family member; why the action is incorrect; and demonstrate the correct method. Assist them to practice the activity until you are certain that they have learned the proper way. Usually, they are grateful for being instructed how to perform activities safely and correctly. If, however, they insist on continuing to perform activities incorrectly, report this to your supervisor and record your observations in the care record. Do not permit family members to assist you if they are unwilling to use the correct, safe procedure.

ASSISTING THE CLIENT TO FALL

If you are with a client who becomes weak or dizzy during a transfer or ambulation, try to ease him or her down to the floor. Grasp the client firmly around the waist, using the gait belt if one is worn. Gently lower the client to the floor by bending your knees and keeping your back straight (Figure 12-30). Do not try to stop a fall because both of you could be injured.

If there is another person in the home, call for help. Check for injuries, and call 9-1-1 or emergency medical services, if necessary. See Chapter 24 for additional information. If there are no obvious injuries, help the client into a comfortable position on the floor. Use pillows, blankets, and so on. Allow the client to rest. You should take a few deep breaths and try to remain calm. Decide if you will be able to safely assist the client to get up, or if you will need additional help. If you do not feel confident about moving your client, do not be pressured into trying. Call your supervisor to report the incident and to get advice on how to proceed.

ORR

ORR

Report the following.
1. What happened: Did client have any complaints or symptoms before the fall?
2. Condition of the client after the fall: Injuries? Complaints? Consciousness? Pulse? Color?
3. Did you call 9-1-1 or emergency medical services? Is the client still on the floor? Did you get the client up to a chair or bed?
4. What assistance will you need to get the client up from the floor if he or she is still there?

Record the fall on the client's record, including all the information above. Complete an incident report form as required by your agency.

INFECTION CONTROL

PREVENTING INFECTION

You will be in close physical contact when moving and lifting clients, so it is important to avoid any risk of infection for both you and your client. Medical asepsis and standard (universal) precautions must be followed. The following are some other hints for preventing infection.

- Be sure the client is clean and dry before moving.
- Offer the bedpan or urinal before moving; tend to elimination needs before getting the client out of bed.
- Protect the seat of the wheelchair with disposable pads or a folded sheet (can be discarded or washed if soiled).
- Wear gloves, as necessary, when there is a possibility of touching body fluids. This may happen when returning clients to bed. Look carefully, before moving, to make sure that the client is not sitting in urine and feces.
- Wear PPE—gown and gloves, as necessary, according to the client's condition and care plan. When in doubt, check with your supervisor.
- Do not let clients cough or sneeze on you during the transfer procedure. Wait until the coughing/sneezing has stopped before moving the client. Also, instruct the client not to cough or sneeze on you but to use a tissue to cover his or her mouth.
- Remember to wash your hands before and after positioning, moving, or transferring the client.

CHAPTER SUMMARY

- Use good body mechanics to prevent injury to yourself and your client.
- Keep your body in good physical condition.
- Wear appropriate clothing and shoes.
- Follow rules for safe moving and lifting.
- Provide position changes in bed, transfers, and ambulation according to the care plan.
- Encourage clients to help as much as possible within their physical abilities. Instruct them how to help.

- If you are unsure about your ability to perform lifting, moving, or transfer activities, notify your supervisor. Do not take any chances that could result in injury to yourself or the client.
- Practice infection control when positioning, moving, and lifting your client.

STUDY QUESTIONS

1. List three tips for maintaining good body mechanics when
   a. Standing
   b. Sitting
   c. Lifting
2. List three effects of immobility.
3. Define the following terms.
   a. Muscle atrophy
   b. Pressure ulcer
   c. Contracture
   d. Bony prominence
4. Explain the use of the following devices.
   a. Trochanter rolls
   b. Bed cradle
   c. Splints
   d. Trapeze
   e. Sliding board
   f. Transfer belt
   g. Turning or lifting sheet
   h. Walker
5. Describe the following positions.
   a. Fowler's position
   b. Supine position
   c. Lateral position
6. List six rules to follow when assisting a client to walk.
7. List 10 safety factors to follow when assisting clients to use walkers, canes, and wheelchairs.
8. Explain how to assist a client who is falling.
9. List three ways to prevent infection when lifting and moving clients.

13

Bedmaking

OBJECTIVES

After you read this chapter, you will be able to:

1. Discuss the importance of a correctly made bed.
2. List five rules for bedmaking.
3. Make an unoccupied bed and an occupied bed.
4. List five rules for infection control when handling linens during bedmaking.

KEY TERM

Incontinent The inability to control urination or bowel elimination

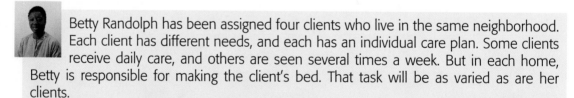

Betty Randolph has been assigned four clients who live in the same neighborhood. Each client has different needs, and each has an individual care plan. Some clients receive daily care, and others are seen several times a week. But in each home, Betty is responsible for making the client's bed. That task will be as varied as are her clients.

Mrs. Santini is an 88-year-old widow who lives alone in a small house. She is recovering from heart failure and needs help with bathing, dressing, and simple housekeeping tasks. Mrs. Santini sleeps in her own double bed in her bedroom. Betty visits three times a week. Mrs. Santini's sister helps on the other days.

Mr. Morowski had a right leg amputation. He is 70 years of age and lives with his wife and son. Mr. Morowski sleeps in a hospital bed in the living room. He can be transferred to a wheelchair. His home has been equipped with a ramp so Mr. Morowski can go outdoors. Betty assists with bathing, dressing, and moving the client daily.

Mrs. Cullen is recovering from shoulder surgery. She needs help with bathing, dressing, and simple household tasks. She is a 64-year-old widow who lives alone in a very small home. Mrs. Cullen hurt her back many years ago. She sleeps in a reclining chair in the living room. Her son and daughter-in-law help out three days a week and on weekends. Betty visits twice a week.

Mr. Tarrant is a 50-year-old hospice client who has cancer. He lives with his partner of many years. The agency has provided a hospital bed with electrical controls, a trapeze, and a footboard. He requires a complete bed bath and linen change daily. His partner has a home-based business and has arranged his schedule to assist the home care aide in any way possible. Betty visits twice a week, and Mr. Tarrant says he will need more help as he gets sicker.

As you can see, Betty will be changing linens on several types of beds and one non-bed. Bedmaking is part of personal care and grooming for all clients. Making sure that the bed is clean, dry, and free of wrinkles contributes to the client's comfort and relaxation. It is an important part of the care plan.

Whenever possible, try to make the bed according to the household custom. If you are unable to follow the client's household custom, you must explain your reasons for the change to your client or family member. However, there will also be times when you need to be flexible. For example, there is no standard procedure for changing the linens on a reclining chair. Ask the client or family how this should be done. Once in a while, you may find that a client's bed or sleeping arrangement is not ideal, but there may be no other choice. CONTACT YOUR SUPERVISOR IF YOU ARE ASKED TO MAKE UP A BED, CHAIR, OR SOFA THAT YOU THINK IS UNSAFE OR DOES NOT MEET YOUR CLIENT'S NEED FOR CARE. Although the size and condition of the bed may vary, you must always be sure that the linens are clean and ready for the client when needed. Whenever possible, use sheets that fit the bed, and prepare it according to the care plan.

TYPES OF BEDS

The following beds are the types you are most likely to find in the home.

REGULAR BEDS

Most of your clients will sleep in the bed they have always used in their home. These beds usually do not have wheels and are not easily moved. If you think that the bed is not in a safe location for your client—near a large window or radiator, for example—discuss your concerns with your supervisor. Perhaps, with the client's or family's permission, it can be moved to another area of the room for safety.

WATER BEDS

The mattress of this bed is filled with water and sits in a special frame. Special fitted sheets may be needed to make this type of bed. Although these waterproof mattresses are made of heavy-duty plastic material, there is still risk of puncture. Do not use any sharp objects, such as scissors and straight or safety pins, near the water bed.

HOSPITAL BEDS

Hospital beds have wheels and can be raised and lowered horizontally. This makes it easier to transfer clients in and out of bed. This adjustable bed also permits the home care aide to work at a comfortable level and to use proper body mechanics. Always keep the hospital bed at its lowest position unless you are working at the bedside. When the bed is raised, there is great risk that the client could be injured trying to

Fig 13-1 Controls for a manually operated hospital bed. Fold under the bed for safety.

Fig 13-2 Controls for an electrically operated hospital bed.

Lock

Fig 13-3 Brakes on a bed wheel.

climb in or out of the bed. Also, because hospital beds are narrower than a regular single bed, it may be easier for the client to fall out of bed.

The metal frame of the hospital bed is made up of three sections so that the head and foot of the bed can be raised or lowered. Some are operated manually by turning a crank at the end of the bed (Figure 13-1). Others are operated electrically by hand-operated controls (Figure 13-2). Many clients will be able to adjust their beds without assistance, but you should make sure they are able to safely operate the controls.

Safety Features of Hospital Beds

Wheel Brakes. Because hospital beds usually have wheels, brakes are needed to keep the beds from moving. Be sure to apply the wheel brakes during transfers, bedmaking, bathing, and other procedures where movement of the bed is not needed. In general, the brakes should be locked at all times and released only when movement of the bed is required. Always remember to relock the brakes (Figure 13-3).

Fig 13-4 **A,** Side rails that attach to the side of the bed. **B,** Straight-backed chairs can be used if side rails are not available.

BOX 13-1 Safety Rules When Using a Hospital Bed

1. Raise bed to a convenient working height before giving care.
2. Keep bed at lowest level at all other times. Bed is ALWAYS at lowest level when client is in or out of it.
3. Lock bed wheels when moving and transferring clients.
4. For a manually operated bed, fold cranks under the foot of the bed when not in use.

If side rails are used
1. Keep side rails raised according to the care plan.
2. Lower rail on side where you are giving care or performing transfer.
3. Raise rail when care or transfer is completed.

Side Rails. These are attached to the bed to prevent the client from falling out of the bed (Figure 13-4, *A*). Side rails are also used by clients to help in moving, turning, and transferring. Some clients prefer to keep the side rails down; others will like the safety and security provided by the raised rails. Follow the directions regarding the use of side rails in the care plan. See Box 13-1 for safety rules when using a hospital bed.

When side rails are not available, two or more straight-backed chairs may be used to provide protection for the client who is using a regular bed. Place the chairs at both sides of the bed with the back of each chair facing the bed (Figure 13-4, *B*).

SPECIAL DEVICES FOR BEDS

BED BOARDS

Bed boards are usually thin, flat pieces of wood cut to fit and placed under the mattress to add extra firmness for clients with back injuries or muscle disorders.

FOOTBOARDS AND BED CRADLES

Footboards and bed cradles are also used on beds, as discussed in Chapter 12. These devices are removed for bedmaking and are replaced after the bottom bed linens have been changed. Be sure that footboards and cradles are properly placed so they will not collapse and injure the client's ankles or feet.

Fig 13-5 Egg crate foam mattress pad.

Fig 13-6 Alternating pressure mattress.

Fig 13-7 Wheelchair gel cushion. (Image courtesy Posey Company, Arcadia, California.)

PRESSURE-RELIEVING DEVICES

A variety of devices are used in an effort to provide comfort and prevent pressure and the development of pressure ulcers. These are placed on top of the mattress. Here are some examples.

- *Foam mattress pads* help to evenly distribute the client's weight in bed. They may have a flat surface, but the egg crate type is most often used (Figure 13-5). Cover both the foam mattress pad and the regular mattress with a bottom sheet only. Do not use any other bottom linens that could interfere with the function of the egg crate mattress pad. Foam mattress pads are treated with a special chemical to retard fire. Washing removes this chemical and makes the mattress pad a fire hazard. Soiled egg crate mattress pads should be discarded and replaced.

- *Alternating pressure mattresses*, which help to distribute weight, are also used. They are made of plastic and have several compartments that are alternately inflated and deflated by an electrical pump (Figure 13-6). This reduces constant pressure on skin surfaces. These mattresses are used for clients who spend most of their time in bed. Always place a sheet between the client's skin and the plastic mattress. No other bottom linens are used. Do not use pins. Check with your supervisor for instructions about the operation of the air mattress.

- *Gel pads* contain a gel-like substance that acts as a layer of cushioning between the client's bony prominences and the surface of the bed/chair (Figure 13-7). Cover the

Fig 13-8 Closed bed.

Fig 13-9 Open bed.

pad with a pillow case to keep the client's skin away from the plastic surface of the pad. Be certain that there are no wrinkles in the pillow case.

Always follow the care plan regarding the use of special devices for beds. DEVICES THAT RELIEVE PRESSURE AND PROVIDE COMFORT DO NOT TAKE THE PLACE OF TURNING AND MOVING CLIENTS AT LEAST EVERY 2 HOURS. POSITIONING, INSPECTING THE SKIN AND BONY PROMINENCES, AND KEEPING CLIENTS DRY AND CLEAN ARE IMPORTANT PRECAUTIONS TO TAKE IN PREVENTING PRESSURE ULCERS.

MAKING THE BED

There are three ways to make a bed:
1. **Closed bed:** Made when the bed will remain empty for a period of time; may be made with or without a bedspread (Figure 13-8)
2. **Open bed:** Made when the bed will become occupied shortly; top linens are fan-folded to the foot of the bed (Figure 13-9)
3. **Occupied bed:** Made while the client is in the bed

REASONS FOR BEDMAKING

There are several reasons for bedmaking and changing linens.
1. To provide comfort for the client
2. To prevent irritation and injury to the client's skin
3. To provide a clean, neat environment

For clients who spend most of their time in bed, the linens are almost like clothing and should be changed at least once daily. These clients may also be very sensitive to wrinkles in the linens or food crumbs, which may irritate the skin and cause pressure ulcers.

Other clients will spend little or no time in bed during the day. Their beds should be straightened and made each day. In this case, however, you may not need to use clean linens every time you make the bed. Before changing the bed linens, find out when they were last changed. Perhaps only the pillowcases need to be changed. Follow the directions in the care plan regarding bedmaking.

REGARDLESS OF HOW MUCH TIME THE CLIENT SPENDS IN BED, LINENS SHOULD BE CHANGED WHENEVER THEY BECOME WET OR SOILED. REMEMBER TO WEAR GLOVES IF YOU WILL COME IN CONTACT WITH BODY FLUIDS WHEN CHANGING THE LINENS.

GENERAL RULES OF BEDMAKING

Whether you are changing linens or just making the bed, here are some general rules to follow when making a client's bed.
- Assemble all items needed before you start to make the bed.
- Practice good body mechanics while making the bed.
- Make the bed according to client's custom.
- Make one side of the bed as much as possible before going to the other side, as this will save time and energy.
- Do not use torn linens.
- Keep bottom linens smooth and free of wrinkles.
- Remove crumbs and food particles from bed linens.
- Change linen when it becomes damp, wet, or soiled.
- Follow rules for infection control (Box 13-2).

MATERIALS NEEDED FOR BEDMAKING

Clients will usually want you to make their bed a certain way. This, of course, will vary from client to client. Some will want only sheets; others will want you to use both sheets and blankets. Some clients may have only one set of linens—those on the bed. You may have to launder these linens while the client is out of bed and then put them back on the bed. Follow the care plan regarding bedmaking. Other clients may have no linens at all; they may be lying on just a bare mattress. Contact your supervisor if your client has no linens or if you do not have enough linens to properly make the bed.

The following materials are usually used to make the client's bed.
- *Mattress pad or cover (optional):* Protects the mattress from being soiled. Made of cotton or plastic.

BOX 13-2   Infection Control Reminders

- Keep all bed linens off the floor.
- Place used linens in laundry container immediately after removing from bed.
- Wash and dry soiled linens as soon as possible.
- Roll soiled linens away from your clothing.
- Do not shake bed linens.
- Hold and fold linens away from your clothing.
- Wash hands before and after changing linens.
- Use gloves when handling linens soiled with body fluids.
- Follow instructions in Chapters 9 and 11 for handling and washing soiled linens.

- *Bottom sheet (flat or fitted):* Provides additional protection for the mattress. Also provides comfort to the client when it is smooth and wrinkle free. Made of cotton, cotton blend, or flannel.
- *Drawsheet (optional):* protects the mattress and bottom sheet. It is placed across the middle third of the bed and can serve as a turning or lifting sheet. It is about half the size of a regular sheet. To make a drawsheet, fold a regular sheet in half, lengthwise. If a plastic drawsheet is used, a cotton drawsheet **must** be placed completely over it to protect the client's skin. Plastic can be very uncomfortable because it retains the body's heat and moisture. Lying directly on a plastic sheet can cause damage to the skin's surface. *NEVER* USE A PLASTIC GARBAGE BAG OR A DRY CLEANER'S BAG. THEY ARE NOT HEAVY ENOUGH TO PROTECT THE BED. THEY CAN ALSO CLING TO THE NOSE OR MOUTH AND KEEP A CLIENT FROM BREATHING.
- *Bed protector/incontinent pad (optional):* Provides added protection to the bottom sheet. It is placed under the client's buttocks and is made of absorbent material, usually with a plastic underside. If the client soils the pad, it can be thrown away. This saves time and energy because bed linens do not have to be removed and replaced each time the client soils the bed. However, bed protectors can be costly. Use according to the wishes of the client/family.
- *Top sheet:* Provides comfort for the client. Because it rests directly on the client, the sheet should not prevent a client from moving the feet or toes. To conserve linens, a clean top sheet can be used as a bottom sheet after the soiled bottom sheet is removed.
- *Blanket (optional):* Provides additional warmth and comfort for the client. Made of cotton, wool, and synthetic blends. When a blanket is used, the top sheet must always be placed between the client and the blanket.
- *Bedspread:* Protects the bed linens when the bed is not in use. Bedspreads are used according to the preference of the client.
- *Pillow protector:* Protects pillow from being soiled. Made of cotton or plastic.
- *Pillowcase:* Provides comfort for the client. Made of cotton, cotton blend, or flannel.

MAKING A CLOSED BED

This type of bed is easier to make than the occupied bed. Whenever possible, get your client out of bed before making the bed. You will save time and energy. Usually, the bed is made in the morning, after the client's bath. The procedure described applies to any size bed: hospital, twin, queen, or king size bed. The supplies you gather will depend on what is available in the home and the client's custom for making the bed (see Procedure 13-1, Making a Closed Bed).

When the client will return to bed soon, an open bed is made using Procedure 13-2, Making an Open Bed.

MAKING AN OCCUPIED BED

This type of bed is made when the client is not able to get out of bed. Follow Procedure 13-3, Making an Occupied Bed.

When making the bed, it is important to do the following.
- Explain what you are going to do before it is done.
- Explain to your client how to help by rolling to one side of the bed at a time.
- Keep the client fully covered with the blanket or top sheet during the procedure; do not expose the client.

PROCEDURE 13-1   Making a Closed Bed

Materials Needed
- Laundry container
- Mattress pad, if used
- Bottom sheet (flat or fitted)
- Plastic drawsheet, if used
- Cotton drawsheet, if used
- Top sheet
- Blanket, if used
- Bedspread, if used
- Pillowcase(s)

Procedure
1. Explain what you are going to do.
2. Wash your hands.
3. Obtain materials listed above, and place them in order of use on a chair near the bed.
4. Place laundry container near bed.
5. Raise bed to convenient working height, and lower both rails.*
6. Place bed in flat position.*
7. Remove pillow(s), and place on chair.
8. Loosen all bed linens: at head, sides, and bottom of bed.
9. Remove each piece of bed linen separately. Fold any linens to be reused (Figure 13-10). Roll each remaining linen into a ball, and discard in laundry container (Figure 13-11).
10. Place clean mattress pad, folded lengthwise, in center of bed. Unfold one half, and roll to center of bed.**

11. Place bottom sheet, folded lengthwise, in center of bed. Unfold one half, and roll to center of bed.
    - *Fitted sheet:* Place ends around corners—top and bottom (Figure 13-12); tuck side of sheet under mattress.
    - *Flat sheet:* Place bottom hem of sheet even with edge of mattress at foot of bed; tuck top of sheet under mattress at head of bed.
12. Miter corner at head end of mattress (see Procedure 13-4).
13. Tuck sheet under side of entire mattress. Work from head to foot of bed.
14. Place plastic drawsheet, folded in half, in center third of bed. Unfold and roll to center of bed.**
15. Place cotton drawsheet, folded in half, in center of bed, covering entire plastic drawsheet (Figure 13-13). Unfold and roll to center of bed.**

Fig 13-11 Roll remaining linen into a ball and discard (Step 9).

Fig 13-10 **A,** Fold top edge of blanket down to bottom edge. **B,** Fold blanket over from far side to near side of bed. **C,** Fold top edge of blanket down to bottom edge. **D,** Place folded blanket over back of chair.

Fig 13-12 Place folded bottom linens lengthwise in center of bed (Step 11).

*Your client may not have an adjustable hospital bed; those steps marked with a single asterisk (*) will not apply.
**Optional; used according to client's needs and care plan.

PROCEDURE 13-1 Making a Closed Bed—cont'd

Fig 13-13 Place cotton drawsheet in center of bed (Step 15).

Fig 13-14 Place top sheet in center of bed (Step 17).

Fig 13-15 Pull through top sheet, blanket, and bedspread (Step 24).

16. Tuck ends of plastic drawsheet and cotton drawsheet under mattress.**
17. Place top sheet, folded lengthwise, in center of bed, with top edge even with top of mattress. Unfold and roll to center of bed (Figure 13-14).
18. Place blanket, folded lengthwise, in center of bed, with top edge even with top of mattress. Unfold and roll to center of bed.**
19. Place bedspread, folded lengthwise, in center of bed, with about 4 inches above top edge of mattress. Unfold and roll to center of bed.**
20. Tuck top sheet, blanket, and bedspread under foot of mattress. Miter corner.
21. Go to other side of bed.
22. Pull through mattress pad and straighten.
23. Pull through all lower linens. Straighten and tuck under mattress. Miter corner of sheet at head end of mattress, or fit top and bottom corners of fitted sheet over mattress corners.
24. Pull through top sheet, blanket, and bedspread. Smooth out wrinkles (Figure 13-15).
25. Tuck top sheet, blanket, and bedspread under foot of mattress.
26. Miter corner at foot end of mattress.
27. Make a cuff at top of bed, and bring top sheet over blanket.
28. Place clean pillowcase on pillow, and place pillow at head of bed.
29. Cover pillow with bedspread.
30. Place bed in lowest position.*
31. Remove laundry container, and bring to washing machine or other location as requested by client or family.
32. Wash your hands.

PROCEDURE 13-2 Making an Open Bed

1. Wash your hands.
2. Obtain materials needed for making a closed bed.
3. Make a closed bed.
4. Fanfold top linens to foot of bed.
5. Wash your hands.

PROCEDURE 13-3   Making an Occupied Bed

Materials Needed
- Laundry container
- Mattress pad, if used
- Bottom sheet (flat or fitted)
- Plastic drawsheet, if used
- Cotton drawsheet, if used
- Top sheet
- Blanket, if used
- Bedspread, if used
- Pillowcase(s)
- Disposable gloves, if needed

Procedure
1. Explain what you are going to do.
2. Wash your hands.
3. Obtain materials listed above, and place them in order of use on a chair near the bed.
4. Provide privacy (close door, shut drapes, pull shades).
5. Place laundry container near bed.
6. Raise bed to comfortable working height, and lock wheels. Lower rail on side where you are working.*
7. Lower head of bed to level comfortable for client, as low as possible.*
8. Loosen top bedding at foot of bed.
9. Remove top bedding, but leave client covered with one blanket or top sheet.
10. Instruct client to hold top sheet while you remove other top linens (Figure 13-16).
11. Fold any linens to be reused, such as blanket. Roll each remaining linen into a ball and discard in laundry container.
12. Help client to roll to side of bed opposite to you and to grasp side rail for support.*
13. Roll each piece of bottom linen to center of bed, and tuck along client's back (Figure 13-17).
14. Smooth mattress pad, if used.**
15. Place clean bottom sheet, folded lengthwise, in center of bed. Unfold one half, and roll to center of bed.
    - *Fitted sheet:* Place ends around corners—top and bottom; tuck side of sheet under mattress.

- *Flat sheet:* Place bottom hem of sheet even with edge of mattress at foot of bed; tuck top of sheet under mattress at head of bed.
16. Miter corner at head end of mattress.
17. Tuck sheet under side of entire mattress. Work from head of bed to foot.
18. Place plastic drawsheet, folded in half, in center third of bed. Unfold and roll to center of bed. Tuck along client's back.**

Fig 13-16 Have client hold sheet while you remove other top linens (Step 10).

Fig 13-17 Roll each piece of bottom linen to center of bed (Step 13).

*Your client may not have an adjustable hospital bed; those steps marked with a single asterisk (*) will not apply.
**Optional; used according to client's needs and care plan.

PROCEDURE 13-3   Making an Occupied Bed—cont'd

Fig 13-18 Place cotton drawsheet in center of bed (Step 19).

Fig 13-19 Provide "toe room" for client's feet (Step 33).

19. Place cotton drawsheet, folded in half, in center of bed, covering entire plastic drawsheet. Unfold and roll to center of bed. Tuck along client's back (Figure 13-18).**
20. Tuck ends of plastic drawsheet and cotton draw sheet under mattress.**
21. Help client to roll toward you, over linens to clean side of bed.
22. Raise rail on side where you have been working.*
23. Go to other side of bed.
24. Lower side rail.*
25. Remove used bottom linens, roll, and discard in laundry container.
26. Pull through all bottom linens. Straighten and tuck under head of mattress. Miter corner of sheet at head end of mattress. Or fit top and bottom corners of fitted sheet over mattress corners.
27. Help client to roll back to center of bed.
28. Place clean top sheet entirely over the client and remove top linen. Discard in laundry container or fold for reuse.
29. Place blanket and bedspread over sheet.

30. Tuck top sheet, blanket, and bedspread under foot of mattress. Miter corner.
31. Raise side rail.*
32. Go to other side of bed. Lower side rail.*
33. Smooth and straighten top sheet, blanket, and bedspread. Tuck them under foot of mattress. Give "toe room" for client's feet (Figure 13-19). Miter corner.
34. Make a cuff at top of bed, and bring top sheet over bedspread.
35. Remove pillow from bed. Remove pillowcase, and discard in laundry container.
36. Place clean pillowcase on pillow, and replace pillow under client's head.
37. Make sure client is safe and comfortable.
38. Place bed in lowest position. (Raise side rail, if indicated.)*
39. Remove laundry container, and bring to washing machine or other location as requested by client or family.
40. Wash your hands.

BOTTOM BEDDING

1. Tuck bottom sheet about 18 inches under the mattress at head of bed (Figure 13-20).
2. Turn side of sheet up over the mattress in a triangle shape (Figure 13-21).
3. Tuck the lower edge of the sheet (hanging down next to the mattress) under the side of the mattress (Figure 13-22).
4. Turn the triangular area of sheet down over the mattress (Figure 13-23).
5. Tuck sheet under the mattress (Figure 13-24).

UPPER BEDDING

Follow the procedure for mitered corners for bottom bedding, omitting the fifth step. The upper sheet hangs freely over the mattress (Figure 13-25).

Fig 13-22 Tuck lower edge of sheet under side of mattress (Step 3).

Fig 13-23 Turn triangular area of sheet down over mattress (Step 4).

Fig 13-20 Tuck bottom sheet under mattress (Step 1).

Fig 13-24 Tuck sheet under mattress (Step 5).

Fig 13-21 Turn side of sheet up in a triangle shape (Step 2).

Fig 13-25 Upper sheet hangs freely over mattress.

CHAPTER SUMMARY

- Bedmaking provides comfort and a clean environment for the client.
- There are several types of beds.
- Make sure the bed is neat, clean, dry, and free of wrinkles and crumbs.
- Procedures for bedmaking may have to be adjusted according to the needs of the client, type of bed, and materials available.

- Practice good body mechanics when bedmaking to avoid the possibility of injury.
- Handle bed linens correctly to avoid the spread of microorganisms. Observe standard (universal) precautions at all times.

STUDY QUESTIONS

1. List three reasons for bedmaking.
2. Describe a hospital bed.
3. Explain the use of the following:
   Footboard
   Alternating pressure mattress
   Bed cradle
4. List five items used in bedmaking.
5. What are five rules to follow when making a bed?
6. List five rules for infection control when handling linens during bedmaking.

14

Personal Care

OBJECTIVES

After you read this chapter, you will be able to:

1. List five reasons why clients may be unable to perform personal care activities.
2. List four purposes of bathing.
3. Discuss six principles to follow when bathing clients.
4. Explain the difference between the following types of baths.
   a. Complete bed bath
   b. Partial bath
   c. Tub bath
   d. Shower bath
5. Discuss the safety factors to be considered while giving personal care.
6. Give two examples of the use of standard (universal) precautions during personal care of clients.
7. List three benefits of range-of-motion (ROM) exercises and four points to remember when assisting with these exercises.
8. Demonstrate procedures for oral hygiene, bathing, grooming, and ROM exercises.

KEY TERMS

Aspiration Breathing in or inhaling a substance into the bronchial tubes and lungs

Emesis basin A kidney-shaped basin that fits against the neck to collect vomitus

Genitalia (genitals) Organs of reproduction, usually external organs

Lubricant A fluid, an ointment, or another substance for reducing friction between parts that rub together and for making a surface slippery; it protects skin and prevents drying

Normal saline solution A solution of table salt and water in the same concentration as in the body

Perineal (perineum) Pertaining to the perineum, the area between the legs; in women, the area between the vagina and the anus; in men, the area between the scrotum and the anus

Surgical incision A cut produced surgically by a sharp instrument creating an opening into an organ or space

Traction To put under tension, by means of weights and pulleys, to straighten or immobilize a body part or to relieve pressure on it

Personal care and grooming are important services provided by the home care aide. Clients are often unable to perform self-care, such as bathing, shampooing, oral hygiene, and skin and nail care. There are many reasons for clients' inability to care for themselves, including

- The effects of illness
- Lack of energy and strength
- Pain and discomfort
- Not being able to reach body parts
- Not being able to obtain, carry, or use supplies needed for personal care
- Anxiety and fear of injury
- Confusion, inability to understand, forgetting what to do and how to do it

A client's inability to perform self-care may be described by using the following terms:

- *Temporary:* will improve with time; performing self-care will return
- *Permanent:* will not change; the client will always need assistance
- *Progressive:* will continue and increase with time

The care plan lists the personal care to be given to your client. If you have any questions, check with your supervisor. Remember to encourage clients to be as independent as possible according to their abilities and limitations. Give as much personal care as needed. Establish a communication system so that the client can call you when needed (Figure 14-1).

ORAL HYGIENE (MOUTH CARE)

Oral hygiene means cleaning the mouth, teeth, gums, and tongue to remove pieces of food and bacteria. This helps prevent tooth decay, gum disease, and mouth odor. Oral hygiene also gives the mouth a clean feeling and a good taste. Because the mouth is the first organ of the digestive system, a clean and healthy mouth is important for good nutrition.

Follow the care plan regarding the type of mouth care and the amount of assistance needed.

Observe the client's mouth, gums, lips, and teeth for any signs of irritation, loose teeth, bleeding gums, or sores. Report unusual findings to your supervisor. Oral hygiene is usually given in the morning on awakening, after meals, and at bedtime.

BRUSHING TEETH

The following are important points to remember when providing mouth care.
1. Wash hands before and after the procedure. Wear gloves. Practice standard (universal) precautions; wear PPE if there is a risk of splashing or spraying.
2. Encourage self-care according to the client's ability and the care plan.

Fig 14-1 Communication systems. Client may call aide using a bell, tapping partially filled water glass with a spoon, or shaking a small can with a few coins inside.

Fig 14-2 Examples of adaptive toothbrushes.

3. Get all of the supplies ready, and let the client brush his or her teeth at the bedside, in the bathroom, or at the kitchen sink.
4. Use a soft-bristled toothbrush.
5. Have the client balloon his or her cheeks in and out to distribute water or mouthwash throughout the mouth and between the teeth.
6. Clients who cannot balloon or swish rinse water and/or mouthwash can turn their heads from side to side (as if to signal "no") to distribute fluid throughout mouth.
7. Gently brush all surfaces of the teeth, mouth, and gums.
8. Apply lubricant to prevent dry, cracked lips.
9. Assist the client to use adaptive toothbrushes (Figure 14-2), if needed.
   Follow Procedure 14-1, Brushing Teeth.

FLOSSING TEETH

Flossing between the surfaces of the teeth helps to remove food particles and other materials that may cause decay, gum disease, and mouth odor. Teeth are usually flossed before brushing. Dentists recommend that flossing be done immediately after breakfast and at bedtime.

There are two types of dental floss: waxed or unwaxed. The waxed floss is smoother, does not fray easily, and glides between the teeth smoothly. The unwaxed floss is thinner and may be more effective in removing food particles where teeth are very close together. Both types of floss are also available with flavoring, such as mint.

Some clients use tiny toothbrushes to clean between the teeth. These are used after regular brushing and usually after each meal. You will need to floss for clients who are unable to do this for themselves. Always wear gloves because there is risk of bleeding from the gums. Wear PPE when necessary. Follow Procedure 14-2, Flossing Teeth.

MOUTH CARE FOR THE UNCONSCIOUS CLIENT

Unconscious clients require frequent mouth care—about every 2 hours. They usually breathe through the mouth and, as a result, have a very dry mouth, tongue, and lips. Because they are unable to drink or swallow, secretions may dry and become crusted, causing odor and providing a place for bacterial growth.

Because these clients cannot swallow, there is a danger of choking and aspiration of fluids into the lungs. To prevent aspiration, place the client in a side-lying position so fluids drain out of the mouth instead of down the throat.

Always explain what you are going to do, and talk to unconscious clients when giving personal care. Clients may be able to hear and understand what is happening, even though they are unable to respond to your communication.

Unconscious clients cannot hold their mouths open during the cleaning procedure. You will need to hold the mouth open by using a padded tongue depressor or a spoon wrapped in gauze. Do not use your fingers because the client may accidentally bite you. Remember, any break in the surface of your skin could permit the entrance of pathogenic organisms and lead to an infection. Wear gloves, and practice standard (universal) precautions.

PROCEDURE 14-1 | Brushing Teeth

Materials Needed
- Toothbrush
- Toothpaste
- Glass of cool water
- Mouthwash (optional)
- Emesis basin or small plastic bowl
- Face towel
- Paper towel
- Disposable gloves
- PPE, as needed

Procedure
1. Explain what you are going to do.
2. Wash hands.
3. Obtain materials listed above.
4. Provide privacy (close door, shut drapes, pull shades).
5. Spread paper towel on work area. Arrange supplies on paper towel.
6. Raise bed to convenient working height. Lower rail on side where you are working.*
7. Assist client to an upright position, or turn on side if unable to sit up.
8. Place face towel under client's chin and over chest.
9. Put on gloves.
10. Assist client with self-care as necessary.
11. Hold toothbrush over emesis basin, and pour a little water over the brush to moisten. Apply the toothpaste.
12. Brush client's teeth and tongue (if he or she is unable to do so) (Figure 14-3, A to D).
13. Have client rinse mouth with water. Hold emesis basin so client can spit into it (Figure 14-4).
14. Have client rinse with mouthwash (optional). Hold emesis basin so client can spit into it.
15. Wipe client's mouth with face towel.
16. Remove face towel.
17. Remove and discard gloves.
18. Make sure client is safe and comfortable.
19. Place bed in lowest position. (Raise side rail, if indicated.)*
20. Clean equipment, and store in proper location.
21. Wipe work surface with paper towel and discard.
22. Place soiled face towel in laundry container to be washed.
23. Wash your hands.
24. Record what you have done. Report any unusual conditions to your supervisor.
    - Bleeding gums
    - Fruity or bad breath
    - Signs of irritation
    - Loose, broken, or chipped teeth
    - Mouth sores

Fig 14-3 Brush client's teeth as shown (Step 12).

Fig 14-4 Hold emesis basin close to client's chin (Step 13).

*Your client may not have an adjustable hospital bed; those steps marked with an asterisk (*) will not apply.

PROCEDURE 14-2 | Flossing Teeth

Materials Needed
- Dental floss dispenser
- Glass of cool water
- Emesis basin or small plastic bowl
- Face towel
- Paper towel
- Disposable gloves
- PPE, as needed

Procedure
1. Explain what you are going to do.
2. Wash your hands.
3. Obtain materials listed above.
4. Provide privacy (close door, shut drapes, pull shades).
5. Spread paper towel on work area. Arrange supplies on paper towel.
6. Raise bed to convenient working height. Lower rail on side where you are working.*
7. Assist client to an upright position, or turn on side if unable to sit up.
8. Place face towel under client's chin and over chest.
9. Put on gloves.
10. Remove 18 inches (44 to 46 centimeters) of floss from dispenser.
11. Wrap floss around the middle finger of each hand to clean upper teeth (Figure 14-5).
12. Hold floss with index fingers to clean lower teeth (Figure 14-6).
13. Insert floss between teeth and use up-and-down, back-and-forth motions to remove any materials between teeth. Proceed from tooth to tooth.
    a. Upper teeth, left to right (Figure 14-7)
    b. Lower teeth, left to right
14. Have client rinse mouth with water. Hold emesis basin so client can spit into it.
15. Wipe client's mouth with face towel.
16. Remove face towel.
17. Remove and discard gloves.
18. Make sure client is safe and comfortable.
19. Place bed in lowest position. (Raise side rail, if indicated.)*
20. Clean equipment, and store in proper location.
21. Wipe work surface with paper towel and discard.
22. Place soiled face towel in laundry container to be washed.
23. Wash your hands.

24. Record what you have done. Report any unusual conditions to your supervisor.
- Bleeding gums
- Gum irritation/sores
- Mouth odor

Fig 14-5 For upper teeth, wrap floss around your middle fingers (Step 11).

Fig 14-6 For lower teeth, hold floss with index fingers (Step 12).

Fig 14-7 Floss teeth in up-and-down, back-and-forth motion (Step 13).

*Your client may not have an adjustable hospital bed; those steps marked with an asterisk (*) will not apply.

Cotton-tipped applicators may be used to clean the surfaces of the mouth. Glycerine swabs are also used, but they can make the mouth feel dry. Sponge (foam) swabs can also be used. Make sure the foam pad is tight on the stick. The client could choke on the pad if it comes off the stick. Clean the mouth and the oral surfaces with mouthwash or normal saline solution. To make normal saline solution, use 1 teaspoon of table salt in 2 cups (500 milliliters) of warm water. Stir to dissolve the salt.

After cleaning, apply a little petroleum jelly or other lubricant to the lips to prevent drying, cracking, and discomfort. If client is receiving oxygen, do not use petroleum jelly. Follow the care plan and instructions from your supervisor regarding any special mouth care needed by your client. See Procedure 14-3, Mouth Care for the Unconscious Client.

DENTURE CARE

Dentures are false teeth that are worn to replace missing natural teeth. A client may have a complete set of false teeth or a partial set. They must be removed from the mouth for thorough cleaning. Any remaining natural teeth are cleaned according to Procedure 14-1. Many clients will be able to clean their own dentures. Gather the supplies needed, and provide assistance as necessary. Dentures are cleaned in the morning and at bedtime and, if necessary, after meals.

Some clients are not able to clean their own dentures. Ask them to remove the dentures and place them in an emesis basin. Sometimes it may be necessary for you to remove the dentures. Wear gloves, and follow the steps listed in Procedure 14-4, Caring for Dentures.

There are important points to remember about denture care.
1. Practice standard (universal) precautions (see Box 14-1, Infection Control Reminders). Wear gloves when handling dentures.
2. Handle dentures very carefully. They are easily broken, and replacement is costly and inconvenient.
3. Use gauze or a clean washcloth to grasp dentures. They are very slippery when wet.
4. Partially fill the sink with warm water to act as a cushion in case you drop the dentures during cleaning.
5. Use warm water to clean dentures. Hot water may damage them.
6. Clean dentures with a toothbrush and toothpaste.

BOX 14-1 Infection Control Reminders

- Use gloves when
    Giving personal care to clients with open sores in mouth or on skin
    Giving perineal care
    Handling clothing, towels, or washcloths soiled with blood or body fluids
    Removing, cleaning, or inserting dentures
    Giving mouth care
    Shaving client with a blade razor
- Wear protective eyewear when giving mouth care or when flossing teeth, if there is risk of splashing or spraying.
- Keep client's clothing, towels, and washcloths off the floor, even when soiled.
- Place soiled clothing in container, and bring to laundry area immediately to be washed.
- Keep client's personal grooming items (e.g., comb, toothbrush, denture box) separate from other family members' items.

PROCEDURE 14-3 Mouth Care for the Unconscious Client

Materials Needed
- Sponge (foam) swabs or cotton-tipped applicators
- Padded tongue depressor
- Glycerine swabs (optional)
- Petroleum jelly or mineral oil for lips (optional)
- Mouthwash
- Glass of cool water
- Emesis basin or small plastic bowl
- Face towel
- Paper towel
- Disposable gloves

Procedure
1. Explain what you are going to do.
2. Wash your hands.
3. Obtain materials listed above.
4. Provide privacy (close door, shut drapes, pull shades).
5. Spread paper towel on work area. Arrange supplies on paper towel.
6. Raise bed to convenient working height. Lower rail on side where you are working.*
7. Place client in a side-lying position.
8. Place face towel and emesis basin under client's chin.
9. Put on gloves.
10. Gently open client's mouth with padded tongue depressor (Figure 14-8).
11. Moisten the swab, and clean all surfaces of mouth: roof of mouth, tongue, gums, lips, inside of cheeks. Rinse and re-wet swab as necessary. Clean teeth with swab (Figure 14-9).
12. Wipe client's mouth with face towel.
13. Remove face towel.
14. Apply lubricant to lips.
15. Remove and discard gloves.
16. Make sure client is safe and comfortable.
17. Place bed in lowest position. (Raise side rail, if indicated.)*
18. Clean equipment, and store in proper location.
19. Wipe work surface with paper towel and discard.
20. Place soiled face towel in laundry container to be washed.
21. Wash your hands.

22. Record what you have done. Report any unusual conditions to your supervisor:
- Mouth sores
- Bleeding gums, lips, or tongue
- Foul odor to breath
- Loose, broken, or chipped teeth

Fig 14-8 **A,** Place two wooden tongue depressors together and wrap gauze around top half. **B,** Tape gauze in place (Step 10).

Fig 14-9 Place client in side-lying position with face towel and emesis basin under chin. Open mouth with padded tongue depressor. Clean all surfaces with swab (Step 11).

*Your client may not have an adjustable hospital bed; those steps marked with an asterisk (*) will not apply.

PROCEDURE 14-4 | Caring for Dentures

Materials Needed
- Toothpaste
- Toothbrush
- Tissues or gauze
- Denture cup or box
- Glass of cool water
- Emesis basin or small plastic bowl
- Paper towel
- Disposable gloves

Procedure
1. Explain what you are going to do.
2. Wash your hands.
3. Obtain materials listed above.
4. Provide privacy (close door, shut drapes, pull shades).
5. Spread paper towel on work area. Arrange supplies on paper towel if procedure will be done at bedside. Otherwise, take supplies for cleaning dentures to sink.
6. Raise bed to convenient working height. Lower rail on side where you are working.*
7. Assist client to an upright position, or turn on side if unable to sit up.
8. Put on gloves.
9. Ask client to remove dentures and place in emesis basin. If you must remove dentures, grasp them with gauze or a tissue (wet dentures are slippery and difficult to grasp). Remove in this manner.
   a. *Upper dentures.* Grasp between thumb and index finger, and move up and down gently until you feel the suction release. Pull down and remove.
   b. *Lower dentures.* Grasp in the same manner, and gently twist sideways and up, lifting them out of the mouth.
10. Assist client to brush dentures. At bedside, client uses water in cup, toothbrush, paste, and so on. At sink, same materials are used.
11. Clean dentures at sink.
    a. Partially fill sink with warm water to act as a cushion, should dentures be accidentally dropped (Figure 14-10, *A*).
    b. Brush with warm water and toothpaste in an up and down motion. Rinse thoroughly (Figure 14-10, *B*).

12. Return dentures to the client for replacement in the mouth, or store in denture cup or box, dry or in solution, according to client's wishes.
13. Remove and discard gloves.
14. Make sure client is safe and comfortable.
15. Place bed in lowest position. (Raise side rail, if indicated.)*
16. Clean equipment, and store in proper location.
17. Wipe work surface with paper towel and discard.
18. Wash your hands.
19. Record what you have done. Report any unusual conditions to your supervisor.
    - Cracked or sharp edges on dentures
    - Loose teeth or broken areas
    - Bleeding gums
    - Foul odor to breath

Fig 14-10 **A,** With toothpaste on brush, hold dentures over sink and brush outside of teeth from side to side and then up and down. **B,** Turn over dentures, and brush insides with an up-and-down motion (Step 11).

*Your client may not have an adjustable hospital bed; those steps marked with an asterisk (*) will not apply.

7. Have client rinse mouth with mouthwash or other solution before replacing the dentures in the mouth.

8. Apply denture adhesive to the false teeth if the client uses this product.

9. Place unworn dentures in a covered denture cup or box, either dry or with solution, according to client's preference. Store in a safe location. Never place dentures in tissues or paper towels because they may be accidentally thrown in the trash.

10. Observe the condition of the client's mouth, and report any unusual findings. Observe the condition of the dentures, and report any cracks, sharp edges, loose teeth, or broken areas.   See Procedure 14-4, Caring for Dentures.

BATHING

Some cultures believe that bathing is a very important part of the healing process. In ancient times, people went to the "baths" to be cured by the warm, soothing waters. Even today, people seek out the soothing, relaxing waters of the spas and mineral baths for relaxation and tension relief. Not all cultures view bathing as particularly helpful during sickness. Some believe that a bath may cause the sick person to become chilled, and, as a result, they may become sicker. If your clients do not want to bathe, try to find out why. They may be afraid of falling in the bathroom, they may have pain, or they may be too tired. **DO NOT FORCE YOUR CLIENT TO BATHE OR CRITICIZE HIM OR HER FOR NOT BATHING. DISCUSS THE SITUATION WITH YOUR SUPERVISOR.**

PURPOSES

The bath has many purposes, including
- Cleansing the skin
- Removing bacteria
- Preventing body odor
- Stimulating circulation
- Moving joints and muscles
- Observing the client's skin (Box 14-2)
- Communicating with the client
- Preventing pressure ulcers
- Providing comfort and a sense of well-being

The frequency of the bath depends on the care plan and the needs of the client. For example, some clients may take a tub bath or shower only twice a week. This includes older adults with very dry skin and clients who are very weak and tire

BOX 14-2	Observing Client's Skin: CHECK FOR
C	Cuts, changes in color (pale, red, blue), cracked
H	Hot to the touch
E	Edema (swelling)
C	Contusions (bruises)
K	Krusty areas, knobby lumps
F	Flaky skin
O	Open sores
R	Redness, rash

easily. Others with limitations, such as those with casts, recent surgical incisions, and traction, will not follow a pattern of daily bathing. Incontinent clients will need to be bathed each time the skin becomes soiled to prevent irritation and breakdown.

GENERAL PRINCIPLES FOR BATHING CLIENTS

There are general principles for bathing clients or assisting them to bathe.
1. Be organized. Have the necessary supplies at hand.
2. Practice standard (universal) precautions when body fluids are present. Wear gloves.
3. Provide privacy. Do not expose the client's body unnecessarily.
4. Prevent chilling. Keep client covered as much as possible, and avoid drafts.
5. Work efficiently.
6. Wash from clean to dirty areas.
7. Change bath water when it becomes too soapy or cool or becomes contaminated with body secretions.
8. Prevent falls by following rules of safety.
9. Use good body mechanics.
10. Keep soap in dish, not in bath water.
11. Encourage client to do as much as possible according to care plan and physical condition.
12. Rinse the skin thoroughly. Wash off soap, which can be drying and irritating.
13. Pat the skin dry. Be gentle.

SKIN CARE PRODUCTS

Many products are available for use on the skin, including the following.
- *Soap* is used to clean the skin. It may be plain, medicated, perfumed, or moisturizing. Plain soap is drying to the skin and is not necessary for every bath. Many older adults have dry skin from aging and may prefer a soap that contains a moisturizer. Use the soap preferred by your client, unless the care plan lists a special product to be used.
- *Bath oil* is placed in the bath water to soften the skin and prevent drying. However, this product can make the tub and client's skin very slippery, increasing the risk of falls. In addition, it is very difficult to clean bath oil from the tub surfaces. Avoid the use of bath oil for your client. Instead, apply a cream or lotion to the skin after the bath.
- *Creams and lotions* are applied to soften the skin and prevent drying. Encourage clients to put on the lotion or cream themselves. Assist them by applying the product to areas they cannot reach. Warm the lotion between your hands before applying to the skin. Gently apply lotion to the surface of the skin. Do not massage or rub in vigorously. Use a small amount, and remove any excess cream or lotion with a towel. Too much lotion makes the skin feel hot and sticky, which is uncomfortable for the client. It may also provide a place for bacteria to live and grow. Use the lotion preferred by your client, unless the care plan lists a special product to be used.
- *Powder* is used to soothe and cool the skin and to prevent friction between two skin surfaces. Do not use a lot of powder but just enough to have a thin layer on the skin. Do not combine powder with creams and lotion; this will cause the powder to crust and cake on the skin, causing irritation and risk of infection. Do not shake powder in the air because inhaled particles may irritate the respiratory tract and cause sneezing.

• *Deodorant* is used to prevent body odor. *Antiperspirants* help stop sweating and reduce body odor. They are applied to the armpits after bathing. Do not apply to irritated or broken skin.

TYPES OF BATHS

Complete Bed Bath

The complete bed bath is given to clients who are unable to get out of bed to bathe themselves. Unconscious, paralyzed, or very weak clients may need to be bathed in bed. Those with casts will not be able to use the tub or shower and may need a bed bath.

Encourage clients to do as much as they can to care for themselves during the bed bath. Check the care plan with your supervisor to determine the level of activity permitted for the client. The complete bed bath may be embarrassing to the client and increase his or her feelings of dependence. Provide privacy, work quickly and efficiently, and talk to the client as you perform the bed bath. Follow the general principles for bathing clients listed earlier and in Procedure 14-5, Giving a Complete Bed Bath.

Partial Bath

In a partial bath, the face, hands, underarms, back, buttocks, and genitalia are washed. This may be done in bed or at the bedside. A partial bath may also be given in the bathroom, at the sink, if this is listed in the care plan. Assemble all of the materials needed for bathing. Oral hygiene may also be done at this time. Place a straight chair in front of the sink so the client can sit while bathing. Help the client as needed. Dressing and grooming are usually done at the bedside.

PROCEDURE 14-5   Giving a Complete Bed Bath

Materials Needed
• Washbasin
• Soap dish and soap
• Orangewood stick (optional)
• Bath blanket (optional)
• Washcloth
• Face towel
• Bath towels (2)
• Paper towels
• Clean clothing (gown, pajamas, or other clothing)
• Oral hygiene materials
• Brush and/or comb
• Other articles used by client (e.g., deodorant, body powder or lotion)
• Disposable gloves

Procedure
1. Explain what you are going to do.
2. Wash your hands.
3. Obtain materials listed above.
4. Provide privacy (close door, shut drapes, pull shades).
5. Raise bed to convenient working height, and lock wheels. Lower rail on side where you are working.*

6. Offer bedpan or urinal (see Procedures 15-1 and 15-2).
7. Lower head of bed to a level comfortable for client, as low as possible.
8. Remove top bedding, and cover client with bath blanket or top sheet.
9. Help client to remove clothing, if needed.
10. Help client to move to side of bed near you.
11. Help client with oral hygiene, if needed.
12. Fill washbasin two-thirds full with warm water (109° to 115° F) (43° to 46° C).
13. Place towel under client's head and a towel over client's chest.
14. Make a mitt with washcloth (Figure 14-11) to be used throughout procedure.
15. Wash eye areas gently with clean water only. Start from inner corner of eye to outer corner of eye. Use opposite corners of washcloth for each eye (Figure 14-12).
16. Ask client if you should use soap or cleansing cream for cleansing the face.
17. Wash face from center outward. Use firm, gentle movements.
18. Wash ears and neck. Rinse and dry using towel on client's chest.

---

*Your client may not have an adjustable hospital bed; those steps marked with a single asterisk (*) will not apply.

PROCEDURE 14-5   Giving a Complete Bed Bath—cont'd

Fig 14-11 Making a washcloth mitt. **A,** Place hand under lower-right corner of washcloth. **B,** Secure washcloth with thumb, and wrap around back of hand. **C,** Continue to fold washcloth over palm of hand, and secure with thumb. **D,** Fold top of washcloth down, and tuck it under the bottom (Step 14).

Fig 14-12 Wash eye, starting from inner corner to outer corner (Step 15).

Fig 14-13 Place client's hand in basin (Step 20).

19. Put a towel, lengthwise, under the arm and a towel near hand on which to place the washbasin.
20. Place client's hand in basin (Figure 14-13); allow it to soak. Wash the arm and armpit (Figure 14-14).
21. Wash, rinse, and dry arm, armpit, and hand. Apply deodorant under arm, if requested. Push back cuticles; clean under nails with orangewood stick. Dry between fingers thoroughly.
22. Follow Steps 19 to 21 for the other arm and hand.
23. Place basin back on bedside table or chair.
24. Put towel over chest and abdomen. Pull bath blanket (top sheet) to thighs (Figure 14-15). Do not expose client when washing chest and abdomen.

Fig 14-14 Wash arm (Step 20).

Continued

PROCEDURE 14-5 Giving a Complete Bed Bath—cont'd

Fig 14-15 Cover chest with a towel (Step 24).

Fig 14-16 Put client's foot in basin while you wash the leg (Step 27).

25. Wash, rinse, and dry chest and abdomen. Cover chest and abdomen with bath blanket (top sheet). Remove towel.
26. Uncover leg. Do not expose genital area. Place towel under the leg and foot. Place another towel near foot, and put basin on towel.
27. Bend client's knee, and put foot in basin; allow it to soak. Wash and dry leg while foot is soaking (Figure 14-16).
28. Wash and dry foot. Clean under toenails. Dry between toes thoroughly.
29. Repeat Steps 26 to 28 for other leg and foot.
30. Place basin back on bedside table or chair.
31. Turn client on side: drape bath blanket (top sheet) to expose back and buttocks.
32. Place towel on bed, tucked lengthwise along neck and shoulders to buttocks.
33. Wash, rinse, and dry neck, shoulders, back, and buttocks. Work from neck to buttocks. Use long strokes for washing the back (Figure 14-17).
34. Give back rub (Procedure 14-7).
35. Change bath water.
36. Turn client on back.
37. Place towel under buttocks. Place basin, soap, and towels within reach. Have client wash genital and rectal areas. Ask client to tell you when finished. If client is unable to wash these areas, complete this part of the bath wearing disposable gloves (Procedure 14-8).
38. Help client to put on gown, pajamas, or other clothing.

Fig 14-17 Wash back from neck to buttocks (Step 33).

39. Comb or brush client's hair (Procedure 14-10).
40. Make sure client is safe and comfortable.
41. Place bed in lowest position. (Raise side rails, if indicated.)*
42. Empty and clean washbasin. Wipe off work area with paper towels and discard them. Place soiled towels and washcloth in laundry container to be washed. Return other supplies to their proper places.
43. Wash your hands.
44. Record what you have done. Report any unusual conditions to your supervisor such as those listed in Box 14-2.

*Your client may not have an adjustable hospital bed; those steps marked with a single asterisk (*) will not apply.

BOX 14-3 Bath and Shower Safety

- Always place rubber or nonskid mat in tub before client enters.
- Be sure bathroom floor is dry to help prevent slips and falls.
- Do not add oil to bathtub water; apply oil to client's skin after the bath.
- Be sure bath water is the proper temperature; adjust water pressure before giving a shower.
- Stay near bathroom while client is bathing.
- Use good body mechanics.
- Be sure bath or shower chairs have rubber suction cups at ends of legs; these will steady the chair and prevent it from sliding.
- Have client use grab bars, if present; do not permit client to use towel bar or tile soap dish as an aid in moving.

Tub Bath

A tub bath is relaxing and soothing, but it can also be a risky procedure because of the danger of burns, falls, and chills. Always make sure there is a rubber mat or nonslip surface in the tub (Box 14-3, Bath and Shower Safety). Tub baths can also cause clients to become weak and tired. The bath should not be any longer than 20 minutes. Tub baths are drying to the skin and are usually given once or twice a week, with partial bathing in between. **NEVER GIVE A TUB BATH UNLESS IT IS WRITTEN IN THE CARE PLAN.** Follow Procedure 14-6, Giving a Tub Bath. Remember to use good body mechanics and be extremely careful when transferring clients into and out of the tub.

No Water Bath

This is a product that comes in a plastic bag. Disposable washcloths are warmed in the microwave oven and used for bathing. Follow the manufacturer's instructions.

Shower

Some clients will prefer a shower to a tub bath. Some homes have bathrooms with shower stalls and/or hand-held shower attachments. It will be easier for the client to step into the shower stall than into a bathtub. There are some important points to keep in mind when helping the client with the shower.

- Obtain necessary materials as listed in Procedure 14-6, Giving a Tub Bath.
- Check to be sure shower chair, if one will be used, is secure and steady.
- Place nonskid mat on shower floor without blocking the drain.
- Turn on water; test and adjust water temperature (109° F or 43° C) and water pressure before client enters the shower.
- Encourage client to use grab bars, if installed, when getting in and out of the shower or tub. Some clients may use a transfer tub bench (Figure 14-18). Assist client to slide along the bench to inside the tub. If needed, assist client to swing legs into the tub.
- If required, assist client to get wet, then turn off water before applying soap to skin; turn on water again to rinse off.
- Avoid chilling; keep the bathroom door and shower curtains closed as much as possible.
- Encourage client to bathe self as much as possible, but give help when needed.
- Use aids to showering, such as soap-on-a-rope and a long-handled back brush or sponge if available.
- Stay with client during entire procedure, if necessary.
- Even if client is able to bathe self, remain close to bathroom so that you will hear if the client calls for help.

Fig 14-18 A transfer bench can be used to help client take a shower. (Courtesy North Coast Medical, Inc., Morgan Hill, California.)

PROCEDURE 14-6   Giving a Tub Bath

Materials Needed
- Soap
- Washcloth
- Bath towels (2)
- Straight chair (optional)
- Slide board (optional)
- Skid-proof bath mat
- Other articles used by client (e.g., deodorant, body powder, lotion)
- Clean clothing
- Disposable gloves, if needed

Procedure
1. Explain what you are going to do.
2. Wash your hands.
3. Obtain materials listed above.
4. Prepare bathroom by placing skid-proof mat on bottom of tub, making sure room is warm and free of drafts, and placing straight chair in bathroom.
5. Provide privacy (close door, shut drapes, pull shades).
6. Help client to undress, put on bathrobe and footwear. Place client in wheelchair, if used. Lock brakes and put footrests in place.
7. Fill tub one-third full of warm water (109° to 115° F) (43° to 46° C).
8. Help client to bathroom and close door.
9. Place client in chair facing tub. If using wheelchair, lock brakes and place footrests out of the way.
10. Help client to lift one foot, then the other over the side of the tub (Figure 14-19).
11. Help client to lower into water, using grab bars for support.
12. Help client to bathe as needed.

Fig 14-19 Assist client into tub (Step 10).

PROCEDURE 14-6	**Giving a Tub Bath—cont'd**

13. Drain water from tub before getting client out of tub.
14. Help client to dry body. Assist client to put on bathrobe, or cover with dry towel.
15. Place straight chair or wheelchair facing tub and place dry towel on side of tub.
16. Help client to sit on towel on side of tub using grab bars. (Reverse Steps 10 and 11.)
17. Help client to stand, get out of tub into straight chair or wheelchair, and put on footwear.
18. Help client to room.
19. Give back rub.
20. Help client to put on clean clothing and return to bed, sofa, and so on. Place in comfortable position.
21. Make sure client is safe and comfortable.
22. Return to bathroom. Clean tub and straighten area.
23. Place soiled towels and washcloth in laundry container to be washed.
24. Wash your hands.
25. Record what you have done. Report any unusual conditions to your supervisor (see Box 14-2).

- Help client to slowly get out of shower. Do not rush. The risk of falling on wet surfaces is great.
- Help client to completely dry off and put on robe or wrap up in bath sheet or large towel. Dressing and grooming may be done at the bedside. NEVER GIVE A SHOWER UNLESS IT IS WRITTEN IN THE CARE PLAN.

BACK RUB

The back rub involves applying lotion to the client's back in long, firm strokes from the buttocks to the shoulders. The back rub has several purposes:
- Stimulates circulation
- Provides relaxation and comfort
- Prevents pressure ulcers

Back rubs are given after the bath and at bedtime. Lotion is used to prevent friction and to soften the skin. Do not use too much. Wipe off any excess with a towel. Do not use alcohol because it is drying and can cause the client to become chilled. Warm lotion between your hands. When giving the back rub, be sure to observe the back and buttocks for any unusual findings. Report them to your supervisor.

The care plan will tell you if there is a reason not to give a back rub. Follow Procedure 14-7, Giving a Back Rub.

PERINEAL CARE

Perineal care refers to cleaning the perineum, the area between the legs. Sometimes the client will refer to this as "washing the privates," "the crotch," or "between the legs." In medical terms, this procedure is also known as *pericare*.

Perineal care is done at least once daily, usually during the bath. Some clients will require more frequent perineal care. These clients include women who have just had a baby and clients who are incontinent. Check the care plan to be sure about the frequency.

Most clients will be able to perform their own perineal care. If not, it is the responsibility of the home care aide. This can be embarrassing for both the client and the aide, because it is a very personal and intimate procedure. Protect the client's privacy, and work quickly, efficiently, and as calmly as possible.

Wear disposable gloves, and always practice standard (universal) precautions. Wear other personal protective equipment as needed. Wash from the cleanest area to the dirtiest area. The urinary meatus is a clean area. Wipe away from this structure toward

PROCEDURE 14-7   Giving a Back Rub

Materials Needed
- Small towel
- Lotion

Procedure
1. Explain what you are going to do.
2. Wash your hands.
3. Obtain materials listed above.
4. Provide privacy (close door, shut drapes, pull shades).
5. Raise bed to convenient working height, and lock wheels. Lower rail on side where you are working.*
6. Lower head of bed to a level comfortable for client, as low as possible.
7. Remove clothing from upper body.
8. Place client on side or abdomen to expose entire back.
9. Put small amount of lotion on your hands. Rub hands together to warm lotion.
10. Use correct body mechanics. Face head of bed, one foot slightly forward, knees bent.
11. Start at the lower back moving upward toward the shoulders. Apply pressure using palms of both hands. Use long, firm but gentle strokes: up, out, and down. Repeat several times (Figure 14-20).
12. Remove excess lotion with towel.
13. Help client to put on clothes.
14. Make sure client is safe and comfortable.
15. Place bed in lowest position. (Raise side rail, if indicated.)*
16. Wash your hands.
17. Record what you have done. Report location and size of any reddened areas or other unusual conditions to your supervisor.

Fig 14-20 Use long, firm but gentle strokes (Step 11).

*Your client may not have an adjustable hospital bed; those steps marked with an asterisk (*) will not apply.

the anus. The perineal area is very sensitive and easily injured. Be gentle. Rinse thoroughly because any remaining soap is extremely irritating to the perineum. Follow Procedure 14-8, Giving Perineal Care.

GROOMING

CARING FOR HANDS AND FEET

Hands and feet need special attention to prevent infection, skin breakdown, odor, and injury. Hand and foot care can be given as part of the bath, or the care plan will give directions for giving care at another time. Some clients have foot problems that require special attention. In these cases, a podiatrist, a doctor trained in the treatment of nail or foot problems, will give the care.

Caring for the hands and feet gives the home care aide a chance to observe the condition of the skin and nails. Record and report the following conditions:

ORR

PROCEDURE 14-8 Giving Perineal Care

Materials Needed

- Washbasin
- Soap dish and soap
- Washcloths (5 or 6) or package of cotton balls or disposable washcloths
- Bath towel
- Waterproof protector pad
- Paper or plastic bag
- Paper towels
- Toilet tissue
- Disposable gloves

Procedure

1. Explain what you are going to do.
2. Wash your hands.
3. Obtain materials listed above.
4. Spread paper towel on work area. Arrange supplies on paper towel.
5. Provide privacy (close door, shut drapes, pull shades).
6. Raise bed to convenient working height. Lower rail on side where you are working.*
7. Fold top bedding to foot of bed and cover client with sheet or blanket.
8. Help client into supine position, and remove clothing from waist down.
9. Position waterproof protector pad under buttocks.
10. Drape the client (Figure 14-21, A and B).
11. Raise side rail.*
12. Fill washbasin two-thirds full with warm water (105° to 110° F) (41° to 43° C).

13. Place basin on work area on top of paper towels.
14. Lower rail on side where you are working.*
15. Fold back the corner of blanket or sheet between client's legs and onto abdomen.
16. Help client to bend knees and spread legs.
17. Put on disposable gloves.
18. Apply soap and water to the washcloth or cotton balls.
19. Give female perineal care.
    a. Separate labia.
    b. Clean downward, with one stroke, from front to back. Use clean washcloth or cotton ball for each stroke. Put used cotton balls in bag, or set aside used washcloths. Repeat this step until area is clean (Figure 14-22).
    c. Rinse area, using same procedure as in Steps 19a and 19b.
    d. Dry area thoroughly.
    e. Fold blanket back between client's legs.
    f. Help client to straighten legs and turn on side away from you.
    g. Separate buttocks and clean rectal area with toilet tissue, if needed (Figure 14-23). Wash area from vagina to anus, using clean

Fig 14-22 Clean in a downward motion, front to back (Step 19b).

Fig 14-21 **A,** Position bath blanket or sheet like a diamond. **B,** Wrap blanket around leg by bringing the corner around under leg and over the top. Tuck corner under the hip.

Fig 14-23 Wash rectal area from vagina to anus (Step 19g).

*Your client may not have an adjustable hospital bed; those steps marked with a single asterisk (*) will not apply. *Continued*

PROCEDURE 14-8   Giving Perineal Care—cont'd

washcloth for each stroke. Repeat this step until area is clean.
h. Rinse area, using same procedure as in Step 19g.
i. Dry area.
20. Give male perineal care.
   a. Gently pull back the foreskin, if client is uncircumcised (Figure 14-24).
   b. While holding penis, clean tip, using circular motion. Start at the urethral opening and work outward. Repeat this step, using a clean washcloth or cotton ball, until the area is clean (Figure 14-25). Put used cotton balls in bag, or set aside used washcloths.
   c. Rinse and dry area thoroughly, using same procedure as Steps 20a and 20b.
   d. Return foreskin to natural position if client is uncircumcised.
   e. Clean shaft of penis using a washcloth with firm but gentle downward strokes. Rinse and dry area thoroughly.
   f. Help client to bend knees and spread legs.
   g. Gently clean scrotum. Wash skin folds carefully. Rinse and dry area thoroughly.
   h. Help client to straighten legs and turn on side away from you.

   i. Separate buttocks, and clean rectal area with toilet tissue, if needed. Wash from scrotum to anus using clean washcloth for each stroke. Repeat this step until area is clean.
   j. Rinse area using same procedure as in Step 20i.
   k. Dry area.
21. Remove soiled bedding, washcloths, and waterproof protector pad, and place in laundry container to be washed.
22. Remove gloves and discard into bag.
23. Straighten bedding; remove sheet or blanket.
24. Make sure client is safe and comfortable.
25. Place bed in lowest position. (Raise side rail, if indicated.)*
26. Empty and clean washbasin. Wipe off work area with paper towels, and discard into bag. Return other materials to their proper place.
27. Wash your hands.
28. Record what you have done. Report any unusual conditions to your supervisor.
   • Redness or irritation of the perineum
   • Drainage from urinary meatus, rectum, or vagina
   • Bruises or rash
   • Odor

Fig 14-24 Gently pull back foreskin (Step 20a).

Fig 14-25 Clean tip of penis in circular motion (Step 20b).

*Your client may not have an adjustable hospital bed; those steps marked with a single asterisk (*) will not apply.

   • Sores, swelling, bruises, or reddened areas on hands and feet and between fingers and toes
   • Changes in coloring of skin and nails
   • Change in temperature of hands and feet: hot or cold to touch.
   IT IS NOT THE HOME CARE AIDE'S RESPONSIBILITY TO CUT THE CLIENT'S NAILS. CUTTING THICK NAILS MAY CAUSE THE NAIL CLIPPER TO SLIP AND ACCIDENTALLY CUT THE SKIN AROUND THE NAIL. THIS CAN BE VERY SERIOUS FOR CLIENTS WHO HEAL VERY SLOWLY OR ARE PRONE TO INFECTION. CHECK WITH YOUR SUPERVISOR ABOUT THE AGENCY'S POLICY ABOUT CUTTING NAILS. Follow Procedure 14-9, Caring for Nails and Feet.

PROCEDURE 14-9 Caring for Nails and Feet

Materials Needed
- Paper towels
- Washbasin
- Emesis basin or small plastic bowl
- Washcloth
- Small towel
- Emery board or nail file
- Bath mat or newspapers
- Orangewood stick (optional)
- Pumice stone (optional)
- Disposable gloves (optional)
- Hand lotion (optional)

Procedure
1. Explain what you are going to do.
2. Wash your hands.
3. Obtain materials listed above.
4. Spread paper towel on work area. Arrange materials on paper towel.
5. Provide privacy (close door, shut drapes, pull shades).
6. Help client into chair or to side of bed.
7. Assist client to remove footwear, if appropriate.
8. Put bath mat, towel, or newspapers under feet.
9. Fill basin with water (100° to 110° F) (38° to 43° C).
10. Place basin on bath mat. Put on gloves (optional). Help client put feet in basin.
11. Allow feet to soak for 10 minutes. Add warm water as needed.
12. Place table or ironing board in front of client at convenient height and close to client. Cover table with hand towel or paper towels (Figure 14-26).
13. Fill emesis basin or small bowl with water (100° to 110° F) (38° to 43° C). Put client's fingers in basin, and soak for 2 to 3 minutes.
14. Clean under fingernails with orangewood stick. Dry fingers thoroughly, and set basin aside.
15. Shape fingernails with emery board or nail file. Push back cuticles gently with washcloth or orangewood stick. Apply hand lotion (optional).
16. Remove table.
17. Remove one foot from basin. Smooth any calloused areas using washcloth or pumice stone.

Dry foot and between the toes thoroughly. Repeat procedure for other foot. Apply lotion, as needed.
18. Remove gloves, if worn, and discard in paper bag.
19. Help client to put on footwear, or help back to bed.
20. Clean equipment, and store in proper location. Discard disposable supplies.
21. Place soiled towels in laundry container to be washed.
22. Wash your hands.
23. Record what you have done. Report any unusual conditions to your supervisor.
   - Sores, swelling, bruises, or redness on hands or feet and between fingers and toes
   - Change in skin temperature or color

Fig 14-26 Place table or ironing board at convenient height (Step 12).

HAIR CARE

Some clients may not be able to do hair care themselves. They will need assistance to brush, comb, wash, and style hair. Hair care is done to:
- Clean the hair and scalp
- Stimulate circulation to the scalp

- Help the client look attractive
- Provide a sense of well-being and comfort

Brushing and Combing

Part the hair, dividing it into at least four sections. Brush from root to end, one section at a time. Follow by combing hair. Encourage clients to do as much of their own hair care as possible. This provides good exercise for the shoulders and upper arms. Follow the care plan, and assist when necessary. Never cut clients' hair, even if there are tangles. Long hair may be braided. Some barbers and beauticians make home visits to groom, cut, and style hair. A family member should be able to arrange for this service. If not, notify your supervisor about your client's wishes.

Hair care is usually done twice daily, once in the morning (usually with the bath or shower) and again at bedtime. However, hair care can be done at any time convenient for the aide and client. Curly, kinky hair may be very dry. You may need to apply oil to the hair before you can brush and comb it. Always ask clients how they care for their hair and what they would like you to do. Some women will have elaborate braids that are left in the hair for several months. In this case, you will need to learn how to wash and care for the scalp from your client and/or a family member. Again, follow the care plan.

ORR Observe the scalp for any scaling, crusting, irritation, bruises, bleeding, lumps, or large areas of missing hair. Report these observations to your supervisor. See Procedure 14-10, Assisting Client with Hair Care.

PROCEDURE 14-10 | Assisting Client With Hair Care

Materials Needed
- Brush
- Comb
- Bath towel
- Other grooming supplies—hair spray, oil, hair tonic (optional)
- Hair pins, barrettes, and so on (optional)
- Mirror (optional)

Procedure
1. Explain what you are going to do.
2. Wash your hands.
3. Obtain materials listed above.
4. Provide privacy (close door, shut drapes, pull shades).
5. Raise bed to convenient working height. Lower rail on side where you are working.*
6. Place client in upright position in bed or in chair, if possible.
7. Place bath towel around client's shoulders. If the client is in bed, place towel under head to cover the pillow.
8. Part hair and separate into sections (Figure 14-27).
9. Brush hair, section by section, working from the root to end of hair (Figure 14-28).

10. Arrange hair according to client's wishes.
11. Remove towel.
12. Make sure client is safe and comfortable.
13. Place bed in lowest position.*
14. Clean supplies, and store in proper location.
15. Place soiled bath towel in laundry container to be washed.
16. Wash your hands.
17. Record what you have done. Report any unusual conditions to your supervisor.
    - Changes in scalp
    - Large areas of missing hair (not baldness)

Fig 14-27 Separate hair into sections (Step 8). Fig 14-28 Brush from root to end of hair (Step 9).

*Your client may not have an adjustable hospital bed; those steps marked with an asterisk (*) will not apply.

Shampooing

Clients may wish to have their hair washed two or three times a week. Some people wash their hair daily. Hair can be washed in bed, at the sink in the kitchen or bathroom, or as part of the shower. Check the care plan to see where and how often the shampoo is to be done. If you are giving a shampoo in the tub, wash the hair last so the client does not have dripping wet hair while bathing. If you are shampooing at the sink, have the client sit in a chair with his/her back to the sink. For a bed shampoo, you will need a plastic trough that drains the water away from the bed. See Procedure 14-11, Giving a Shampoo. A dry shampoo may also be used. Follow instructions on the container.

SHAVING

Men usually shave their beards daily. Women may shave their legs and underarms when necessary. Most clients will shave themselves. This provides good exercise for the shoulders and upper arms. Assist clients, as necessary, according to the care plan.

Electric or blade razors may be used. CORDED (PLUG IN) ELECTRIC RAZORS SHOULD NOT BE USED WHEN THE CLIENT IS RECEIVING OXYGEN BECAUSE THERE IS DANGER THAT AN ELECTRICAL SPARK COULD CAUSE A FIRE. Rechargable electric razors may be used. Blade razors should not be used when the client is taking certain types of medications because of danger of bleeding or infection. Wear disposable gloves when using a blade razor to shave a client.

Soften facial hairs with warm water before shaving. Beards and moustaches should be washed with soap and water, dried, and brushed or combed. Check with the client regarding any special care for facial hair. Trimming may be done by the client with special clippers, or the barber may visit.

Shaving may be done at the sink, bedside, or in bed. Gather all materials needed, and place within the client's reach. Follow Procedure 14-12, Shaving the Male Client.

CARING FOR EYEGLASSES, CONTACT LENSES, AND HEARING AIDS

Eyeglasses

Some people need glasses to read; others need them every minute of the day to see. Be careful when handling glasses; they are very expensive and break easily. Clean glasses with soap and cool water or lens cleaner, and dry them with a soft tissue. Unworn glasses should be stored in an eyeglass case that is always kept in the same location.

Contact Lenses

Contact lenses are worn directly on the surface of the eye. Some lenses require special cleaning and storage; other lenses are disposable and need no special care. Clients usually care for their own lenses.

Hearing Aids

Most hearing aids operate on batteries that must be replaced as needed. Also, hearing aids need to be turned on to work. Very tiny aids are worn in the ear canal (Figure 14-31, A). Some clients may wear a disposable hearing aid. These are worn in the ear canal and last for several months (Figure 14-31, B). There are no batteries to be replaced; the aids themselves are replaced when necessary. Behind-the-ear hearing aids have two parts: an ear mold and a behind-the-ear battery and control portion (Figure 14-31, C).

PROCEDURE 14-11   Giving a Shampoo

Materials Needed
- Shampoo
- Conditioner, optional
- Comb
- Brush
- Bath towel
- Washcloth (folded)
- Handheld shower attachment
- Hair dryer
- For bed shampoo
  Waterproof bed protector
  Trough
  Basin or bucket
  Pitcher of warm water

Procedure
1. Explain what you are going to do.
2. Wash your hands.
3. Obtain materials listed above.
4. Provide privacy (close door, shut drapes, pull shades). Remove eyeglasses, hearing aids. Store properly.
5. Raise bed to convenient working height. Lower rail on side where you are working.*
6. Position client for shampoo—at sink, in tub or shower, or in bed with trough under head and neck (Figure 14-29, A and B).
7. Brush and comb hair.
8. Have client hold folded washcloth over eyes to protect from shampoo.
9. Wet hair, from front to back, with warm water (100° F) (38° C).
10. Put a small amount of shampoo in palm of your hand.
11. Apply shampoo to scalp; lather from front to back, rubbing gently.
12. Rinse thoroughly with warm water.
13. Repeat Steps 10 to 12.
14. Apply conditioner, according to directions, as desired.
    (CAUTION: Conditioner can make the bottom of the tub slippery. Rinse conditioner down drain before assisting client to step out of tub.)
15. Wrap client's head in bath towel.
16. Bath/shower stall: Help client out, and assist with drying body and hair.
17. Bed shampoo: Remove trough from bed. Towel-dry hair.
18. Dry hair using dryer, if available. Arrange hair according to client's wishes.
19. Make sure client is safe and comfortable. Replace eyeglasses and hearing aids, if appropriate.
20. Place bed in lowest position. (Raise side rail, if indicated.)*
21. Clean materials, and store in proper location.
22. Place soiled bath towel in laundry container to be washed.
23. Wash your hands.
24. Record what you have done. Report any unusual conditions to your supervisor.
    - Sores on scalp
    - Redness

Fig 14-29 **A,** Firm, plastic trough. **B,** Inflatable trough (Step 6).

*Your client may not have an adjustable hospital bed; those steps marked with an asterisk (*) will not apply.

PROCEDURE 14-12   Shaving the Male Client

Materials Needed

- Razor (blade or electric)
- Shaving cream or soap (for blade razor)
- Shaving brush (optional)
- Mirror
- Aftershave lotion
- Tissues
- Bath towel
- Face towel
- Washcloth
- Washbasin or sink
- Warm water (for blade razor)
- Disposable gloves

Procedure

1. Explain what you are going to do.
2. Wash your hands.
3. Obtain materials listed above.
4. Provide privacy (close door, shut drapes, pull shades).
5. Raise bed to convenient working height. Lower rail on side where you are working.*
6. Place client in an upright position in bed (or assist to sit by bathroom sink, if possible).
7. Shaving with a blade razor
   a. Put on disposable gloves.
   b. Wet washcloth with warm water (115° F) (46° C). Place on client's face for a few minutes. Remove.
   c. Apply shaving cream, and lather the face.
   d. Hold the skin taut, and shave in the direction of hair growth (Figure 14-30).
   e. Rinse the blade razor when necessary.
   f. Rinse skin, and dry with towel.
   g. Assist client to apply aftershave lotion (optional).
8. Shaving with an electric razor
   a. Put on disposable gloves.
   b. Make sure face is clean and dry. Do not apply shaving cream or water to the face.
   c. Turn on razor.
   d. Hold skin taut, and shave in the direction of hair growth.
   e. Turn off razor.
   f. Assist client to apply aftershave lotion (optional)
9. Remove towel.
10. Remove and discard gloves.
11. Make sure client is safe and comfortable.
12. Place bed in lowest position. (Raise side rail, if indicated.)*
13. Clean materials, and store in proper location.
14. Place soiled bath towel in laundry container.
15. Wash your hands.
16. Record what you have done. Report any unusual conditions to your supervisor.

Fig 14-30 Shave in direction of hair growth (Step 7d).

*Your client may not have an adjustable hospital bed; those steps marked with an asterisk (*) will not apply.

When caring for clients' hearing aids
- Do not let any liquid get into the hearing aid; keep the battery section dry.
- Handle gently; hearing aids are fragile.
- Remove before shampooing, using a hair dryer, or applying hair spray.
- Clean gently with dry tissue or damp cloth. Use special tool to remove ear wax from disposable aids.
- Ear wax may be removed from ear molds of behind-the-ear aids with an applicator dampened with water and a little soap.

Fig 14-31 Hearing aids. **A,** In-the-ear hearing aid. **B,** Disposable in-the-ear hearing aid. **C,** Behind-the-ear hearing aid.

Fig 14-32 **A,** Long-handled shoehorn reduces bending and discomfort. **B,** Clothing with Velcro makes it easy to undress.

Hearing aids are very expensive and difficult to fit. Handle carefully, and do not drop them. Store them in the special container provided, and keep in the same location.

HELPING THE CLIENT TO DRESS AND UNDRESS

When clients dress in regular clothing, rather than in bedclothes, during the day, they usually feel better. Being dressed and well groomed contributes to one's self-esteem. To some, it is a sign of getting back to the normal routines of daily life. Most clients will need some help with dressing and undressing. Some will only need their clothing placed within easy reach, so that they can dress themselves without any further help. Others will need more help. Clothing for clients who need help to dress should be easy to put on and take off, such as shirts or dresses with zippers, snaps, or Velcro, instead of buttons.

Special Aids to Help with Dressing

There are special aids that can be used to help make dressing easier. A long-handled shoehorn (Figure 14-32, *A*) allows the person to put on shoes without bending over.

Elastic shoelaces make it easier to slip the foot into or out of the shoe without tying or untying the shoelaces. Velcro strips sewn on garment closures eliminate the need to button and unbutton shirts, pants, and trousers (Figure 14-32, *B*). The occupational therapist may teach the client ways to make dressing easier with the use of these and other special aids.

Preparing to Dress the Client

It is important to ask the client what he or she wants to wear, whenever possible. Choosing what to wear gives the client a sense of being in control. Clothes should be
- Easy to put on and take off
- Comfortable, not too tight or binding
- The correct size (or one size larger) for ease in dressing
- Suitable for the home environment
- Suitable for weather conditions, if client is going outdoors
  The following guidelines should be followed when helping the client to dress.
- Lay out clothing in proper order according to client's dressing practices (underwear first, then outer wear, socks, and shoes).
- Follow client's dressing practices when helping to put on clothing.
- Encourage client to dress himself or herself, as much as possible.
- Do not rush; getting dressed can be hard work; muscles stretch and joints bend with each movement.
- Put clothing on weak side first.
- Remove clothing from strong side first.
  Follow Procedure 14-13, Helping Client to Dress, and Procedure 14-14, Helping Client With an Intravenous (IV) Line to Remove Used Clothing and Apply Clean Clothing.

RANGE-OF-MOTION EXERCISES

In Chapter 5, the types of body joints were described. Each joint performs a certain movement. Hinge joints, such as the elbow and knee, cause movement back and forth. Ball and socket joints, such as the shoulder and hip, cause a circular movement. Joints move because muscles are attached by means of tendons.

Range-of-motion (ROM) exercise means moving the joint through the desired motion. During an illness, the body is usually not as active, so the muscles and joints may not be used as much. If a joint is not moved through its normal ROM, the muscles weaken. Then the joint stiffens and, with time, cannot move. This condition is called a *contracture*. To prevent this from happening, muscles need to be exercised, and joints need to be moved through their normal ROM. ROM exercises help to improve muscle tone, increase circulation, and prevent deformities. An excellent time to perform these exercises is during bathing.

There are two main types of ROM exercises.
1. Active: The client performs the exercise without help.
2. Passive: The home care aide moves the body part without help from the client.

The care plan will indicate the exercise to be done and how frequently each exercise is to be repeated. Head and neck exercises are usually not performed by the home care aide. Also, hip exercises for older adults and small children are usually done by the physical therapist or nurse because of the danger of injury to the client. The following are important points to remember when helping with ROM exercises.
- Support the body part being moved above and below the joint.
- Move the part in a slow, steady manner.
- Move the joint through as complete a range as possible.

PROCEDURE 14-13   Helping Client to Dress

Materials Needed
- Outer clothing
- Underwear
- Socks
- Shoes

Procedure
1. Explain what you are going to do.
2. Wash your hands.
3. Obtain materials listed above.
4. Arrange clothing in order of use.
5. Provide privacy (close door, shut drapes, pull shades).
6. Lower bed to lowest position. Lower rail on side where you are working.*
7. Help client to sit on side of bed, if possible. If client must stay in bed, place in supine position.
8. Help client to put on undershirt or bra, shirt, or pajama top.
   a. Over-the-head-type garment: Place injured arm into garment first (Figure 14-33). Pull neck of garment over client's head. Guide other arm into garment.
   b. Front-button or zipping type garment: Place injured arm through sleeve first. Bring shirt to the back of client, and guide the other arm into the sleeve (Figure 14-34).
9. Help client to put on underwear, slacks, shorts, or pajama bottoms. If leg is injured, place into garment first, then the other leg. Help client to stand at side of bed and pull up clothing to the waist. If client is in bed, help client to lift buttocks while you pull up the garments.
10. Help client to put on socks or stockings and footwear.
11. Make sure client is safe and comfortable.
12. Place bed in lowest position. (Raise side rail, if indicated.)*
13. Wash your hands.
14. Record what you have done. Report any unusual conditions to your supervisor.
   Note: To help client to undress, reverse the procedure. Injured arm or leg is removed from garment last.

Fig 14-33 Dress injured arm first (Step 8a).

Fig 14-34 Begin with injured arm (Step 8b).

*Your client may not have an adjustable hospital bed; those steps marked with an asterisk (*) will not apply.

ORR
- Stop the exercise if the client complains of pain or shows signs of severe discomfort; report these findings to your supervisor.
- Stop if you feel resistance or tightness in the joint.
   Follow Procedure 14-15, Helping with Range-of-Motion Exercises in Bed: General Procedure.

PROCEDURE 14-14   Helping Client With an Intravenous (IV) Line to Remove Used Clothing and Apply Clean Clothing

Materials Needed
- Clean clothing

Procedure
1. Explain what you are going to do.
2. Wash your hands.
3. Obtain clean clothing.
4. Arrange clothing in order of use.
5. Provide privacy (close door, shut drapes, pull shades).
6. Lower bed to lowest position. Lower rail on side where you are working.*
7. Help client to sit on side of bed, if possible. If client must stay in bed, place in supine position.
8. Help client to remove used garment from arm without IV.
9. Gather up sleeve of garment on arm with IV. Slide sleeve over the IV site and tubing. Remove client's arm and hand from sleeve.
10. Slide your hand along tubing to IV bag, keeping sleeve gathered.
11. Remove IV from pole. Slide bag and tubing through the sleeve. **Keep bag above client's arm.** Do not pull on the tubing. Place used clothing on chair (Figure 14-35).
12. Hang bag back on the pole.
13. Gather the sleeve of clean garment that is to be put on the arm with the IV.

Fig 14-35 **A,** Pajama top is removed from arm without IV. Other sleeve is gathered up and slipped over IV site and tubing. **B,** Gathered sleeve is slipped over tubing and up to intravenous bag. **C,** Remove intravenous bag from pole and pass through sleeve. **D,** To dress client, start with IV arm first. Gather sleeve of shirt, slip over intravenous bag, and back up to shoulder.

*Your client may not have an adjustable hospital bed; those steps marked with an asterisk (*) will not apply.

Continued

PROCEDURE 14-14   Helping Client With an Intravenous (IV) Line to Remove Used Clothing and Apply Clean Clothing—cont'd

14. Remove the IV bag from the pole. Make sure the bag is above the client's arm.
15. Slip sleeve and garment shoulder over the bag. Place bag back on the pole.
16. Slide the gathered sleeve over the tubing, hand, arm, and intravenous site.
17. Adjust garment over client's shoulders, and help client to put other arm through other sleeve.
18. Check that IV is working properly (see Chapter 18).

19. Assist client to remove other garments and put on clean garments, as needed.
20. Make sure client is safe and comfortable.
21. Place soiled garments in laundry container.
22. Place bed in lowest position. (Raise side rail, if indicated.)*
23. Record what you have done. Report any unusual conditions to your supervisor.

*Your client may not have an adjustable hospital bed; those steps marked with an asterisk (*) will not apply.

PROCEDURE 14-15   Helping With Range-of-Motion Exercises in Bed: General Procedure

1. Explain what you are going to do and how the client can help.
2. Wash your hands.
3. Provide privacy (close door, shut drapes, pull shades).
4. Raise bed to convenient working height. Lower rail on side where you are working.*
5. Fold top bedding to foot of bed. Cover client with sheet or blanket.
6. Help client to move to side of bed near you. Make sure client is in correct supine position.
7. Repeat each exercise as listed in the care plan.
8. Exercise upper body, both sides. Then exercise lower body, both sides.

9. Help client to center of bed, replace top bedding, and remove sheet or blanket covering client.
10. Make sure client is safe and comfortable.
11. Place bed in lowest position. (Raise side rail if indicated.)*
12. Wash your hands.
13. Record what you have done. Report any unusual conditions to your supervisor or physical therapist, such as
    • Complaints of pain or severe discomfort
    • Resistance or tightness in joint

SHOULDER AND ARM EXERCISES
(Figure 14-36)

Directions: Hold client's wrist and hand with one hand. With the other hand, grasp client's arm above the elbow.

Movement
  a. Move arm, with palm down, forward and upward along side of head and downward to the side. Repeat with palm up.
  b. Move arm with palm down, away from body, sideways, to above the head and return. Repeat with palm up.

Fig 14-36 Range-of-motion exercises for the shoulder and arm.

*Your client may not have an adjustable hospital bed; those steps marked with an asterisk (*) will not apply.

| PROCEDURE 14-15 | **Helping With Range-of-Motion Exercises in Bed: General Procedure—cont'd** |

FOREARM AND ELBOW EXERCISES
(Figure 14-37)

Directions: Rest client's upper arm on bed with forearm raised upright and elbow bent. Support client's wrist and hand.

Movement: Move lower arm down, then up, with palm down. Repeat with palm up.

Directions: Rest client's upper arm on bed with forearm upright. Support client's wrist with one hand and client's hand with the other.

Movement: Twist palm toward client, then away.

Fig 14-37 Range-of-motion exercises for the forearm and elbow.

WRIST EXERCISES (Figure 14-38)

Directions: Hold client's wrist with one hand. Use other hand to

Movement
  a. Move hand forward, then backward.
  b. Move hand from one side to the other.

Fig 14-38 Range-of-motion exercises for the wrist.

FINGER EXERCISES (Figure 14-39)

Directions: Hold client's wrist with one hand. With other hand

Movement
  a. Bend fingers (make a fist), then straighten.
  b. Spread fingers and thumb apart, then bring together.

Fig 14-39 Range-of-motion exercises for the fingers.

THUMB EXERCISES (Figure 14-40)

Direction: Hold client's hand and fingers with one hand. With other hand grasp thumbs.

Movement
  a. Move thumb across palm of hand and straighten, then return to side.
  b. Touch each finger tip with thumb.
  c. Bend thumb into palm and return to straightened position.
  d. Move thumb using wide, circular motion.

Fig 14-40 Range-of-motion exercises for the thumb.

Continued

HIP, LEG, AND KNEE EXERCISES
(Figures 14-41 and 14-42)

Directions: Support client's leg with one hand under knee and other at the heel.

Movement
   a. Bend knee and raise toward chest, then lower.
   b. Raise leg straight up as high as possible, then lower leg gently.

**Directions:* Support client's leg with one hand under knee and other hand under ankle.

Movement
   a. Move leg outward, away from body as far as possible. Return to starting position.
   b. Move leg across the other leg as far as possible, and return to starting position.

**Directions:* Place one hand over top of knee and grasp. Place other hand over top of ankle and grasp.

Movement: Turn leg so toes are pointed inward, then outward.

Directions: Support client's leg with one hand just above the knee and the other hand at the ankle.

Movement: Bend the knee, and slide the heel toward the buttocks as far as possible. Then straighten knee to starting position.

Fig 14-41 Range-of-motion exercises for the hip and leg.

Fig 14-42 Range-of-motion exercises for the knee.

FOOT AND ANKLE EXERCISES (Figure 14-43)

Directions: Support ankle by placing client's heel in palm of one hand with other hand just above the ankle.

Movement
   a. Bend foot up toward the leg, then down, away from leg.
   b. Turn foot outward, sole facing away from body, then turn foot inward toward body.

Fig 14-43 Range-of-motion exercises for the foot and ankle.

TOE EXERCISES (Figure 14-44)

Directions: Hold client's foot with one hand. Use the other hand to do the following.

Movement: Bend toes down toward the ball of the foot, then bend toes back to front of foot.

Fig 14-44 Range-of-motion exercises for the toes.

**These exercises cause the ball and socket joint of the hip to rotate. Do not perform these exercises unless indicated in the client's care plan. Older adults and young children may be severely injured by these exercises.

CHAPTER SUMMARY

- Clients may be unable to perform self-care because of the effects of illness, pain and discomfort, lack of strength and energy, fear of injury, anxiety, or confusion.
- The home care aide may assist the client to perform the following personal care activities.
  - Oral hygiene (brushing and flossing teeth, denture care)
  - Bathing
  - Grooming (caring for hands and feet, hair care, shampooing, and shaving)
  - Dressing and undressing
  - Care of eyeglasses, contact lenses, and hearing aids
- Bathing is done to cleanse the skin, remove bacteria, prevent body odor, stimulate circulation, move joints and muscles, prevent pressure ulcers, and provide comfort and a sense of well-being.

- Bathing provides the opportunity to communicate with the client, observe his or her skin, and perform range-of-motion (ROM) exercises.
- It is important to be aware of safety hazards that may arise when performing personal care activities.
- The home care aide needs to be alert to possible safety hazards (to client and self) when performing personal care activities. Be sure to practice safety principles discussed in this chapter and Chapter 8.
- Always use standard (universal) precautions when giving personal care to clients.
- Respect the client's need for privacy when performing personal care activities. Some of these procedures can cause embarrassment for the client.
- ROM exercises are used to improve muscle tone, increase circulation, and prevent deformities.

STUDY QUESTIONS

1. List five reasons why clients may not be able to perform personal care activities.
2. Describe how you would care for the following:
   a. False teeth
   b. Eyeglasses
   c. Hearing aids
3. List four purposes of bathing.
4. List six principles to follow when bathing clients.
5. Explain the difference between the following:
   a. Complete bed bath
   b. Partial bath
   c. Tub bath
   d. Shower bath

6. List three safety practices to follow for each of the following procedures:
   a. Tub bath
   b. Shower
   c. Denture care
7. Describe three personal care procedures where standard (universal) precautions must be followed.
8. List five important points to remember when performing ROM exercises.

15

Elimination

OBJECTIVES

After you read this chapter, you will be able to:

1. Describe the normal characteristics of urine and feces.
2. List six ways to promote normal urinary and bowel elimination.
3. Discuss the care needed for clients with urinary incontinence.
4. Describe the care needed for clients with catheters.
5. Discuss common bowel problems.
6. Discuss the care of clients with a colostomy or ileostomy.
7. Give five examples of the use of standard (universal) precautions when handling body waste.
8. Demonstrate the procedures in this chapter.

KEY TERMS

Diagnose(d) To determine the type and cause of an illness or a condition based on a variety of information

Diuretic(s) Drug or other substance that causes an increase in the production and excretion of urine

Dysuria Difficult or painful urination

Elimination Process of removing waste products from the body

Flatus Air or gas in the intestine that is released through the anus

Impaction The presence of a large, hard mass of feces in the rectum or colon

Output All fluids lost from the body that can be measured

Sedative(s) Substance, procedure, or measure that has a calming effect

Elimination of body wastes takes place in a number of ways:
- Perspiration, through the skin
- Carbon dioxide and moisture from the lungs
- Urine from the kidneys
- Bowel movements from the digestive system

Normal elimination is usually so automatic that we do not even think about it. Clients, however, may have problems with elimination for many reasons.
- Clients who are physically limited and cannot walk to the bathroom because it is upstairs, outside, or down the hall

- Clients with diseases that affect elimination
- Clients who take medications that influence elimination

URINARY ELIMINATION

URINARY SYSTEM REVIEW

- The *kidneys* filter blood, remove waste and impurities, regulate the salt and water in the body, and manufacture urine.
- The *ureters* are tubes that connect the kidneys to the urinary bladder.
- The *bladder* is a muscular organ that stores urine until it is eliminated from the body.
- The *urethra* is a tube from the bladder to the outside of the body.
- The *urinary meatus* is the external opening of the urethra.
- The *process of urination* is a complex one that involves several body systems: nervous, muscular, and urinary.

Urine is the liquid waste produced by the kidneys. The amount of urine a person produces differs according to age, illness, activity, medications taken, fluid intake, body temperature, and amount of other types of output. However, the amount of urine produced by the kidneys is usually about the same as the amount of fluid intake each day.

The medical terms for passing urine are *void, voiding, urinate, urinating, urination,* and *micturition.* Most English-speaking adults are familiar with the words *urine* and *urinate,* although many people will use the term *pass water* for emptying the urinary bladder. If your client speaks another language, try to find out the term used for the elimination of urine. Children, too, often have their own terms to describe urination. Again, try to find out what term the client uses, and use it whenever possible.

IN SOME CULTURES, HEALTH MATTERS REGARDING ELIMINATION ARE CONSIDERED VERY PRIVATE AND ARE NOT DISCUSSED WITH STRANGERS. SOMETIMES CLIENTS MAY REFUSE CARE BECAUSE IT MAKES THEM FEEL SO UNCOMFORTABLE OR BECAUSE SUCH INTIMATE CONTACT WITH STRANGERS IS NOT ACCEPTABLE IN THEIR CULTURE. Respect differences among cultures, and be willing to learn about the reasons for your client's behavior. You may find that some male clients object to having a female aide assist with procedures involving elimination. Some women, too, may be embarrassed by the type of personal care involved with elimination. However, helping your client to use the bathroom, commode, bedpan, or urinal as needed is part of your job. Discuss any embarrassing situations with your supervisor, and be sure to report any problems your client may have with elimination.

CHARACTERISTICS OF NORMAL URINE/URINATION

- Urine is clear and has a light yellow color. A high fluid intake will make urine a very pale yellow; a low fluid intake will make a darker, concentrated urine. Certain drugs may also cause a change in color.
- Normal urine may have a slight acidic odor or none at all; certain foods and drugs may produce other odors.
- The amount of urine will vary, but the normal adult will produce and eliminate about 1 to 1½ quarts (1000 to 1500 milliliters) daily.
- The frequency of urination will also vary. Some adults will urinate every 2 to 3 hours during the day; others will not void as often. The bladder is able to hold urine for longer periods during sleep.
- Urination is done with ease and without pain or discomfort; see Box 15-1 for suggestions on how to help clients maintain normal urination.

BOX 15-1 **Helping Clients Maintain Normal Urination**

- Make sure the path to the bathroom is direct and free of clutter.
- Place a commode, urinal, or bedpan at the bedside.
- Offer toileting at times when the client usually needs to void.
- Keep a walker or crutches nearby so they can be used when needed.
- Attend to the client's need to void immediately; do not make the client wait.
- Give the client adequate amounts of fluids: eight glasses of fluid per day.
- Reduce intake of fluids and foods that irritate the urinary bladder and increase urinary frequency, such as coffee, tea, colas, alcohol, chocolate, and large amounts of sugar.
- Provide privacy.
- Give clients enough time to urinate, but do not let them sit on the bedpan, toilet, or commode for too long.
- Position the client in the normal voiding position (standing for men; sitting for women) whenever possible.

CHARACTERISTICS OF ABNORMAL URINE/URINATION

- Urine is dark and cloudy; it may appear to contain blood, shreds of mucus, or other substances.
- Odor may be present; there may be a strong smell.
- Amount of urine may be much greater or much less than what is considered normal, about 1 to 1½ quarts (1000 to 1500 milliliters); immediately report anything above what is normal or anything less than 600 milliliters in a 24-hour period.
- Frequency may increase or decrease; observe, record, and report changes in voiding patterns and the presence of any dysuria. Frequent voiding of small quantities of urine may indicate abnormal emptying of the bladder. Be sure to let your supervisor know the frequency of the voiding and the amount voided.

URINARY ELIMINATION PROBLEMS

URINARY RETENTION

The inability to urinate or to completely empty the bladder is called *urinary retention*. This may occur after perineal surgery, childbirth, or prostate disease and with some diseases of the nervous system. If your client is unable to void or frequently voids small quantities of urine, report this to your supervisor *immediately*.

URINARY INCONTINENCE

The inability to control the release of urine from the bladder is called *urinary incontinence*. Although it is not a disease, it can be a symptom of other problems. For example, illness may cause some clients to become incontinent. It is estimated that about 13 million Americans (mostly women) experience incontinence at some time in their lives. Many are too ashamed or embarrassed to discuss this with a health care professional. Instead, they use pads or absorbent undergarments without having their conditions properly diagnosed and treated.

There are several types of urinary incontinence (Box 15-2). Incontinence may be caused by many factors.

- Inability to get to the bathroom fast enough
- Inability to remove clothing fast enough to use the commode or toilet due to injury or disability

BOX 15-2 Types of Urinary Incontinence

STRESS INCONTINENCE

Leakage of small amounts of urine during "stressful" activities, such as laughing, sneezing, coughing, lifting heavy objects, or certain types of exercise

URGE INCONTINENCE

Involuntary loss of urine when the "urge" to void occurs; person is "unable to make it to the toilet in time"

OVERFLOW INCONTINENCE (DRIBBLING)

Involuntary loss of urine that occurs when urine is being retained and the bladder is overfilled

- Having to wait too long for the bedpan or urinal
- Urinary tract infection
- Disease conditions of the nervous system and other disorders
- Medications, such as diuretics and sedatives
- Immobility, being confined to a bed or wheelchair
- Emotional disorders, including depression
- Confusion, forgetting to void, forgetting how to void
- Stool impaction
- Weakening of pelvic floor muscles resulting from birth of several children
- Urinary retention, which may cause overflow

Managing Urinary Incontinence

If your client has been incontinent for some time, the care plan will tell you what to do. If this is a new symptom, you must report it *immediately*. The client's condition will be assessed by the nurse and doctor, and a plan to treat or manage the symptoms will be developed. The treatment is based on the cause of the incontinence. Sometimes surgery or medications may be necessary to correct the problem. However, there are several treatments frequently used in home care: bladder training, habit training, pelvic muscle exercises, absorbent products, and catheters.

The incontinent client is at great risk for skin breakdown caused by irritation from the urine and bacterial growth in the warm, moist environment. Check the skin for rash and redness at least every 2 hours. Record and report abnormal findings to your supervisor.

Give perineal care each time the client is incontinent. Wash all the skin that has been in contact with the urine, using mild soap, warm water, and soft washcloths. Dry the skin gently, and apply cream or ointment according to the care plan. Because you will be coming in contact with body fluids, you must wear gloves when giving skin care and when changing and washing contaminated linens.

Bladder Training

Bladder training is a program of education, scheduled voiding, praise, and encouragement. The nurse or physical therapist, together with the client, establishes the schedule of voiding. This causes the bladder to be "trained" to hold more urine for a longer amount of time. Fluid intake, output, and voiding patterns are recorded daily, usually by the client. This information is used to evaluate the success of the training program and to make changes as necessary. The home care aide helps clients to carry out the program according to the care plan by doing the following.

- Encouraging clients to follow the schedule
- Teaching clients or family members to record intake and output accurately
- Following suggestions to help clients to maintain normal urination (see Box 15-1)
- Providing privacy and following procedures for use of bedpan, urinal, and commode
- Praising clients for success in the program
- Encouraging clients not to give up or become discouraged if incontinence occurs

Bladder training may take several months, with repeated visits from the therapist or nurse to provide continuing instruction. Be sure to record progress, or lack of progress, and notify your supervisor.

Habit Training

Habit training is a program of timed voiding. Both the client and the nurse develop the schedule for voiding. This should be as close to the person's natural pattern of urination as possible. Clients void at specific times, such as on awakening, before and after meals, and at bedtime. The bladder is not trained to hold more urine; rather the client is encouraged to void at times when he or she would usually use the bathroom. Assist the client by following the care plan and the suggestions for bladder training.

Pelvic Muscle Exercises

Also called *Kegel* exercises, pelvic muscle exercises strengthen the muscles of the pelvic floor. Urine leakage can be improved and often prevented by the use of these exercises. They are easy to do and are taught by a nurse or therapist. These are resistance exercises used mostly by women (also by men after prostate surgery). The exercises are performed by "drawing in" the muscles of the perineum as if to control voiding and bowel movements. Encourage the client to practice the exercises according to the care plan. Report any problems to your supervisor.

Absorbent Products

These products include pads, briefs, and underpads (placed under the client's hips to keep the bed dry). Absorbent products often give a false sense of security because the client no longer worries about having an "accident." This may delay diagnosis and effective treatment of incontinence. Protective absorbent products, when used improperly, may lead to skin breakdown and urinary tract infection. Odor control is another problem. Absorbent products should be changed every 2 to 3 hours. Perineal care is given, and all soiled skin areas are cleansed. For clients in bed, the changing schedule is every 2 hours. Observe the skin, and report any abnormal findings to your supervisor. Underpads and briefs are available in disposable and washable, reusable forms. Disposable products are convenient, but expensive. Reusable products (Figure 15-1, *A* and *B*) must be laundered according to the directions in Chapter 9, pp. 133–134. Always wear gloves when handling soiled absorbent products.

Fig 15-1 **A,** Reusable undergarment. **B,** Reusable underpad for use in bed.

Catheters

Catheters are tubes used to remove and/or insert fluids into a body cavity. Some clients will be taught by the professional nurse to perform intermittent self-catheterization to remove urine.

Indwelling catheters remain in the body and may be used for clients who retain urine or who are incontinent. They carry great risk of urinary tract infection. External collecting devices (condom catheters) are used by men. Care of the client with an indwelling catheter and external collecting devices is discussed later in the chapter.

CARING FOR THE CLIENT

ASSISTING WITH THE BEDPAN AND URINAL

Bedpans and urinals are used by clients who are unable to get to the toilet to eliminate body wastes. Men will use a urinal for voiding (Figure 15-2). There are two types of bedpans: the regular, large pan and the fracture pan (Figure 15-3, *A* and *B*), a smaller version used for clients with problems of mobility in bed. Bedpans and urinals can be made of metal or plastic. Metal bedpans are very cold, so warm them by rinsing with warm tap water. Wear gloves when removing and emptying the bedpan. You need to wear gloves when giving the bedpan if there is any risk of contact with body fluids. Check to see if the client or linens are soiled with urine or feces before providing the bedpan or urinal. Cover the bedpan with newspaper or a washable cloth when carrying it to the client and then into the bathroom to be emptied.

Be sure to give clients privacy when using the bedpan or urinal. Do not let them sit on the bedpan too long, because this causes pressure and damage to the tissues of the hips and buttocks. Empty bedpans and urinals immediately after use to avoid odors and growth of bacteria. Be careful when emptying bedpans and urinals to avoid splashing body fluids on clothing or skin. Rinse with cold water, clean thoroughly, and disinfect according to Chapter 11, pp. 180–182. Store properly when not in use. Do not keep on the table or under the bed.

See Procedure 15-1, Giving and Removing a Bedpan, and Procedure 15-2, Giving and Removing a Urinal.

ASSISTING CLIENTS TO USE THE COMMODE

Commodes are placed near the bedside to be used by clients who are very weak or are unable to get to the bathroom because it is inaccessible or because they are too slow to

Fig 15-2 A urinal.

Fig 15-3 **A,** Regular bedpan. **B,** Fracture pan.

PROCEDURE 15-1   Giving and Removing a Bedpan

Materials Needed

- Bedpan
- Bedpan cover
- Toilet tissue
- 2 pairs disposable gloves
- Paper towels

Procedure

1. Explain what you are going to do.
2. Wash your hands.
3. Obtain materials listed above.
4. Provide privacy (close door, shut drapes, pull shades).
5. Raise bed to convenient working height.*
6. Warm bedpan with warm tap water. Dry with paper towels.
7. Take bedpan to bedside, and place on chair or bed.
8. Lower rail on side where you are working.*
9. Assist client to lie on back. Elevate head of bed slightly.
10. Fold back upper linens.
11. Instruct client to bend knees and raise buttocks. Assist as needed (Figure 15-4, A). If bed or client is soiled, put on gloves.
12. Slide the bedpan under the client (Figure 15-4, B).

13. When the client cannot raise the hips to get onto the bedpan, do the following.
    a. Turn the client on his or her side, facing away from you.
    b. Position the bedpan firmly against the buttocks.
    c. Turn the client on to his or her back, while holding the bedpan in place under the buttocks.
14. Cover client with top sheet to avoid chilling and exposure.
15. Raise side rail, and place bed in sitting position.*
16. Prop up client with pillows if the bed is not adjustable.
17. Make sure bedpan is in correct position.
18. Give toilet tissue, and ask client to call when finished.
19. Leave room. Remove gloves, if using. Discard gloves.
20. Wash your hands.
21. Return to room when client calls.
22. Lower rail on side where you are working.*
23. Put on gloves.
24. Place client in flat position and remove bedpan in same manner used to give the bedpan.
25. Cleanse perineal area with toilet tissue if necessary, wiping from front to back.
26. Raise side rail.*

Fig 15-4 **A,** Instruct the client to bend knees and raise buttocks (Step 11). **B,** Slide the bedpan under the client (Step 12).

*Your client may not have an adjustable hospital bed; those steps marked with an asterisk (*) will not apply.

PROCEDURE 15-1 | Giving and Removing a Bedpan—cont'd

27. Cover bedpan, take to bathroom, and empty contents. Measure output if necessary. Observe contents.
28. Rinse bedpan with cold water, clean, and disinfect following instructions in Chapter 11, p. 182.
29. Remove and discard gloves.
30. Wash your hands.
31. Put bedpan away.

32. Lower rail on side where you are working.*
33. Help client to wash his or her hands.
34. Make sure client is safe and comfortable.
35. Place bed in lowest position. (Raise side rail, if indicated.)*
36. Wash your hands.
37. Record what you have done. Report any unusual elimination to your supervisor.

PROCEDURE 15-2 | Giving and Removing a Urinal

Materials Needed
- Urinal
- Cover
- Disposable gloves

Procedure

1. Explain what you are going to do.
2. Wash your hands.
3. Obtain materials listed above.
4. Provide privacy (close door, shut drapes, pull shades).
5. Take urinal to bedside, and place on chair or bed.
6. Assist client to stand. If client cannot stand, place client on his back.
7. Fold back upper linens.
8. Give urinal to client so he can position it properly.
9. If client is unable to position urinal, put on gloves and position it for him.
10. Cover client with top sheet to avoid chilling and exposure.

11. Leave room. Remove gloves, if using. Discard gloves.
12. Wash your hands.
13. Return to room when client calls.
14. Put on gloves.
15. Remove the urinal in the same manner you gave it to the client.
16. Cover urinal, take to bathroom, and empty contents. Measure output if necessary. Observe urine.
17. Rinse urinal with cold water, clean, and disinfect following instructions in Chapter 11, p. 182.
18. Remove and discard gloves.
19. Wash your hands.
20. Put urinal away.
21. Help client to wash his hands.
22. Make sure client is safe and comfortable.
23. Wash your hands.
24. Record what you have done. Report any unusual urine or urination to your supervisor.

"make it in time." These commode chairs should be stable and be wide enough for large clients to sit comfortably (Figure 15-5). If the commode has wheel brakes, lock them before transferring the client to the commode chair using the transfer techniques discussed in Chapter 12. Provide privacy. Place toilet tissue within reach. Instruct the client to call you when finished. Return the client to bed, wash his or her hands, and provide perineal care (see Procedure 14-8, Giving Perineal Care) as needed. Empty the commode in the toilet: wear gloves. If there is a risk of splashing, wear eye protection. Clean according to directions in Chapter 9 to avoid the presence of bacteria and offensive odor. Be sure to wash your hands.

INTAKE AND OUTPUT (I&O)

Measuring the client's fluid intake and output is an important part of the care plan and helps to determine the effectiveness of treatment. For example, clients with kidney, heart, and liver disease may retain fluid in the tissues (edema). Some may take diuretics

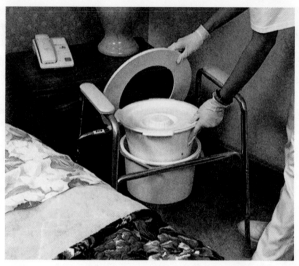

Fig 15-5 The bedside commode has a toilet seat and a removable pail.

to increase the production of urine and to promote fluid loss from the tissues. THE LOSS OF TOO MUCH FLUID CAN CAUSE DEHYDRATION, A SERIOUS MEDICAL PROBLEM THAT CAN LEAD TO DEATH.

Occasionally, the doctor may restrict the fluid intake to a specific amount. All fluid intake must be measured to make sure the client does not go over the restricted amount.

Fluid Intake

Intake of the following is to be measured and recorded when the care plan calls for I&O (measuring and recording of fluid intake and output):

- *All liquids taken in by mouth:* Water, tea, coffee, milk, juice, soda, and soup
- *Semisolid foods:* Ice cream, sherbet, ice pops, pudding, Jello, custard, creamed soups, and creamed cereals
- *Intravenous fluids*
- *Tube feedings*

Fluid Output

Measure and record the amount of the following:

- *Urine:* Measure urine that is voided and from catheter drainage.
- *Feces:* Only liquid feces can be measured. For formed stool, the quantity is described as a large, medium, or small amount.
- *Vomitus:* If the client vomits into an emesis basin, it can be measured; otherwise, describe the amount as a large, medium, or small quantity. In addition to measuring the vomitus, describe its appearance. Report vomiting to your supervisor.
- *Drainage from wounds:* This is reported according to the care plan. Follow instructions from your supervisor. Large amounts of drainage must be reported.

Remember: The fluids listed as output are body fluids. You must wear gloves when handling these materials and when changing and washing the client and soiled linens. Review Chapters 9 and 11.

Measuring Intake and Output

Intake and output is measured in milliliters (mL) or cubic centimeters (cc) (1 mL equals 1 cc). These are metric system measurements. One fluid ounce equals about 30 mL. One pint is about 500 mL, and a quart is 1000 mL. Fluids are measured in a special pitcher called a "graduate" that has markings to show the amount being measured. A graduate is like a measuring cup and is marked in both the metric system and the

BOX 15-3 | **Examples of the Capacity of Serving Containers**

Teacup	6 ounces	180 milliliters
Juice glass	4 ounces	120 milliliters
Water glass	8 ounces	240 milliliters
Iced tea glass	12 ounces	360 milliliters

household system. Most plastic emesis basins, urinals, and commode pails have these markings for measuring output.

You will need to know how much fluid is held by containers in which liquids are served to your client. Fill serving containers, cups, glasses, and bowls with water to measure their contents. For example: Fill a drinking glass with water. Pour the water into a graduate or measuring cup. Measure the amount. Prepare a list of the contents of various containers used for fluid intake. Box 15-3 lists some examples of container capacity. The sizes of bowls, cups, glasses, and mugs vary greatly, so always measure to be sure of the exact capacity of each container. NEVER USE THE SAME GRADUATE TO MEASURE BOTH INTAKE AND OUTPUT.

The graduate for measuring output should be left in the bathroom.

When output is to be measured, clients cannot use the toilet as usual for elimination; they use the urinal, bedpan, and/or commode. A special insert known as specimen collector, or a "hat," may be placed under the toilet seat to collect the urine (Figure 15-6). These containers are usually marked for ease in measuring urinary output. Tell your client not to put toilet tissue into the bedpan, commode, or "hat" because it can interfere with accurate measurement of urine.

Clients and family members may need to be taught to measure and record intake and output. Follow the care plan, and make sure they know how to do this properly.

Recording Intake and Output

Record the amount of intake and output immediately after measuring it. Use the I&O form provided by your agency. Put it in a convenient place as a reminder to measure intake and output. A total is added up for each day (Figure 15-7). Procedure 15-3 lists the steps for measuring and recording intake and output.

CARE OF A CLIENT WITH AN INDWELLING CATHETER

An indwelling or retention catheter remains in the bladder and provides constant drainage of urine. The catheter is inserted by the nurse. It is not the responsibility of

Fig 15-6 A specimen collector ("hat") is placed in the toilet to collect the urine.

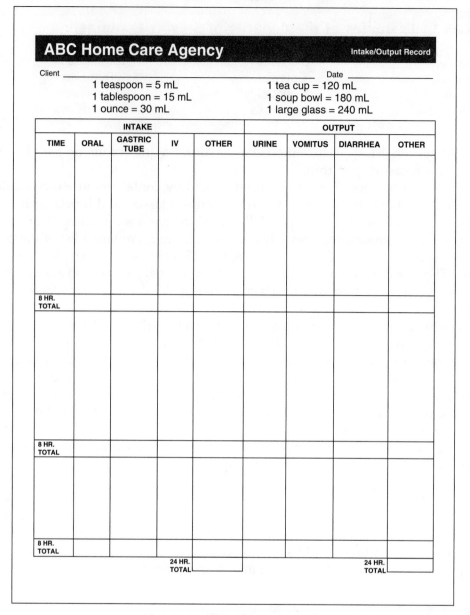

Fig 15-7 Intake and output record.

the home care aide to insert or remove indwelling catheters. A balloon, inflated with sterile solution, holds the catheter in place and prevents it from slipping out of the bladder (Figure 15-8, *A* and *B*). The catheter is connected to a drainage tube and collection bag.

Long-term use (more than 2 to 4 weeks) of indwelling catheters can lead to urinary tract infection and damage to the bladder and urethra. Therefore, catheters are used only when absolutely necessary.

The inside of the catheter and drainage system is sterile and should never come in contact with any other objects. Do not insert anything into the catheter or drainage tubing or let any part of the system come in contact with the floor. **KEEP THE COLLECTION BAG BELOW THE LEVEL OF THE URINARY BLADDER TO PREVENT BACKFLOW OF URINE INTO THE BLADDER.** Attach the collection bag to the bed frame; keep it free from linens and side rails. Do not attach catheter drainage bag tubing to the side rails or other moveable parts of the bed. Clients are often ashamed and embarrassed when visitors see the urine collection bag. Try to cover it with bed linens or a lap robe when the client has visitors.

PROCEDURE 15-3 | Measuring and Recording Intake and Output

Materials Needed

- Measuring cups or graduates; separate measuring containers are needed for intake and output
- List of serving containers, which you measured earlier (see Box 15-3)
- Pencil
- Paper
- Intake and output (I&O) form
- Disposable gloves

Intake

1. Wash your hands.
2. Obtain materials listed above.
3. Measure each remaining liquid separately after client finishes eating or drinking. Pour into measuring cup.
4. Hold at eye level, and measure the amount left.
5. Subtract the remaining amount from the amount of the original full serving.
6. Repeat for each liquid and record.

7. Rinse, clean, dry, and store container used to measure intake.
8. Wash your hands.
9. Record the amount of fluid intake and the time on the I&O form.

Output

1. Wash your hands.
2. Put on gloves.
3. Empty bedpan, urinal, commode pail, "hat," or emesis basin into a graduate if original container is not marked for measuring.
4. Measure amount of liquid, and discard into toilet.
5. Rinse, clean, disinfect, dry, and store container used to measure output.
6. Remove and discard gloves.
7. Wash your hands.
8. Record the amount of fluid output and the time on the I&O form.
9. Report any unusual output to your supervisor.

Fig 15-8 **A,** An indwelling catheter in the female bladder. An inflated balloon prevents the catheter from slipping out of place. **B,** An indwelling catheter in the male bladder.

A   B

The following are some guidelines to remember when caring for clients with catheters.

1. Always practice standard (universal) precautions. Wear gloves when there is a chance of coming in contact with body fluids.
2. Make sure urine is draining freely into the collection bag. Check for kinks in the tubing.
3. Tape the catheter to the thigh or abdomen (males). Be sure it is connected to the drainage tubing and collection bag or leg bag (Figure 15-9).
4. Pin connecting tubing to lower bed linen. Arrange in a coil to prevent dangling and drainage problems (see Figure 15-9).
5. Empty the collection bag according to the care plan. Be careful when emptying the drainage bag to avoid splashing on clothing or in eyes.
   Wear face mask and goggles, if necessary. Record the amount, color, odor, and clarity of the urine.

ORR

6. Provide perineal and catheter care daily, or more frequently if indicated in the care plan. Keep catheter and tubing clean.
7. Record and report the following to your supervisor:
   a. Leakage of urine around the catheter
   b. Client complaints of pain, burning, irritation, pressure, and feeling the urge to void
   c. Discharge from the urinary meatus or vagina
   d. Abnormal quantity or appearance of urine
   e. Leaks in the drainage tubing or collection bag
8. When moving the client, also move the tubing and bag apparatus.
9. Leg bags are not used when clients are lying in bed because of the possibility of backflow of urine into the bladder and the risk of urinary tract infection. At bedtime, the leg bag is removed and the regular drainage system is connected.
10. Whenever the catheter is separated from the drainage tube, it must be handled in a manner that will prevent it from being contaminated. Follow Procedure 15-4, Care of the Client with an Indwelling Catheter, and Procedure 15-5, Emptying a Catheter Drainage Bag.

A   B

Fig 15-9 Securing catheters. **A,** The drainage tubing is coiled on the bed and secured to the bottom linens so urine flows freely. The catheter is taped to the inner thigh. Enough slack is left on the catheter to prevent friction at the urethra. **B,** The catheter is secured to the man's abdomen. (From Sorrentino SA: *Mosby's textbook for long-term care nursing assistants,* ed 6, St. Louis, 2011, Mosby.)

PROCEDURE 15-4   Care of the Client With an Indwelling Catheter

Materials Needed
- Materials for perineal care (See Procedure 14-8, p. 249)
- Cotton balls or gauze
- Disposable gloves
- Waterproof protector pad
- Plastic or paper bag

Procedure
1. Explain what you are going to do.
2. Wash your hands.
3. Obtain materials listed above.
4. Provide privacy (close door, shut drapes, pull shades).
5. Put on gloves.
6. Perform perineal care (see Procedure 14-8).
7. Female client: Separate labia to visualize the urinary meatus. Male client: Retract foreskin (if uncircumcised).
8. Moisten cotton balls or gauze with soap and water.

PROCEDURE 15-4   Care of the Client With an Indwelling Catheter—cont'd

9. Wash catheter tube in a downward motion away from the urinary meatus for approximately 4 inches (20 cm) (Figure 15-10). Use one cotton ball or gauze pad for each stroke. Rinse with water in the same manner. Discard used cotton balls or gauze into bag.
10. Tape and position catheter properly (see Figure 15-9).
11. Remove waterproof protector pad. Replace top linens.
12. Make sure client is safe and comfortable.
13. Clean materials, and store in proper location.
14. Remove and discard gloves.
15. Wash your hands.
16. Record what you have done. Report any unusual conditions to your supervisor.
    - Leakage of urine around catheter
    - Complaints of pain, burning, or irritation
    - Feeling the urge to void

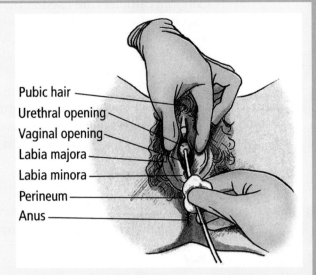

Pubic hair
Urethral opening
Vaginal opening
Labia majora
Labia minora
Perineum
Anus

Fig 15-10 Wash catheter tube in a downward motion (Step 9).

PROCEDURE 15-5   Emptying a Catheter Drainage Bag

Materials Needed
- Disposable gloves
- Measuring container or graduate

Procedure
1. Explain what you are going to do.
2. Wash your hands.
3. Obtain materials listed above.
4. Provide privacy (close door, shut drapes, pull shades).
5. Put on gloves and other personal protective equipment as needed.
6. Place measuring container under drainage tube of collection bag.
7. Open clamp on drainage tube so urine can empty into graduate (Figure 15-11). The drainage tube must not touch the insides of the graduate or any other surface, including the floor.
8. Close clamp, and replace drainage tube in holder on collection bag.
9. Measure urine, and then discard in toilet.
10. Rinse, clean, disinfect, and store graduate.
11. Remove and discard gloves.
12. Wash your hands.
13. Record what you have done. Note the amount, color, and clarity of the urine. Report any unusual conditions to your supervisor.

Fig 15-11 Open clamp on drainage tube (Step 7).

CARE OF A CLIENT WITH A CONDOM CATHETER

Condom catheters are used in place of indwelling catheters to reduce the risk of urinary tract infections. The catheter goes over the penis and is connected to a drainage system, usually a leg bag (Figure 15-12). Velcro or self-adhesive holds the condom in place. The catheter is changed daily, and perineal care is given.

In some states, the home care aide may perform this procedure, whereas in others it is the responsibility of the nurse. Follow your agency policy and the rules that apply in your state (see Procedure 15-6, Applying a Condom Catheter). This procedure can be extremely embarrassing for the client. Do not expose him any more than necessary. Provide privacy, and have a professional, matter-of-fact attitude when giving this care.

PROCEDURE 15-6 | Applying a Condom Catheter

Materials Needed
- Materials to give perineal care (see Procedure 14-8, p. 249)
- Condom catheter and collection bag
- Velcro band
- Disposable gloves
- Small plastic bag

Procedure
1. Explain what you are going to do.
2. Wash your hands.
3. Obtain materials listed above.
4. Provide privacy (close door, shut drapes, pull shades).
5. Help client to lie on back.
6. Put on gloves.
7. Cover client with sheet or bath blanket as for perineal care.
8. If condom catheter is present, remove gently and place in plastic bag.
9. Give perineal care (see Procedure 14-8).
10. Attach collection bag to leg or bed frame.
11. Apply protective coating to the skin of the penis if using a self-adhesive condom catheter.
12. Hold penis firmly. Roll the condom catheter onto penis with drainage opening at the urinary meatus.
13. Secure edge of condom catheter in place with Velcro band. Be careful not to constrict the penis.
14. Connect catheter tip to drainage tubing (Figure 15-12).
15. Make sure tubing is in correct position and that tip of catheter is not twisted.
16. Make sure client is safe and comfortable.
17. Discard used supplies in plastic bag.
18. Remove and discard gloves.
19. Wash your hands.
20. Record what you have done. Report any unusual conditions to your supervisor.

Fig 15-12 Connect catheter tip to drainage tubing (Step 14).

BOWEL ELIMINATION

There are many terms used to describe the process of eliminating solid waste (feces) from the body. The correct term, *defecation,* may not be familiar to your client. The terms *bowel movement* or "BM" are more commonly understood. Another word for feces is *stool.* It is important that you understand the words your client uses for defecation and feces. However, use the correct terms, not slang, when discussing elimination with your client.

DIGESTIVE SYSTEM REVIEW

In Chapter 5, information about the organs of the digestive system and how they function was provided, including the following:
* The digestion of food is completed in the small intestine.
* The substances not absorbed in the small intestine (i.e., seeds, food fiber, other waste products, water) pass into the large intestine.
* The large intestine absorbs water and stores semisolid waste materials (feces) until they are eliminated.
* The powerful action of muscles (peristalsis) in the lower part of the large intestine helps to move the feces during defecation.
* The anal sphincter muscles control the opening and closing of the anus during the process of defecation.
* The process of defecation is a complex one that involves several body systems: nervous, muscular, and digestive.

MAINTAINING HEALTHY BOWEL HABITS

Eliminating waste products helps to keep the body functioning properly (Box 15-4). Principles of maintaining healthy bowel habits include the following:

Maintaining an Established Routine
Some clients have well-established bowel habits. Knowing your client's habits is very important. For example, Lucille has a BM every day after breakfast. As Lucille's home care aide, you plan to provide the time for her to maintain this habit.

Maintaining Privacy
Defecation is a very private act. Some clients will resist the urge to defecate if they think their privacy is at risk. It is the home care aide's responsibility to be

---

BOX 15-4 Helping Client Maintain Normal Bowel Elimination

* Make sure the path to the bathroom is direct and free of clutter.
* Place commode at the bedside.
* Offer toileting according to the client's established pattern of bowel movements.
* Keep a walker or crutches nearby so they can be used when needed.
* Attend to the client's need to defecate immediately; do not make the client wait.
* Give the client adequate amounts of fluids: eight glasses of fluid per day.
* Give the client a diet containing fiber: fruits, vegetables, and whole grains.
* Provide privacy.
* Give clients enough time to defecate, but do not let them sit on the toilet or commode for too long.
* Encourage activity and exercise, within the limits of the client's ability and the care plan.

sensitive to clients' concerns and to provide the privacy needed to carry out this body function.

Encouraging Fluids and a Well-Balanced Diet

Fluids are essential to keep the body functioning properly. The large intestine absorbs water as waste products pass through. With sufficient amounts of water, feces are soft and easy to eliminate. In Chapter 10, the importance of a well-balanced diet was discussed. Foods high in natural fiber, such as fruits, vegetables, and whole grains, provide bulk. Bulk helps to stimulate peristaltic action of the muscles of the digestive system, and defecation occurs more easily. When the amounts of fluids, fruits, vegetables, and whole grains in the diet are limited, problems with defecation can occur. Feces become hardened and difficult to eliminate. Encourage your client to drink fluids and eat foods high in fiber content, according to the diet ordered by the doctor.

Encouraging Activity and Exercise

Activity and exercise help the body systems work more efficiently, including the digestive system. Inactivity, due to illness, usually makes the digestive system sluggish. The large intestine is not as active, and the process of defecation may be slowed. Help your client to be as active as possible.

BOWEL ELIMINATION PROBLEMS

Some clients spend most of their time in bed or have limited exercise and activity. Others may be taking a variety of medications or have a poor appetite. All of these situations will make eating well-balanced meals with fiber and bulk more difficult. As a home care aide, you will need to recognize and report the problems listed here.

All night long, Winston Campbell had diarrhea. "I can't count how many bowel movements he had," Alex tells Betty Randolph. "I was up all night taking care of Winston: washing him, and changing and washing sheets. I am so tired."

As soon as Betty heard this, she called her supervisor, Mrs. Quick, who immediately came to the home. "It's a good thing you called me right away because diarrhea can be a very serious problem." Mrs. Quick did a nursing assessment and then called in her observations to Winston's doctor.

Betty and Mrs. Quick bathed Winston and then gave him perineal care. He complained, "I am so sore down there." "Yes," Mrs. Quick said, "diarrhea is very irritating to the skin. It is important that you are clean and dry." She and Betty showed Alex how to gently wash and dry Winston's irritated skin and then to apply a soothing, protective ointment to the area. "Oh, that feels so much better," said Winston.

"That's good," said Betty, "and these disposable linen protectors should help to keep the bottom sheets dry and clean."

"Well, I just hope I don't have any more diarrhea. It's no fun—and we are both exhausted," Winston added.

"Diarrhea can be a serious problem, so let's see what treatment the doctor recommends," advised Mrs. Quick. "In the meantime, drink plenty of fluids to replace those you have lost. Try to get some rest, and I'll let you know what the doctor has to say."

DIARRHEA

Diarrhea occurs when feces move through the intestines so fast that the water is not absorbed. The stool in diarrhea is not formed but is watery. The client may have frequent urges to defecate. These urges may be so strong that the client is unable to control the release of the stool. Complaints of cramping and soreness around the anus due to the frequent bowel movements are not unusual.

BOWEL (FECAL) INCONTINENCE

The inability to control the release of feces and *flatus* (gas) from the anus is called *bowel incontinence*. There are many causes, such as disease, nervous system disorders, weakness of the anal sphincters, or the inability to get to the bathroom or commode quickly enough when the urge to defecate comes. No matter what the cause, this condition is usually very embarrassing for the client.

CONSTIPATION

Constipation occurs when feces remains in the large intestine for long periods of time. Water from the feces continues to be absorbed, and the stool becomes dry and hard. Elimination is painful because the stool is hard to pass. The stool may be large or in small, marble-like pieces.

FECAL IMPACTION

This condition occurs when feces are held in the rectum for so long that they become too hard and dry to pass without help. Small amounts of liquid feces may pass around the hardened feces and leak out of the anus. The client may complain of abdominal discomfort or pain, of a full feeling in the rectum, or even of rectal pain. Treatment may include the use of medications or enemas. Sometimes a nurse must remove the impacted stool with a gloved finger. FECAL IMPACTION CAN BE AVOIDED BY REPORTING THE LACK OF BOWEL MOVEMENTS TO YOUR SUPERVISOR. IT IS MUCH EASIER TO TREAT CONSTIPATION THAN TO TREAT A FECAL IMPACTION.

CARING FOR THE CLIENT

HELPING THE CLIENT TO REESTABLISH BOWEL ROUTINE

A member of the home care team, such as the nurse or physical therapist, may perform procedures and assist with exercises to help the client with bowel elimination. The home care aide also plays an important role in helping the client return to normal bowel function. These activities include the following:

- Giving the bedpan or helping the client to the commode or bathroom as soon as the client requests—do not delay.
- Recording each time the client defecates; after several days of recording the frequency and time of bowel movements, you may see that your client has a regular pattern of bowel movements. For example, many clients will have the urge to defecate after a meal; be sure to offer the bedpan or help the client to the commode based on this pattern.
- Providing adequate time to defecate; do not rush your client or give the impression that you are in a hurry for the client to finish.

- Encouraging the client to drink water and other fluids and to eat high-fiber foods.
- Reporting changes in bowel habits to your supervisor, such as diarrhea, constipation, or other signs of problems.

OBSERVING AND RECORDING FECES

It is important to carefully observe feces eliminated by the client. This waste product can tell a lot about the health of the entire digestive system. The following should be recorded:

- *Frequency:* The amount of bowel movements (once daily, two or three times daily; every 2 to 3 days); the frequency varies with each client. Find out what is normal for your client.
- *Amount of each bowel movement:* Large amount, small amount; the amount varies with each client because of food and fluids consumed.
- *Consistency:* Normal feces are formed, soft, and shaped like the rectum.
- *Color:* Normal feces are light to dark brown; this color may vary according to the foods eaten.
- *Odor:* Feces have a characteristic odor; foods eaten can also affect the odor.
- *Flatus:* During defecation, flatus may be passed with feces; eating gas-forming foods, such as cabbage, onions, beans, or Brussels sprouts, can increase the amount of flatus.

In addition to the list above, notice the behavior of your client. Defecation should be easy and should not cause pain or discomfort. Other factors can affect the frequency, consistency, color, and odor of feces.

- *Medications:* Some types of vitamins can cause the feces to become darker in color; other medications may cause more frequent or fewer bowel movements.
- *Other treatments:* Cancer treatments, such as chemotherapy and radiation, may affect one or more characteristics of bowel movements.
- *Emotions:* Worry, anxiety, and fear can affect the bowel and cause changes in the frequency of bowel movements.

ALWAYS CHECK WITH YOUR SUPERVISOR IF YOU NOTICE CHANGES IN YOUR CLIENT'S BOWEL MOVEMENTS.

THE CLIENT WITH AN OSTOMY

Ostomy is a term that means "to form a new opening." This is performed by making a surgical opening in the bladder or small or large intestine. You may care for clients who have had surgery where part of the intestine is brought out through the abdominal wall. An artificial opening, called a *stoma,* is made so that fecal material, flatus, or urine can be expelled through the stoma rather than through the anus or urethra. This surgical procedure may be performed when there is cancer, other diseases, or severe injury to the intestines or bladder. Ostomies can be temporary, meaning that the bowel will be reconnected after healing takes place. Or, the ostomy can be permanent, meaning that the diseased or injured part of the bowel was removed.

When part of the large intestine is brought out through the abdominal wall, the surgical opening is called a *colostomy*. When part of the small intestine is brought out through the abdominal wall, the surgical opening is called an *ileostomy*.

The care needed for an ostomy depends on the location of the surgical opening. If the surgery has been performed on the small intestine (ileostomy), less water can be absorbed by the intestines. Therefore, the bowel contents will have a more liquid appearance. If the surgery has been performed farther down in the large intestine (colostomy), more water can be absorbed from the feces. The appearance of the feces will be more formed and normal.

Fig 15-13 A closed colostomy drainage pouch. (Courtesy ConvaTec, a Bristol-Myers Squibb Company, Princeton, NJ.)

Fig 15-14 A drainable ostomy pouch. (Courtesy ConvaTec, a Bristol-Myers Squibb Company, Princeton, NJ.)

An appliance, usually called a pouch or "bag," will be attached to the stoma to collect fecal material. There are two types of pouches: a closed pouch, which must be changed after each use (Figure 15-13), and a drainable pouch, which has a removable clamp to empty the contents of the pouch (Figure 15-14). This type of pouch is usually changed every 3 to 5 days. However, the pouch should be changed more often if it becomes loose around the stoma or if the skin around the area becomes irritated. Some clients who have had a colostomy for some time may not wear any pouch around the stoma. The colostomy is regulated to eliminate feces like a normal bowel movement, so the pouch is no longer necessary. Instead, a gauze pad is worn over the stoma to provide protection from clothing.

HELPING THE CLIENT TO CARE FOR THE OSTOMY

The client usually is taught how to care for the ostomy before leaving the hospital. The caregiver may also be shown how to help the client. Even so, there may be times when the home care aide will need to assist the client to care for the ostomy. The care plan will give directions about what needs to be done. Be sure to wear gloves when performing ostomy care to protect yourself. Some of the duties the home care aide may perform include caring for the skin around the stoma, disposing of fecal material, and cleaning the ostomy pouch.

The following information about caring for the ostomy is taught to the client or caregiver. However, the home care aide may need to assist when necessary.

Skin Care

Remove any fecal material on the stoma with toilet paper, and discard in plastic trash bag or flush in toilet. Wash the skin around the stoma thoroughly, but gently, with soap and warm water. Pat dry.   If you notice any redness or irritation, notify your supervisor, who will give further directions for skin care.

Disposing of Fecal Material from Pouch

If possible, have the client sit backward on the toilet or commode. He or she holds the pouch and places it between the legs. The bar clamp is removed, and the client empties the contents into the toilet. Some clients find it easier to empty the contents into a container first and then into the toilet.

Those with poor eyesight or difficulty handling the bar clamp usually need help with opening and closing it. Wear gloves and other personal protective equipment, if needed, when assisting the client to empty the pouch.

The pouch should be emptied when one-third to one-half full. If the pouch is allowed to fill completely, the weight of the pouch can cause it to loosen from the skin.

Cleaning the Pouch

Most pouches are odor proof, if cleaned properly. Each time the pouch is emptied, put on gloves and follow these directions.
1. Remove the pouch from the appliance attached to the skin.
2. Fold back the end of the pouch (like a cuff) before emptying to prevent additional fecal material from collecting at the bottom, causing odors.
3. Empty contents into toilet.
4. Rinse inside of pouch with warm water.
5. Wipe the last 2 inches (10 cm) of pouch with toilet tissue to remove any fecal material.
6. Uncuff the end of the pouch and put on the clamp.

PROVIDING EMOTIONAL SUPPORT

Adjusting to the ostomy and its care can be difficult for both the client and the family. It is not unusual for some clients to be sad, withdrawn, or even angry during this time. YOUR ATTITUDE TOWARD CARING FOR THE CLIENT IS VERY IMPORTANT. WHEN GIVING CARE, USE A POSITIVE APPROACH. DO NOT GIVE THE SLIGHTEST IMPRESSION THAT YOU ARE DISTURBED OR DISGUSTED ABOUT GIVING OSTOMY CARE. IF YOUR CLIENT WANTS TO TALK ABOUT THE SURGERY OR HAS CONCERNS ABOUT CARING FOR THE OSTOMY, LISTEN CAREFULLY.   Record your client's concerns, and report them to your supervisor.

Remember, clients are usually embarrassed to be eliminating through an opening in the abdomen. Your thoughtful, caring attitude can help the client to adjust to the day-to-day activities of living with an ostomy.

STANDARD (UNIVERSAL) PRECAUTIONS AND MEDICAL ASEPSIS

Standard (universal) precautions and medical asepsis must be followed when handling body fluids, feces, and soiled linens and clothing. Review the rules listed in Box 15-5.

BOX 15-5   Standard (Universal) Precautions and Medical Asepsis Rules When Handling Body Wastes

- Wash hands before and after wearing gloves.
- Wear gloves when
  - There is risk of contact with urine, feces, sputum, mucous membranes, vomitus, blood, or drainage from wounds
  - Assisting clients with toileting who have diarrhea, incontinence of urine and/or feces, or an ostomy
  - Measuring client's output
  - Handling clothing or bed linens soiled with body fluids
- Dispose of body wastes carefully; avoid splashing when disposing of contents of bedpan, urinal, or commode; if splashing occurs, clean area immediately.
- Empty bedpans and urinals immediately after use; clean and disinfect properly.
- Follow procedures listed in Chapters 9 and 11 for cleaning clothing and bed linens that have been soiled with body wastes.
- Wear goggles if there is danger of splashing body fluids in your eyes. Use personal protective equipment as needed.
- Place soiled disposable materials in plastic bags; remove immediately and discard.
- Double-bag any soiled linens or clothing; launder as soon as possible.

CHAPTER SUMMARY

- Illness, injury, and/or disability may cause clients to have problems with elimination.
- The home care aide can promote normal urinary and bowel elimination.
- Body waste is eliminated as perspiration, carbon dioxide, urine, and bowel movements.
- Many clients are embarrassed when someone who is not a family member helps to meet their needs for elimination.

- Good skin care is essential to prevent skin breakdown in incontinent clients.
- Standard (universal) precautions are required when handling body fluids, feces, and contaminated linens and clothing.
- Observing, recording, and reporting changes in the client's elimination is an important duty of the home care aide.

STUDY QUESTIONS

1. Describe normal urine and feces.
2. List six ways the home care aide can promote normal urinary and bowel elimination.
3. What is urinary incontinence? What special care is needed by incontinent clients?
4. What is an indwelling catheter? When are indwelling catheters used?
5. List five guidelines to remember when caring for a client with an indwelling catheter.
6. Describe three common bowel problems.
7. Mr. Halpern has a colostomy. Discuss three ways the home care aide can assist him with colostomy care.
8. List five examples of the use of standard (universal) precautions when handling body wastes.

Collecting Specimens

OBJECTIVES

After you read this chapter, you will be able to:

1. Discuss three reasons for collecting specimens.
2. List five general rules for specimen collection.
3. Practice standard (universal) precautions and medical asepsis when collecting and handling specimens.
4. Demonstrate procedures for collecting urine, stool, and sputum specimens.
5. Assist clients to perform blood sugar monitoring.

KEY TERMS

Analysis Determining the substances present in a specimen

Calculi Stones formed in the body due to the accumulation of mineral salts

Diabetes Disease resulting from lack of insulin secreted by special cells of the pancreas; causes blood sugar level to be elevated

Lancets Short pointed blades used to obtain blood from capillaries

Parasites Organisms that live in or on another organism

SPECIMENS

Specimens are small amounts of body tissue or fluids that are collected for examination and analysis in the medical laboratory. Tests are performed on the specimens for the following reasons:

- Evaluate the health of organ systems
- Determine the cause of illness
- Identify infecting microorganisms
- Evaluate results of treatment
- Observe client's progress
- Check for presence of abnormal substances, chemicals, drugs, and cells

Brigid Kennedy complained of frequent and painful voiding. Her home care aide, Anna Petrova, noted that Brigid's urine was cloudy and had a dark color. Anna reported these observations to her supervisor. The agency nurse visited Brigid to assess her condition. Anna was told to collect a urine specimen and to be sure that Brigid drinks eight glasses of fluid a day.

When clients are unable to leave home, specimens are obtained and taken to the medical laboratory according to agency policy. A few tests can be done in the home; for example, urine is strained for the presence of stones. Specimen collection may be embarrassing for the client. Remember to provide privacy when collecting any specimen.

Avoid confusion and mix-up by properly labeling the specimen container with the following:

- Client's name and address
- Date
- Time of specimen collection

Be sure the specimen container is tightly sealed and placed in a plastic bag for transportation to the laboratory. It is important that specimens are collected properly. Follow the general rules listed in Box 16-1.

The usual specimens collected in the home are urine, stool, and sputum. When handling these body substances, all rules of standard (universal) precautions and medical asepsis must be followed (Box 16-2). Always wear disposable gloves when collecting and handling specimens.

BOX 16-1   General Rules for Obtaining and Handling Specimens

- Follow the agency's directions for collecting specimens from clients.
- Complete all information requested on the label (Figure 16-1).
  Client's name
  Address
  Date
  Time specimen was collected
- Be sure all information is spelled correctly and is readable.
- Place label on the container, not on the lid.
- Collect the specimen at the time specified.
- Use a clean container for each specimen.
- Use the proper container for the specimen.
- Do not touch the inside of the container or the lid.
- Put the lid on the container immediately.
- Place the container in a plastic bag.
- Follow directions for storing the specimen.
- Store the specimen immediately.
- Inform the client or family member where the specimen is stored.
- Follow the agency's instructions about sending the specimen to the laboratory.

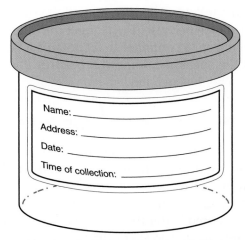

Fig 16-1 Specimen container with label.

> **BOX 16-2** **Standard (Universal) Precautions and Medical Asepsis Rules for Obtaining and Handling Specimens**
>
> - Wash hands before putting on gloves.
> - Always wear gloves when obtaining a urine, stool, or sputum specimen.
> - Pour urine into container carefully; do not splatter or allow urine to contaminate the outside of the container.
> - Wear goggles or other personal protective equipment when there is risk of splashing urine.
> - Do not fill the urine specimen container to the top, to avoid the chance of spilling over.
> - Place stool specimen in container or on stool card carefully; avoid contaminating the outside of the container.
> - Have client cough directly into the sputum specimen container; wear a mask, if necessary.
> - Remove and discard gloves after placing specimen in container, securing the lid, and cleaning and storing materials.
> - Place specimen container in plastic bag and seal.
> - Wash hands after removing gloves, goggles, or mask.
> - Dispose of used lancets according to agency policy and community regulations.
> - Do not handle used lancets. Assist client to discard them into proper container.

URINE SPECIMENS

Urine specimens are analyzed to determine the presence of
- Normal contents
- Abnormal contents, such as blood, bacteria, and protein

Results of laboratory tests help in making the diagnosis and establishing a treatment plan. Repeated or "follow-up" analysis of urine is used to determine the effectiveness of the treatment and to evaluate the client's condition.

When you collect a urine specimen from a client who is on intake and output (I&O), measure the amount of urine in the specimen and record it on the I&O form.

ROUTINE URINE SPECIMEN

A routine urine specimen may be collected any time the client voids. The urine may be voided into the bedpan, urinal, commode, or specimen-collecting pan ("hat") placed in the toilet (see Figure 15-6). Tell your client not to discard toilet paper into the voided specimen because it will affect the quality of the specimen. Do not collect a urine specimen from a container that contains a bowel movement. This will also affect the quality of the specimen. Follow Procedure 16-1, Collecting a Routine Urine Specimen. Assist the client as needed.

"CLEAN CATCH" OR MIDSTREAM URINE SPECIMEN

This specimen is collected to determine the presence of bacteria in the urine. Before voiding, the perineal area is cleansed. The "clean" urine specimen is collected in the middle of the voiding process. First, the client begins to void. Then, the client stops voiding, and the specimen container is positioned to "catch" the urine when voiding is restarted. After the specimen is collected, voiding is stopped again, and the container is removed. The client finishes voiding.

Many clients are unable to perform this procedure without assistance. You will assist by cleaning the perineum and positioning the specimen container properly. Always wear gloves. The agency will provide a special kit that contains all the materials

PROCEDURE 16-1   Collecting a Routine Urine Specimen

Materials Needed

- Bedpan, urinal, commode, or urine collector ("hat") for toilet
- Bedpan cover
- Urine specimen container and lid
- Label for specimen container
- Disposable gloves
- Graduate
- Small plastic bag (sandwich bag size)
- Small paper bag (lunch bag size)
- PPE, if needed

Procedure

1. Explain what you are going to do.
2. Wash your hands.
3. Obtain materials listed above.
4. Label container, and place in bathroom.
5. Put on gloves.
6. Assist client to bathroom or commode, or offer a bedpan or urinal (see Procedures 15-1 and 15-2).
7. Remind client not to drop toilet paper into specimen. Ask client to discard toilet paper into wastebasket.
8. Have client void into commode, bedpan, urinal, or "hat."
9. Take bedpan, urinal, or commode pail into bathroom.
10. Pour urine into graduate and then into specimen container until three-fourths full. Discard remaining urine into toilet.
11. Put lid on specimen container.
12. Place container into a plastic bag and then into a paper bag.
13. Clean materials, and store in proper location.
14. Remove and discard gloves.
15. Wash your hands.
16. Help client, as needed, back to bed or chair.
17. Store specimen in refrigerator.
18. Record what you have done. Report any unusual conditions to your supervisor.

necessary for collecting a clean catch urine specimen. Follow Procedure 16-2, Collecting a "Clean Catch" or Midstream Urine Specimen.

24-HOUR URINE SPECIMEN

Twenty-four-hour specimens are collected to evaluate the body's elimination of certain chemicals and hormones. Your agency will provide a large container for storing the collected urine. This is kept in the refrigerator or stored in a bucket of ice to prevent growth of the bacteria in the specimen. Sometimes a preservative may be added to the container for the same purpose. When you begin to collect the specimen, discard the first voided specimen because it was produced by the kidneys during the previous 24-hour period. Then save all other urine for the next 24 hours. Add each additional specimen to the large container, and keep it cold. The last voided specimen is also added to the container, per the following example.

- Tuesday, 8:00 AM, voided 250 mL; DISCARD and begin 24-hour collection
- Wednesday, 8:00 AM, voided 300 mL; INCLUDE in 24-hour specimen

Always explain the procedure to both the client and the family. Usually, you will not be in the home for a 24-hour period, and the client and caregiver need to know what to do with the urine. Be sure they understand. If there are any problems, check with your supervisor. Follow Procedure 16-3, Collecting a 24-Hour Urine Specimen.

STRAINING URINE

Urine is strained to detect the presence of calculi that can develop in the urinary tract. They can be very large or as small as grains of sand. A client who has large stones may

PROCEDURE 16-2   Collecting a "Clean Catch" or Midstream Urine Specimen

Materials Needed
- Midstream urine specimen kit (from agency)
- Disposable gloves
- Bedpan, urinal, or commode
- Small plastic bag (sandwich bag size)
- Small paper bag (lunch bag size)
- PPE, if needed

Procedure
1. Explain what you are going to do.
2. Wash your hands.
3. Obtain materials listed above.
4. Open kit (Figure 16-2). Remove contents, and label container.
5. Assist client to bathroom or commode, or offer a bedpan or urinal (see Procedures 15-1 and 15-2).
6. Tell client how to perform procedure. Be sure client understands what to do and how to do it. Instruct client to call you when finished.
7. If assistance is necessary, put on gloves.
8. Give perineal care using towelettes in specimen kit.
9. Keep labia separated until specimen has been collected so that urine will not flow over skin surfaces. In uncircumcised males, the foreskin is retracted until the specimen has been collected.
10. Collect the specimen.
    a. Ask client to begin voiding into urinal, bedpan, commode, or toilet.
    b. Instruct client to stop voiding.
    c. Hold specimen container under urinary meatus, but do not allow it to touch the skin surface. Do not touch the inside of container with your hands.
    d. Ask client to restart voiding.
    e. Catch enough urine to fill the container about halfway.
    f. Ask client to stop voiding.
    g. Remove container.
    h. Instruct client to finish voiding.
11. Put lid on specimen container. Be careful not to touch inside, to keep the specimen clean.
12. Place container into a plastic bag and then into a paper bag.
13. Assist client to complete toileting, if necessary.
14. Clean materials, and store in proper location.
15. Remove and discard gloves.
16. Wash your hands.
17. Help client, as needed, back to bed or chair.
18. Store specimen in refrigerator.
19. Record what you have done. Report any unusual conditions to your supervisor.

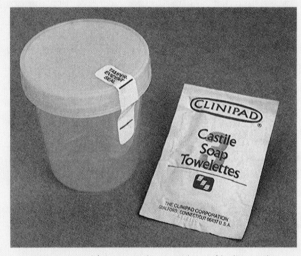

Fig 16-2 Midstream urine specimen kit (Step 4).

have to have them removed surgically. Very small stones may be passed when the client voids. When the care plan calls for urine to be strained, ALL the urine is poured through a paper filter or 4-by-4–inch gauze dressing to remove any calculi. If any stones are found, they are saved for laboratory examination.

Be sure to explain the procedure to the client and family members because they will need to strain the urine when you are not in the home. Show them what to do, and ask them to demonstrate the procedure to you. If there are questions or problems, notify your supervisor. For clients on I&O, measure and record the amount of urine in each strained specimen. Also, remind your client not to put toilet tissue into the specimen and to defecate separately from urinating. Follow Procedure 16-4, Straining Urine.

PROCEDURE 16-3 Collecting a 24-Hour Urine Specimen

Materials Needed

- 24-Hour urine container with biohazard label (with preservative, if needed)
- Container lid and label
- Bucket with ice, if needed
- Disposable gloves
- Graduate or funnel
- PPE, if needed

Procedure

1. Explain procedure to client and family.
2. Wash your hands.
3. Obtain materials listed above.
4. Label container.
5. Arrange urine container in bucket of ice in the bathroom (Figure 16-3). Place preservative in container, if needed.
6. Place a sign saying "Save All Urine" in bathroom near toilet.
7. Put on gloves.
8. Have client void first specimen. Discard. Record time.
9. Remove and discard gloves. (Wear gloves each time you handle another urine specimen. Wash hands after removing gloves. Discard gloves.)
10. Collect all urine for the next 24 hours. Pour into specimen container.
11. Remind client not to have a bowel movement when urinating. If feces comes in contact with the urine, the entire procedure will have to be repeated.
12. Record I&O if needed.
13. Add each urine specimen to the container immediately following voiding. Pour into graduate and then into large container to avoid spilling and splashing (Figure 16-4). A funnel may also be used.
14. Add ice to the bucket as necessary to keep the specimen cold.
15. At the end of 24 hours, have client void as before. Place final specimen in large container.
16. Record what you have done. Report any unusual conditions to your supervisor.
17. Keep specimen on ice until ready for transfer to laboratory.
18. Remove container from ice, and dry outside of container. Place in large plastic grocery bag for delivery to laboratory.

Fig 16-3 Place urine container in a bucket of ice (Step 5).

Fig 16-4 Add each urine specimen to the container (Step 13).

PROCEDURE 16-4   Straining Urine

Materials Needed

- Graduate
- Strainer (disposable paper filter or 4-by-4–inch gauze)
- Specimen container
- Disposable gloves
- Goggles (if needed)
- PPE (if needed)

Procedure

1. Explain procedure to client and family.
2. Obtain materials listed above, and place in bathroom.
3. Place sign saying "Strain All Urine" near toilet.
4. Wash your hands.
5. Put on gloves and goggles, if needed.
6. Have client void into bedpan, urinal, commode, or urine collector ("hat") in toilet.
7. Transfer urine into graduate.
8. Place strainer or gauze over specimen container.
9. Pour urine through strainer and into specimen container (Figure 16-5).
10. Inspect filter paper or gauze. If stones are present, wrap them in the filter material and place into the specimen container for transport to the laboratory. Label container. Store in refrigerator according to directions in Procedure 16-1.
11. If no stones are found, discard urine. Discard used disposable materials. Clean used reusable materials, and prepare for reuse the next time the client voids.

Fig 16-5 Pour urine through the strainer (Step 9).

12. Remove and discard gloves. Remove goggles. Use gloves each time you handle a urine specimen.
13. Wash your hands.
14. Record what you have done. Report any unusual conditions to your supervisor.

STOOL SPECIMENS

Small amounts of stool are collected for laboratory examination for the presence of blood, fats, microorganisms, parasites, and other abnormal contents. Only a small amount of stool is needed for examination; about 2 tablespoons is sufficient.

In some cases, a tiny amount of stool is applied to a card. This is a test for occult (hidden) blood. Follow the directions on the card.

Do not use stool that has come in contact with urine. Sometimes a warm specimen is needed. In that case, the specimen must be transported to the laboratory quickly. Follow your supervisor's instructions regarding delivery of the stool specimen. Follow Procedure 16-5, Collecting a Stool Specimen.

SPUTUM SPECIMENS

Sputum is thick mucus produced by the respiratory tract when disease or infection is present. Sputum specimens are obtained to check for the presence of blood, bacteria, and abnormal cells. The client coughs up sputum from the trachea and bronchi. Sputum

PROCEDURE 16-5 | Collecting a Stool Specimen

Materials Needed
- Stool specimen container and label
- Tongue depressor
- Bedpan, commode, or "hat"
- Toilet paper
- Disposable gloves

Fig 16-6 Use a tongue depressor to place stool in specimen container (Step 8).

Procedure
1. Explain what you are going to do.
2. Wash your hands.
3. Obtain materials listed above.
4. Label container.
5. Assist client to bathroom or commode, or offer bedpan.
6. Ask client not to urinate, if possible, while having the bowel movement.
7. Put on gloves.
8. Transfer stool to specimen container using tongue depressor (Figure 16-6), and put on lid.
9. Flush remaining feces down toilet, and assist client to complete toileting, as necessary.
10. Remove and discard gloves.
11. Wash your hands.
12. Help client, as needed, back to bed or chair.
13. Store specimen according to agency policy or supervisor's directions.
14. Record what you have done. Report any unusual conditions to your supervisor.

specimens are usually easier to collect in the morning because this material collects in the lungs during sleep. Be sure that you collect sputum, not saliva (the fluid found in the mouth). Rinse the client's mouth with plain water to remove saliva. Encourage the client to cough sputum directly into the specimen container, close the lid, and then place the container into a plastic bag. If you handle the specimen, wear gloves. NEVER LET A CLIENT COUGH ON YOU. Follow Procedure 16-6, Collecting a Sputum Specimen.

ASSISTING CLIENTS TO SELF-MONITOR BLOOD SUGAR LEVELS

Clients with diabetes may monitor their blood sugar (glucose) levels. They use a small electronic monitor called a "glucometer" (Figure 16-7, *A*). The client collects a sample of his or her capillary blood on a specially treated dipstick. The sample is inserted into the glucometer, which displays the amount of sugar in the blood. This procedure is the client's responsibility. If necessary, the agency nurse will teach the client how to perform this test and will evaluate his or her accuracy in performing the test. You may need to take the equipment to the client so he or she can perform the test. Observe the results, and assist the client to record them in the blood sugar diary. This diary contains a record of blood sugar levels for each day. Clients may monitor their blood sugar several times a day. You may be asked to write the results in the client care record. Report abnormal blood sugar levels as instructed by your supervisor and the care plan.

Teach the client to dispose of used lancets and blood collection strips (Figure 16-7, *B*) according to agency and local community policies. Do not handle lancets because of the risk of skin puncture. Both lancet and strip are contaminated with the client's blood. Dispose of any other used materials, such as cotton balls, in the correct manner. Review Chapter 11 for safe disposal of materials. Return glucometer to proper storage area.

PROCEDURE 16-6   Collecting a Sputum Specimen

Material Needed
- Sputum specimen container with lid
- Label
- Tissues
- Small plastic bag (sandwich bag size)
- Small paper bag (lunch bag size)
- Disposable gloves
- Disposable mask (if needed)
- Glass of water and emesis basin

Procedure
1. Explain procedure to client.
2. Wash your hands.
3. Obtain materials listed above.
4. Label container.
5. Provide privacy.
6. Put on gloves.
7. Assist client to rinse mouth with plain water.
8. Have client hold sputum specimen container in one hand and tissue in the other.
9. Instruct client to take a deep breath, hold it for a second, and then cough into tissue. Do not let client cough on you. Use disposable mask, if needed. Have client repeat the coughing two or three times to loosen the sputum deep in the respiratory tract.
10. When client has loosened sputum, have client cough sputum directly into the specimen container. Approximately 2 tablespoons of sputum will be needed.
11. Do not touch the inside of the container. Keep the outside clean and free of any sputum.
12. Put lid on specimen container.
13. Place container into a plastic bag and then into a paper bag.
14. Remove and discard gloves.
15. Wash your hands.
16. Record what you have done. Report any unusual conditions to your supervisor.
17. Specimen is sent to laboratory according to agency policy.

Fig 16-7 **A,** A glucometer with a blood sample in place and normal reading. **B,** To reduce risk of infection from bloodborne pathogens, be sure lancets and dipsticks are disposed of properly. (From Sorrentino SA: *Mosby's textbook for long-term care nursing assistants,* ed 6, St. Louis, 2011, Mosby.)

CHAPTER SUMMARY

- Specimens are small samples of body tissues and fluids that are examined in the medical laboratory for the presence of normal and abnormal contents.
- The results of laboratory tests are used to determine the cause of illness and to evaluate the client's progress.

- Usual specimens collected by home care aides are urine, stool, and sputum.
- Proper labeling of specimen containers includes client's name, address, and date and time of specimen collection.
- Practice standard (universal) precautions and medical asepsis when collecting and handling specimens.

STUDY QUESTIONS

1. What are three reasons for collecting specimens?
2. List five rules to follow when collecting specimens.
3. Give two examples of the use of standard (universal) precautions and medical asepsis when collecting the following specimens:

a. Routine urine specimen
b. Clean catch urine specimen
c. 24-Hour urine specimen
d. Stool specimen
e. Sputum specimen

17

Measuring Vital Signs

Temperature, pulse, respirations, and blood pressure are called the vital signs. They give information about essential body processes: circulation, breathing, and heat regulation. See Box 17-1 for a review of the circulatory and respiratory systems.

Home care aides measure temperature, pulse, and respirations. Some agencies may also require you to measure blood pressure. This will vary according to the agency and state. Vital signs are taken and recorded according to the client's plan of care.

Take the vital signs while the client is at rest. Exercise and activity can cause the vital signs to increase. Other factors that influence vital signs are sleep, age, anxiety, fear, pain, illness, foods and fluids, and medications.

BOX 17-1 **Circulatory and Respiratory Systems Review**

- The heart is a muscular organ that pumps blood through the arteries to all parts of the body.
- The heartbeat has two parts:
  Systole: When the heart muscle is contracting
  Diastole: When the heart muscle is resting
- The act of breathing has two parts:
  Inhaling: When oxygen is taken into the body
  Exhaling: When carbon dioxide is expelled from the body
- The heart and lungs are located in the chest cavity.

BOX 17-2 **Vital Signs: Normal Adult Ranges**

TEMPERATURE

Oral	97.6° to 99.6° F (36.5° to 37.5° C)
Axillary	96.6° to 98.6° F (36.0° to 37.0° C)
Tympanic	98.6° to 100.6° F (37.0° to 38.1° C)
Rectal	98.6° to 100.6° F (37.0° to 38.1° C)

PULSE RATE
60 to 100 beats per minute

RESPIRATORY RATE (RESPIRATIONS)
12 to 20 respirations per minute

BLOOD PRESSURE

Systolic	100 to 120
Diastolic	70 to 80

TEMPERATURE

Temperature is the amount of heat produced by the body as it uses food for energy. Normally, the amount of heat produced should be the same as the amount of heat lost from the body. Heat leaves the body through urine, feces, exhaling, and skin surfaces. When heat produced by the body is not removed through normal means, it builds up in the body. This increase in body temperature is called a **fever**.

Measuring body temperature is an important way to observe the client's response to illness and treatment. Pulse and respirations are usually measured at the same time the temperature is taken.

Some factors may change the reading of the body temperature for a short time and include the following:

- Drinking hot or cold liquids
- Eating hot or cold foods
- Smoking
- Taking a hot or cold bath or shower
- Exercising

If your client has participated in any of these activities, wait 15 minutes before taking the temperature.

There is a vast difference in normal temperature from person to person. Some older adults may have a very low normal temperature. It is important to know what is normal for each person. This is part of the information collected by the nurse during the first visit to the client (Box 17-2).

LOCATION

Temperature may be taken in several areas of the body.
- Oral temperature (mouth)
- Axillary temperature (armpit)
- Tympanic temperature (ear canal)
- Rectal temperature (rectum)

Follow the care plan's directions for taking your client's temperature. **SPEAK WITH YOUR SUPERVISOR IF YOU ARE UNSURE ABOUT HOW YOUR CLIENT'S TEMPERATURE SHOULD BE TAKEN.**

THERMOMETERS

A **thermometer** is an instrument used to take the temperature. There are several different kinds of thermometers: oral, rectal, electronic, tympanic, and disposable. They may be made of plastic or paper.

In the past, glass thermometers filled with mercury were used. However, mercury is a hazardous chemical that is harmful to humans, animals, and the environment. Since 2001, 20 states have banned mercury thermometers for medical use. Several substitutes are used in thermometers. These may be alcohol and galistan (an earth-friendly mercury substitute). These solutions may have a red, blue, or silvery color and are readily seen in the stem of the thermometer.

The client should have his or her own personal thermometer, not one shared with others. If a thermometer is brought from the agency for a single use, a disposable one is best to avoid any risk of transmission of infection.

READING A THERMOMETER

Regular Thermometer

The thermometer has three important parts (Figure 17-1).
1. Bulb or tip where the solution is stored
2. Solution (red, blue, or silvery color)
3. Stem or tube that contains the scale for reading the temperature

The heat of the body causes the solution to expand and rise in the stem. Long lines on the tube mark 94° to 108° F (34° to 42° C). Short lines indicate two tenths of a degree. An arrow marks the normal adult oral temperature of 98.6° F (37.0° C).

Read the thermometer in the following manner:
1. Hold the thermometer at eye level, handling only the end of the stem.
2. Find the column of solution. Turn the thermometer slowly until you see the colored line along the scale.

Fig 17-1 **A,** A Fahrenheit thermometer with a long or slender tip. The temperature measurement is 98.6° F. **B,** Centigrade thermometer with a stubby tip (rectal thermometer). The temperature is 37.0° C. **C,** Fahrenheit thermometer with a pear-shaped tip. The temperature measurement is 99.2° F. (From Sorrentino SA, Remmert LN: *Mosby's textbook for nursing assistants,* ed 8, St. Louis, 2012, Mosby.)

Fahrenheit Thermometer
   a. Find the mark to indicate 94° F. Each long line marks 1 degree of temperature.
   b. Only every other degree is labeled with a number: 94° F, 96° F, 98° F, and so on.
   c. Between each long line are four short lines. Each represents two tenths of 1 degree (2/10 or 0.2) (see Figure 17-1).

Celsius (Centigrade) Thermometer
   a. Find the mark to indicate 35° C. Each long line marks 1 degree of temperature.
   b. Each degree is marked with a number: 35° C, 36° C, 37° C, and so on.
   c. Between each long line are nine short lines. Each line represents one tenth of 1 degree (1/10 or 0.1) (see Figure 17-1).

3. Read the temperature at the point where the solution ends.

   A NOTE OF CAUTION: IF YOUR CLIENT HAS A GLASS MERCURY THERMOMETER, NOTIFY YOUR SUPERVISOR. THE THERMOMETER SHOULD BE DISCARDED ACCORDING TO THE ACCEPTABLE PROCEDURES FOR HAZARDOUS WASTE REMOVAL IN YOUR LOCALITY.

Electronic Thermometer

This thermometer gives a digital (number) reading of the results. If the battery is working, you will see the results in the readout area. The letter *F* after the reading indicates the Fahrenheit scale of measurement, and the letter *C* indicates the Celsius (centigrade) scale (Figure 17-2).

Disposable (Single-Use) Thermometer

The last dot on the thermometer to change color indicates the temperature reading (Figure 17-3). This thermometer comes in a Fahrenheit or a Celsius scale. Wait 10 seconds after removing the thermometer from the client's mouth before you read

Fig 17-2 An electronic thermometer; note the "On/Off" button.

Fig 17-3 A disposable Fahrenheit thermometer. This example reads 98.6° F. The last colored dot shows the correct temperature.

PROCEDURE 17-1 | Cleaning a Thermometer

Materials Needed
- Thermometer
- Cotton balls or tissues
- Soap and cold water
- Disposable gloves

Procedure
1. Wash your hands.
2. Obtain materials listed above.
3. Put on disposable gloves.
4. Wet cotton ball (or tissue) with soap and water.
5. Hold thermometer by stem over sink or wastebasket.

6. Begin at stem end. Wash from stem to bulb end, twisting cotton ball firmly.
7. Discard used cotton ball.
8. Rinse thermometer with a clean, wet cotton ball using the same twisting, downward movement.
9. Repeat washing and rinsing.
10. Dry with a tissue, wiping in same downward movement.
11. Discard tissue.
12. Store thermometer properly.
13. Remove and discard gloves. Wash hands.

it. Other single-use thermometers may be applied directly to the skin surface, usually the forehead. They are read in the same manner.

CLEANING A THERMOMETER

Thermometers are cleaned before and after each use. Handle the thermometer by its stem only. For both regular and home use electronic thermometers, follow Procedure 17-1, Cleaning a Thermometer.

SHAKING DOWN A REGULAR THERMOMETER

The solution in a thermometer should be below 95° F or 35° C before you take the temperature. To get an accurate reading, shake down the solution.
- Grasp the thermometer firmly by the stem end with your thumb and two fingers.
- Stand away from areas where you might hit the thermometer and break it.
- Shake the thermometer with a movement that snaps the wrist, as in a vigorous shaking to remove water from the hands.
- Shake over a bed or sofa if there is danger of dropping the thermometer.

TAKING AN ORAL TEMPERATURE

The usual way to take the temperature is by mouth. The thermometer is left in the mouth for 3 minutes. Electronic thermometers signal with a "beep" when the reading is complete. Single-use thermometers will give results in 60 seconds.

For certain clients, taking an oral temperature is not recommended.
- Unconscious, restless, or confused clients
- Mouth breathers
- Clients receiving oxygen
- Paralyzed clients
- Clients with sore mouths
- Children younger than 5 years of age

Remember, if your client has had something hot or cold to eat or drink or has smoked, wait 15 minutes before taking the temperature. Follow Procedures 17-2, 17-3, and 17-4, Taking an Oral Temperature with Regular, Electronic, or Single-Use Thermometers.

PROCEDURE 17-2 | Taking an Oral Temperature (With a Regular Thermometer)

Materials Needed
- Oral thermometer
- Tissues or cotton balls
- Watch with sweep second hand
- Pencil
- Paper
- Disposable gloves (optional)

Procedure
1. Explain what you are going to do. (Remind client not to eat, drink, or smoke for 15 minutes.)
2. Have client lie down or rest in a chair.
3. Wash your hands.
4. Obtain materials listed above.
5. Put on disposable gloves (optional).
6. Clean thermometer (see Procedure 17-1).
7. Shake down thermometer to 95° F (35° C), if necessary.
8. Place thermometer under client's tongue, as far back as possible, into either heat pocket (Figure 17-4).
9. Tell client to keep mouth closed and not to talk.
10. Leave thermometer in place for 3 minutes. (You may take the pulse and respirations at this time.)
11. Remove thermometer.
12. Wipe thermometer with tissue from stem end to bulb end. Discard tissue. Do not touch any part of the thermometer that has been in the client's mouth.
13. Read the thermometer and then place it on a tissue.
14. Write the temperature (pulse and respirations) on the paper.
15. Clean and dry thermometer.
16. Shake down thermometer to 95° F (35° C).
17. Store thermometer in holder in proper location.
18. Remove and discard gloves (optional). Wash hands.
19. Record temperature on client record. Indicate (O) for oral temperature.
20. Report abnormal temperature to your supervisor.

Fig 17-4 Place thermometer under the tongue into the heat pocket (Step 8).

PROCEDURE 17-3 | Taking an Oral Temperature (With an Electronic Thermometer)

Materials Needed
- Electronic thermometer
- Tissues or cotton balls
- Pencil
- Paper
- Disposable gloves (optional)

Procedure
1. Explain what you are going to do. (Remind client not to eat, drink, or smoke for 15 minutes.)
2. Have client lie down or rest in a chair.
3. Wash your hands.
4. Obtain materials.
5. Put on disposable gloves (optional).
6. Clean thermometer (see Procedure 17-1).
7. Turn on thermometer.
8. Wait until the thermometer reads "0" or shows "- - -" on the digital display window (Figure 17-5).
9. Place thermometer under client's tongue, as far back as possible, into either heat pocket.
10. Tell client to keep mouth closed and not to talk.
11. Leave thermometer in place until you hear it "beep." (You may take pulse and respirations at this time.)

PROCEDURE 17-3   Taking an Oral Temperature (With an Electronic Thermometer)—cont'd

12. Remove thermometer.
13. Wipe thermometer with tissue from stem end to bulb end. Discard tissue.
14. Read the thermometer and then place it on a tissue.
15. Write the temperature (pulse and respirations) on the paper.
16. Clean and dry thermometer.
17. Turn off thermometer.
18. Store thermometer in holder in proper location.
19. Remove and discard gloves (optional). Wash hands.
20. Record temperature on client record. Indicate (O) for oral temperature.
21. Report abnormal temperature to your supervisor.

Fig 17-5 With the "° F" sign flashing, the thermometer is ready to take a temperature.

PROCEDURE 17-4   Taking an Oral Temperature (With a Single-Use Thermometer)

Materials Needed
- Single-use thermometer
- Watch with sweep second hand
- Tissues
- Pencil
- Paper

Procedure
1. Explain what you are going to do. (Remind client not to eat, drink, or smoke for 15 minutes.)
2. Have client lie down or rest in a chair.
3. Wash your hands.
4. Obtain materials listed above.
5. Remove thermometer from wrapper.
6. Place thermometer under client's tongue, as far back as possible, into either heat pocket.
7. Tell client to keep mouth closed and not to talk.
8. Leave thermometer in place for at least 1 minute. (You may take pulse and respirations at this time.)
9. Remove thermometer. Do not touch any part of thermometer that has been in the client's mouth. Wait 10 seconds, and read the last colored dot on the thermometer. Place thermometer on a tissue.
10. Write the temperature on the paper.
11. Discard thermometer.
12. Wash your hands.
13. Record temperature on client record, and indicate (O) for oral.
14. Report abnormal temperature to your supervisor.

TAKING AN AXILLARY TEMPERATURE

Axillary temperatures are taken when the oral method cannot be used. This method may be used for adults, children, and infants. It is the least accurate method of measuring temperature. However, it is preferred over the rectal temperature because it is not damaging to body tissue. Also, because there is no contact with body fluids, there is a reduced risk of infection.

The axilla (armpit) is dried before beginning the procedure. Hold the thermometer in contact with the skin surfaces. This will ensure an accurate reading. Have your client sit or lie down during the procedure. The thermometer remains in place for 10 minutes, the single-use thermometer for 3 minutes. The electronic thermometer remains in place until a "beeping" sound is heard, about 2 to 3 minutes (see Procedure 17-5, Taking an Axillary Temperature).

PROCEDURE 17-5   Taking an Axillary Temperature

Materials Needed
- Thermometer: Regular, electronic, or single use
- Watch with sweep second hand
- Dry towel or washcloth
- Tissues
- Pencil
- Paper

Procedure
1. Explain what you are going to do.
2. Have client lie down or rest in a chair.
3. Wash your hands.
4. Obtain materials listed above.
5. Clean thermometer (see Procedure 17-1).
6. Shake down thermometer to 95° F (35° C). Turn on electronic thermometer, or remove single-use thermometer from wrapper.
7. Provide privacy (close door, shut drapes, pull shades).
8. Remove client's arm from sleeve. Expose axilla.
9. Dry axilla with towel or washcloth.
10. Place thermometer in axilla so that it is in contact with skin. Put client's arm across chest to hold thermometer in place (Figure 17-6). For infant or child, hold arm in place as necessary.
11. Leave thermometer in place.
    Regular: 10 minutes
    Electronic: Until "beep" is heard
    Single use: 3 minutes
    (You may take pulse and respirations at this time.)
12. Remove thermometer.
13. Wipe with tissue from stem end to bulb, if regular or electronic thermometer is used. Then discard tissue.
14. Read the thermometer, and then place it on a tissue.
15. Write the temperature on the paper.
16. Help client put arm back in sleeve.
17. Turn off electronic thermometer, if used.
18. Clean and dry thermometer. Discard single-use thermometer.
19. Shake down thermometer.
20. Store thermometer in holder in proper location.
21. Wash your hands.
22. Record temperature on client record. Indicate (A) for axillary temperature.
23. Report abnormal temperature to your supervisor.

Fig 17-6 Place thermometer in the armpit (axilla) (Step 10).

TAKING A TYMPANIC (EAR) TEMPERATURE

A tympanic thermometer (Figure 17-7) measures the temperature of the client's eardrum. It may be used when the oral method cannot be used and is effective for taking a child's temperature. The advantages of using this type of thermometer are that it is comfortable and records the temperature quickly (1 to 3 seconds). However, if the client has drainage from the ear or has had recent ear surgery, this thermometer should not be used.

The end of the thermometer is called a *probe* and has a removable cover that is discarded after use. Before inserting the probe with cover into the ear canal, check the following:

- Check the battery because a low battery may give an incorrect temperature reading.
- For hearing aids, remove the aid from the ear to be used.
- The right mode (infant-toddler or child-adult) is set on the thermometer.

Fig 17-7 Tympanic thermometer. (Courtesy American Diagnostic Corp., Hauppauge, New York.)

THEN
- Pull the top of the ear up and back to straighten the ear canal in an adult.

OR
- Pull the earlobe down and back in a child younger than 2 years of age.

The probe with cover should be inserted gently into the ear canal. When the temperature has been measured, the thermometer will indicate this by means of a flashing light or sound. After taking the temperature, discard the probe cover and return the thermometer to the base unit for recharging (see Procedure 17-6, Taking a Temperature Using a Tympanic Thermometer).

TAKING A RECTAL TEMPERATURE

Rectal temperatures are taken when the oral and axillary routes cannot be used. Rectal temperatures are not taken when clients have diarrhea, rectal disease or surgery, and certain types of heart and blood diseases.

A rectal thermometer is used. The end of the stem is colored red. **RECTAL THERMOMETERS ARE USED IN THE RECTUM ONLY. THEY ARE NEVER TO BE USED IN THE MOUTH.** If a single-use thermometer is used, its transparent plastic cover is left on while the temperature is taken. Both types should be lubricated for ease in insertion and to prevent damage to rectal tissues. Electronic thermometers are usually not appropriate for taking rectal temperatures. Gently insert the tip of the thermometer into the rectum. Do not push if you have difficulty inserting the thermometer. Always hold the thermometer in place to prevent it from breaking or being lost in the rectum. Follow Procedure 17-7, Taking a Rectal Temperature.

REPORTING CHANGES FROM NORMAL TEMPERATURE

ORR   Notify your supervisor if your client's temperature is above the normal range listed in Box 17-2. When a fever is present, a client may have other symptoms, such as headaches, chills, and sweating. Keep the client warm with extra clothing or blankets. Remove these if the client sweats and complains of feeling hot. Change wet clothing

PROCEDURE 17-6 | Taking a Temperature Using a Tympanic Thermometer

Materials Needed
- Tympanic thermometer with probe cover
- Pencil
- Paper

Procedure
1. Explain what you are going to do.
2. Have client lie down or rest in a chair.
3. Provide privacy (close door, shut drapes, pull shades).
4. Wash your hands.
5. Obtain materials listed above.
6. Ask client to turn head so ear is in front of you.
7. Pull top of ear up and back to straighten the ear canal in adults (Figure 17-8, *A*), or pull earlobe down and back for children younger than 2 years of age (Figure 17-8, *B*).
8. Gently insert tympanic thermometer probe with cover into the ear canal (Figure 17-8, *C*).
9. Read the measurement when you see a flashing light or hear a tone.
10. Remove thermometer probe from ear canal.
11. Discard probe cover directly into wastebasket.
12. Write the temperature on the paper. Indicate (T) for tympanic temperature.
13. Return thermometer to base unit for recharge.
14. Wash your hands.
15. Record what you have done. Report any abnormal temperature to your supervisor.

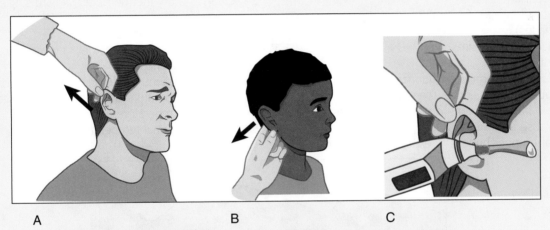

A   B   C

Fig 17-8 **A,** In adults, pull top of ear up and back (Step 7). **B,** Pull earlobe down and back for children younger than 2 years of age (Step 7). **C,** Gently insert thermometer probe with cover (Step 8).

as needed. Make sure the client drinks fluids. Check with your supervisor before increasing the fluid intake.

PULSE

The pulse is caused by the beating of the heart. With each beat, the heart forces blood to flow out through the arteries of the body. The pulse rate, then, shows the number of heartbeats that are felt in an artery during 1 minute. The pulse rate can be slower or faster depending on several factors.
- *Exercise:* Immediately after climbing stairs, the rate will be higher than when sitting and watching television
- *Age:* Infants have higher pulse rates than adults
- *Fever:* Elevated temperature and elevated pulse rate usually go together

PROCEDURE 17-7 | Taking a Rectal Temperature

Materials Needed

- Rectal thermometer or single-use rectal thermometer with wrapper
- Watch with sweep second hand
- Toilet tissue
- Disposable gloves
- Water-soluble lubricant
- Pencil
- Paper

Procedure

1. Explain what you are going to do.
2. Put client in bed.
3. Wash your hands.
4. Obtain materials listed above.
5. Clean thermometer (see Procedure 17-1).
6. Shake down thermometer to 95° F (35° C), if necessary.
7. Provide privacy (close door, shut drapes, pull shades).
8. Place client in Sims' position.
9. Put on gloves.
10. Place small amount of lubricant on toilet tissue. Lubricate bulb end of thermometer.
11. Fold back top linens, and remove clothing to expose anal area.
12. Raise upper buttock to expose anus (Figure 17-9).
13. Gently insert thermometer 1 inch (2.5 cm) into the rectum.
14. Hold thermometer in place for 3 minutes (Figure 17-10).
15. Remove thermometer.
16. Wipe thermometer with toilet tissue from stem end to bulb end. Place soiled tissue on several folded layers of toilet tissue.
17. Place thermometer on clean toilet tissue.
18. Cleanse excess lubricant and feces from anal area using toilet tissue.
19. Replace clothing and cover client.
20. Discard soiled toilet tissue into toilet.
21. Remove and discard gloves. Wash hands.
22. Read the thermometer, and then place it back on tissue.
23. Write the temperature on the paper.
24. Clean and dry thermometer. Discard single-use thermometer.
25. Shake down thermometer to 95° F (35° C).
26. Store thermometer in holder in proper location.
27. Wash your hands.
28. Make sure client is safe and comfortable.
29. Record temperature on client record. Indicate (R) for rectal temperature.
30. Report abnormal temperature to your supervisor.

Fig 17-9 Raise upper buttock (Step 12).

Fig 17-10 Hold thermometer in place for 3 minutes (Step 14).

- *Excitement or fear:* Causes the heart to beat faster
- *Pain:* May also cause the heart to beat faster
- *Medications:* Some are used to slow down the pulse rate; others are used to raise the pulse rate

FORCE AND RHYTHM

When taking the pulse, you will also need to note its force and rhythm. The force shows the strength of each beat. A strong pulse is usually easy to feel. A weak pulse is usually hard to feel. The rhythm, or pattern of beats, should be regular. This means that the time between each beat is the same. An irregular pulse is caused by the heart beating unevenly or skipping beats. It is very important to note the force and rhythm of the pulse rate. Record and report weak and/or irregular pulse rates to your supervisor (Box 17-3).

TAKING A RADIAL PULSE

Usually, the pulse is taken on the radial artery. This artery is located on the palm side of the wrist at the base of the thumb. Using your three middle fingers, press against

---

BOX 17-3 **Report to Your Supervisor ...**

CHANGES IN VITAL SIGNS

Temperature

- Increased (Fever)
  Oral: Above 99.6° F (37.5° C)
  Rectal: Above 100.6° F (38.1° C)
  Axillary: Above 98.6° F (37° C)
  Tympanic: Above 100.6° F (38.1° C)
- Decreased:
  Oral: Below 97.6° F (36.5° C)
  Rectal: Below 98.6° F (37° C)
  Axillary: Below 96.6° F (36° C)
  Tympanic: Below 98.6° F (37° C)
- Major change from what is "normal" for your client

Pulse

  Below 60 beats per minute
  Above 100 beats per minute
  Change in rhythm or force of beats

Respirations

  Below 12 respirations per minute
  Above 20 respirations per minute
  Changes in pattern or depth of respirations
  Difficulty breathing
  Noisy breathing

Blood Pressure

  Any blood pressure reading that is not within normal range or is changed from what is "normal" for your client
  According to instructions in care plan

PROCEDURE 17-8   Taking a Radial Pulse

Materials Needed
- Watch with sweep second hand
- Pencil
- Paper

Procedure
1. Explain what you are going to do.
2. Ask client to sit or lie down.
3. Wash your hands.
4. Obtain materials listed above.
5. Locate radial pulse. Use your middle three fingers to press down on radial artery (Figure 17-11).
6. Note the following:
   Strong or weak
   Regular or irregular
7. Count the beats for 1 minute.
8. Write the pulse rate on the paper. Also note the strength and regularity of beats.
9. Make sure client is safe and comfortable.
10. Record pulse on client record.
11. Report any abnormal pulse conditions to your supervisor.

Fig 17-11 Locate radial pulse (Step 5).

the wrist bone to feel the blood pumping through the radial artery. Do not use your thumb to take the client's pulse. Your thumb has its own artery, and you may mistake your pulse for the client's. Take the pulse for 1 full minute, and note the rate, force, and rhythm of the beats (see Procedure 17-8, Taking a Radial Pulse).

Do not take your client's pulse immediately after any physical activity such as climbing stairs or using the bathroom. Wait for 15 minutes before taking the pulse to get an accurate reading.

The normal pulse rate is

Adults: 60 to 100 beats per minute

Record and report the following abnormal conditions to your supervisor immediately.

Adults	Rate	Force	Rhythm
	Above 100	Weak	Irregular
	Below 60	Weak	Irregular

RESPIRATIONS

The act of inhaling oxygen and exhaling carbon dioxide is called *respiration*. During one respiration, the chest usually rises as air enters the lungs (inhalation) and falls as air is pushed out of the nose and mouth (exhalation). The rate of respirations means the number of times the chest rises and falls during a 1-minute period. You may find that some clients use their abdominal muscles rather than chest muscles to help them breathe. In these cases, the chest may not rise and fall. Rather, the abdomen rises and falls with each breath.

The rate of respirations is one way to tell the health of the respiratory system. Because both the circulatory and respiratory systems work closely together, the pulse and respiratory rates are affected by similar factors. For example, running to the bus stop causes the heart rate to increase (pulse) and breathing (respirations) to also increase. Exercise, age, fever, excitement or fear, and medications influence the respiratory rate.

In healthy persons, the normal respiratory rate for adults is 12 to 20 respirations per minute.

DEPTH, PATTERN, AND EFFORT OF RESPIRATIONS

When taking the client's respirations, also note the depth, pattern, and effort of breathing while counting each respiration. In normal respirations, both sides of the chest rise and fall equally. The respirations are regular in pattern and depth; they are quiet and without effort. Use the following guidelines when observing your client's respirations.

Rate

Normal	12 to 20
Abnormal	Under 12 or over 20

Depth

Normal	Both sides of chest rise and fall equally
Shallow	Breath is short
Deep	Breath is long and deep

Pattern

Regular	Each inhalation and exhalation is at the same rate
Irregular	May have periods where no breath is taken, followed by rapid or slow, shallow breaths

Noise

Normal	Breathing is quiet
Abnormal	Raspy, gurgling, wheezy breathing

Effort

Normal	Breathing is easy, without effort
Abnormal	Breathing is difficult, painful, or takes great effort

Report any changes from normal respirations to your supervisor immediately (see Box 17-3).

TAKING RESPIRATIONS

Count the client's respirations when he or she is resting. Wait 15 minutes after exercise or activity to allow the respiratory system time to adjust to normal. Have client sit or lie down so that you can see the chest rise and fall. For abdominal breathers, you may need to rest your hand on the abdomen and notice the rise and fall of your hand.

Respirations can be controlled to some extent by the client, especially if he or she knows you are taking the respirations. This may result in an incorrect count. So, do not tell the client when you are taking respirations. After taking the pulse, just keep your fingers on the pulse while watching the rise and fall of the client's chest. In this way the client will think that you are still taking the pulse. Follow Procedure 17-9, Taking Respirations.

PROCEDURE 17-9 | Taking Respirations

1. Continue holding client's wrist after taking the pulse.
2. Do not tell the client that you will count the respirations.
3. Count each rise and fall of the chest or abdomen as one respiration (Figure 17-12).
4. Count respirations for 1 minute.
5. Observe for the following.
   Deep or shallow breathing
   Painful or difficulty breathing
   Noisy breathing
6. Record the respirations on the paper, noting the information listed above.
7. Make sure client is safe and comfortable.
8. Wash your hands.
9. Record respirations on client record.
10. Report any abnormal respirations to your supervisor.

Fig 17-12 Count each rise and fall of the chest (or abdomen) (Step 3).

MEASURING BLOOD PRESSURE

Blood pressure is the force of the blood that pushes against the walls of the blood vessels. When taking the client's blood pressure, you are measuring the force of the blood flowing through the arteries. This force is caused by the heart pumping blood into the arteries. It is this force that makes the blood circulate to all parts of the body.

The amount of pressure in the arteries depends on two factors: the client's heart rate, and how easily blood flows through the blood vessels.

TWO READINGS

When taking your client's blood pressure (BP), you are measuring two pressures.
- **Systolic pressure:** The force of the blood pushing against the walls of large arteries when the heart is contracting. This is the higher reading and is listed first, <u>120</u>.
- **Diastolic pressure:** The force of the blood pushing against the walls of the arteries when the heart is resting. This is the lower reading and listed below the systolic reading, 80.

FACTORS AFFECTING BLOOD PRESSURE

Like the client's temperature, pulse, and respirations, blood pressure also is affected by many factors. For example, pain, anxiety, and fear can cause an increase in blood pressure. Exercise can also cause the blood pressure to rise due to the increased effort of the heart to pump blood to the body. This rise is usually only temporary. Have the client sit and rest for 15 minutes before taking the blood pressure (see Box 17-4, Guidelines for Taking Vital Signs).

Illnesses of the circulatory system may cause the blood pressure to become higher or lower. Clients with disease conditions that affect the heart, blood, or blood vessels will usually have their blood pressure taken regularly. These conditions include:

> **BOX 17-4**   **Guidelines for Taking Vital Signs**
>
> - Take vital signs when client has been resting for 15 minutes.
> - Take vital signs when client is sitting or lying down.
> - Wait for 15 minutes before taking the temperature, if your client has been
>   Smoking
>   Exercising
>   Drinking hot or cold liquids
>   Eating hot or cold foods
> - Ask client not to talk while you take the vital signs.
> - Take the temperature while taking the pulse and respirations.
> - Record vital signs immediately after taking them, using paper and pencil; transfer this information to the client's care record.
> - Record the method of taking the temperature: (O) oral, (R) rectal, (A) axillary, or (T) tympanic.

- **Hypertension:** High blood pressure
- **Hypotension:** Low blood pressure
- Certain heart diseases
- Kidney diseases
- Problems with pregnancy

Your supervisor will explain what to look for when taking your patient's blood pressure. It is important to know your client's usual blood pressure. The normal adult blood pressure is considered to be below $\frac{120}{80}$.

Notify your supervisor when the pressure is higher or lower than the "usual" reading for your client.

EQUIPMENT NEEDED

There are two items that are needed to take a blood pressure reading: the stethoscope and the blood pressure cuff. Your agency or the client will have these available for you to use.

Using a Stethoscope

The stethoscope is an instrument used to listen to sounds produced in the body. Invented in the early 1800s, it is said to be one of the 10 greatest contributions to medical science. By hearing the sounds of the heart, arteries, lungs, abdomen, and other body cavities, health care professionals are able to diagnose illnesses more easily.

Basically, the stethoscope makes body sounds easier to hear. It magnifies sound like a hearing aid. The three parts of the stethoscope are as follows (Figure 17-13).

1. *Earpieces:* Block out outside noises and receive sound from the tubing
2. *Metal* and *plastic tubing:* Connect earpieces to chest piece (diaphragm) or bell. Sound travels through the tubing to the earpieces.
3. *Chest piece (diaphragm)* or *bell:* Transmits sound to the tubing when placed over a part of the body
   a. Chest piece (diaphragm), a round, flat piece
   b. Bell, a bell-shaped piece
   The following are tips to follow when using a stethoscope.
- Wipe earpieces and chest piece with antiseptic wipes before and after using to prevent spread of pathogens.

Fig 17-13 The parts of the stethoscope.

Fig 17-14 The blood pressure cuff.

- Turn off radio and television, and reduce other background noises (if possible) before using stethoscope.
- Ask the client not to talk or move during the procedure.
- Warm the chest piece (diaphragm) or bell with your hands before placing it on the client's body.
- Do not touch the metal or plastic tubing after earpieces are inserted; the noise will be very irritating to you.
- Store the stethoscope in the proper location after use.

Using the Blood Pressure Cuff

The blood pressure cuff is an instrument placed over an artery to measure the pressure of the blood. There are four parts to this instrument (Figure 17-14).

1. *Dial:* Shows numbers from 20 to 300 and has a pointer. Each line represents 2 millimeters (mm) of mercury. This part can also be called the *gauge* or *scale*.
2. *Cuff:* Contains a cloth-covered rubber bag that can be inflated. The cuff fits around the client's arm with the rubber bag positioned over the artery.
3. *Valve:* A thumbscrew opens and closes the valve. The valve controls the air that goes in and out of the cuff.
4. *Bulb:* Allows air to enter the rubber bag in the cuff when the bulb is squeezed.

TAKING THE BLOOD PRESSURE

Taking an accurate blood pressure requires a great deal of skill. Several skills are involved, and all are used at the same time.

Hearing: The sounds of the blood in the artery

Seeing and Reading: The pointer on the dial

Handling: The thumbscrew and squeezing the bulb to inflate and deflate the rubber bag in the cuff

Remembering: The readings so they can be accurately recorded when you finish taking the blood pressure.

See Procedure 17-10, Measuring Blood Pressure, and Box 17-5 for steps and reminders for measuring blood pressure.

If you are not sure of the blood pressure reading, deflate the cuff. Wait 5 minutes before taking it again.

PROCEDURE 17-10 | Measuring Blood Pressure

Materials Needed
- Blood pressure cuff
- Stethoscope
- Antiseptic wipes
- Paper
- Pencil

Procedure
1. Explain what you are going to do.
2. Have client lie down or rest in a chair.
3. Wash your hands.
4. Obtain materials listed above.
5. Wipe stethoscope earpieces and chest piece (diaphragm) or bell with antiseptic wipes.
6. Place client's arm in a position that is level with the heart, palm up, supported by a pillow(s), table, or arm of chair (Figure 17-15).
7. Expose client's upper arm. Remove clothing so that area is bare.
8. Squeeze blood pressure cuff to expel any air. Close the valve of the bulb.

9. Find the brachial artery by feeling the pulse at the inner side of the elbow (Figure 17-16).
10. Wrap cuff around client's arm, at least 1 inch above the bend in the arm. Make sure cuff is secure and even. Position rubber bag over the artery (Figure 17-17).
11. Put stethoscope earpieces in your ears.
12. Place fingers over radial pulse. Inflate cuff until you cannot feel the radial pulse. Inflate cuff 30 mm beyond the point at which you last felt the pulse.

Fig 17-16 Find brachial artery (Step 9).

Fig 17-15 Position client's arm so it is at level with the heart (Step 6).

Fig 17-17 Cuff should be 1 inch (2.5 cm) above bend in client's arm (Step 10).

PROCEDURE 17-10   Measuring Blood Pressure—cont'd

13. Place stethoscope chest piece (diaphragm) or bell over the brachial artery (Figure 17-18).
14. Keep your eyes on the dial, and begin to deflate the cuff slowly and evenly (2 to 4 mm per second) by turning the valve of the bulb counterclockwise.

Fig 17-18 Place stethoscope chest piece over the brachial artery (Step 13).

15. Note the first sound you hear, and read the dial at this point. This is the systolic pressure reading.
16. Keep your eyes on the dial, and continue to deflate the cuff. Note the last sound you hear, and read the dial at this point. This is the diastolic pressure reading.
17. Deflate cuff completely. Remove stethoscope and cuff from the client's arm.
18. Write the blood pressure on the paper.
19. Assist client, as needed, to desired position.
20. Clean earpieces and chest piece (diaphragm) or bell of stethoscope with antiseptic wipes. Discard used wipes.
21. Return all materials to proper storage place.
22. Wash your hands.
23. Record blood pressure results on client record.
24. Report any abnormal blood pressure reading to your supervisor.

BOX 17-5   Reminders When Measuring Blood Pressure

- Ask client not to talk during the procedure.
- Turn off radio and television, and reduce other background noises (if possible).
- Remove clothing from the client's arm.
- Wrap the cuff snugly around the client's arm; make sure the edge of the cuff is above the bend in the arm and the rubber bag is over the artery.
- Place the dial in the holder attached to the cuff; make sure you have a clear view of the dial.
- Do not take the blood pressure in the client's arm that
  Is injured or paralyzed
  Has a cast
  Has an intravenous infusion or a site for intravenous infusion
  Is on the same side as a mastectomy
- Record your results immediately using paper and pencil, including the time blood pressure was taken; remember to transfer this information to the client's care record.

THE ELECTRONIC (AUTOMATIC) BLOOD PRESSURE MONITOR

Clients who have hypertension often purchase an electronic device to monitor their blood pressure at home between visits to the physician. It is easy to use and gives accurate readings. These small machines include an arm cuff that is attached by tubing to the device (Figure 17-19). When the START button is pressed, the cuff automatically inflates. The digital display panel indicates the blood pressure and pulse after the cuff is deflated. See Box 17-6 for tips when using electronic blood pressure monitoring equipment. Contact your supervisor if you have questions about using this monitoring device.

Fig 17-19 Electronic (automatic) blood pressure monitor. (Courtesy Omron Healthcare, Inc., Lake Forest, Illinois.)

BOX 17-6   **Using an Electronic (Automatic) Blood Pressure Monitor**

- Follow Steps 1 to 4 and Steps 6 and 7 of Procedure 17-10.
- Place machine on table next to client.
- Apply cuff as in Figure 17-17.
- Make sure tubing is attached to the machine.
- Turn on the machine using the "On/Off" button.
- Symbol appears on the digital panel when ready to inflate cuff.
- Press the "Start" button.
- Remind client to remain still during the procedure.
- The cuff deflates automatically.
- Blood pressure reading (systolic and diastolic) and pulse reading are displayed on the digital panel.
- Turn off the machine using the "On/Off" button.
- Follow Steps 18 and 19 and Steps 21 to 24 of Procedure 17-10.

BOX 17-7   **Infection Control Rules When Taking Client's Vital Signs**

- Wash your hands before and after taking vital signs.
- Use client's own personal thermometer, not that of another family member.
- Wash regular or electronic thermometer before and after use.
- Clean thermometer from stem to bulb.
- Discard cotton balls or tissue after cleaning thermometer.
- Do not touch any part of the thermometer that has been in the client's mouth or rectum.
- Use rectal thermometer to take rectal temperature only.
- Wipe stethoscope's earpieces and chest piece with antiseptic wipes before and after use.
- Wear gloves when there is risk of coming in contact with the client's body fluids.

PREVENTING INFECTION

It is important to prevent the spread of infection when taking the client's vital signs. Infection may be spread by improper cleaning of equipment and by contact with the client's body fluids. Follow the infection control rules listed in Box 17-7 when taking the client's vital signs.

CHAPTER SUMMARY

- Vital signs give information about essential body processes: circulation, breathing, and heat regulation.
- Temperature, pulse, respirations, and blood pressure are the vital signs.
- The range of normal vital signs varies from person to person and is influenced by many factors, including sleep, age, fear, anxiety, food and fluid intake, medications, and activity.

- Home care aides observe, record, and report vital signs according to the care plan.
- Home care aides are expected to know the normal range of vital signs for adults.
- Practice measures to avoid the spread of infection when taking vital signs.

STUDY QUESTIONS

1. Explain the meaning of the term *vital signs*.
2. List four vital signs and three factors that may affect each.
3. List the normal adult range for
   a. Oral temperature
   b. Axillary temperature
   c. Rectal temperature
   d. Tympanic (ear) temperature
   e. Pulse
   f. Respirations
   g. Blood pressure
4. Describe the procedure for taking
   a. Oral temperature
   b. Axillary temperature
   c. Tympanic (ear) temperature
   d. Pulse
   e. Respirations
   f. Blood pressure
5. Discuss three ways the home care aide prevents the spread of infection when taking vital signs.

18

Special Procedures

OBJECTIVES

After you read this chapter, you will be able to:

1. List seven guidelines to follow when performing or assisting with special procedures.
2. Explain the difference between assisting clients to take medications and administering medications.
3. Discuss the role of the home care aide in assisting clients to take medications.
4. List 10 guidelines to follow when assisting clients to take medications.
5. Give two desired effects of hot applications and two desired effects of cold applications.
6. Describe five safety rules to follow when applying heat or cold.
7. Discuss six safety precautions to follow when oxygen is used by the client.
8. Describe four conditions that must be reported to the supervisor when the client is receiving intravenous infusions.
9. Identify three responsibilities of the home care aide for each of the following:
   - Client needing clean, dry dressing
   - Client wearing elastic stockings
   - Client wearing elastic bandages
10. Demonstrate procedures listed in this chapter.
11. Identify three ways the home care aide can prevent the spread of infection when performing special procedures.

KEY TERMS

Antiembolism stockings Elastic stockings worn to prevent the formation of blood clots in the legs

Compress (compresses) Gauze, washcloths, or small towels applied to a body area; may be moistened with hot or cold solution

Constrict To narrow

Dilate Expand or open wider

Embolus Blood clot that travels through the circulatory system until it lodges in a distant blood vessel

Humidifier Equipment used to increase the amount of moisture in an oxygen delivery system

Medications Substances used in the treatment of disease or illness; drugs

Nasal cannula Two-pronged device that delivers oxygen; short prongs are inserted into client's nostrils

Thrombus Blood clot

Trauma Injury caused by external force or violence

As a home care aide, you perform client care procedures according to the care plan. Most of these will be personal care procedures in which you assist clients with grooming, hygiene, elimination, and mobility.

The procedures in this chapter are not routine. They are special because they are important in the treatment of a client's condition. Some of the procedures are done by the home care aide, such as applications of heat and cold and changing dressings, according to agency policy. Other procedures, such as the administration of medications, will be done by the client. The home care aide assists the client to carry out these procedures according to the care plan. Certain special procedures, such as oxygen administration and intravenous therapy, are done by a health care professional. Your role is to observe the progress of the therapy and to report any problems or client complaints. IN SOME STATES, HOME CARE AIDES ARE NOT PERMITTED TO PERFORM SPECIAL PROCEDURES. BE SURE YOU KNOW WHAT YOU ARE ALLOWED TO DO.

GUIDELINES FOR SPECIAL PROCEDURES

The following guidelines apply to all special procedures.
1. Follow the care plan.
2. Know your limits; do only what you have been taught.
3. Notify your supervisor if you are not sure that you are permitted to perform a certain procedure.
4. Observe the immediate effects of the procedure on the client.
5. Observe any changes in the client's condition as a result of a special procedure.
6. Record on the client's care record what you have done and observed.
7. Report any unusual symptoms to your supervisor.

MEDICATIONS

Medications (drugs) are substances used in the treatment of disease or illness. They are very powerful and cause many effects. For example, a medication taken for pain relieves the pain. However, that medication may also cause drowsiness, nausea, and constipation. These symptoms are known as *side effects* or *adverse effects*. Many of these side effects are predictable, and the care plan or medication sheet will include which side effects to expect and which to report. Some side effects are so serious that the medication must be stopped until the physician is notified.

Medications come in many different forms, both solid and liquid. They are available as tablets, capsules, ointments, drops, lotions, suppositories, and other forms (Table 18-1). Clients may take

- Over-the-counter (OTC) drugs and herbs, which can be bought without a prescription (e.g., aspirin, Tylenol, vitamins, minerals)
- Prescription (Rx) drugs, which are available through a pharmacist according to the doctor's order

HOWEVER, THERE MUST BE A WRITTEN ORDER FROM THE PHYSICIAN FOR EACH MEDICATION THAT YOU ASSIST THE CLIENT TO TAKE. THIS INCLUDES BOTH PRESCRIPTION AND OTC DRUGS.

ASSISTING WITH MEDICATIONS

Most clients are able to take medications by themselves. Some may need assistance from the home care aide because they are unable to reach the medicines or get them

TABLE 18-1 | Types of Medication

SOLIDS

Capsules	Small gelatin containers that hold medication.

Lozenges	Flat disks containing medication in a flavored base. Lozenges are held in the mouth, where they dissolve and slowly release medication.

Tablets	Dry, powdered drugs that have been formed into small disks.

Ointments	Semisolid material containing medication. These are applied externally.

Suppositories	Solid form of medication for insertion into a body cavity, usually the rectum or vagina. Body temperature causes the suppository to melt and medication is released.

Transdermal disks or patches	Medication is located on a disk or strip that is applied to unbroken skin. Drug is absorbed through the skin over a 24-hour period.

Transdermal gels	Medication is applied to unbroken skin and rubbed in.

LIQUIDS

Elixirs	Medication is dissolved in a liquid containing alcohol or water and flavorings.
Suspensions	Medication is suspended in a liquid and may be labeled "Shake before using."
Syrups	Medication is dissolved in a concentrated sugar solution.
Drops	Liquid form of medication in a special container that allows one drop at a time to be administered. Usual types are eyedrops, ear drops, and nasal sprays.

OTHER

Metered-dose inhalers (MDIs)	Small cylinders (used with a special delivery system) containing a drug that is inhaled through the mouth in specifically measured (metered) doses.

out of the container. "Assist" means to help; "administer" means to give. HOME CARE AIDES NEVER ADMINISTER MEDICATIONS OF ANY TYPE, PRESCRIPTION OR OTC. THEY ASSIST CLIENTS TO TAKE THEIR OWN MEDICATIONS. YOU ARE LEGALLY RESPONSIBLE FOR YOUR OWN ACTIONS. As a home care aide, you are not licensed or certified to administer medication of any type. Only registered nurses (RNs), licensed practical nurses (LPNs), and licensed vocational nurses (LVNs) are permitted to administer medications according to the regulations of the state Nurse Practice Act. Never assume this responsibility. Always follow your agency's policies and state laws to protect yourself and your employer.

When assisting clients to take medications, you may
- Bring medication containers to the client.
- Loosen and remove container lids.
- Supervise the client as he or she pours the medication into hand, spoon, or cup.
- Steady the client's hand while pouring medications; direct hand as needed for eye-drops, nasal sprays, and so on.
- Bring prepoured medications and prefilled syringes to the client according to the care plan and medication sheet (Figure 18-1).
- Record what medications the client has taken.
- Watch for desired effect of medication.
- Watch for and report side effects according to the care plan and medication sheet.

The nurse will teach the client about the medications he or she is taking. Clients should be able to follow the medication sheet and take drugs accurately. They should know the drug's desired effect, when and how to take the drug, any side effects to watch for, and foods or other medications to avoid or omit. If your client does not know this information, notify your supervisor.

Medications may be prepoured by the nurse, client, or family member and stored in a "reminder" device (Figure 18-2). These containers help clients to remember what they have taken and what medications remain to be taken each day. If the client is unable to prepour, a nurse or family member may do so. This is not the responsibility of the home care aide.

SIX "RIGHTS" OF ASSISTING WITH MEDICATIONS

To assist clients to take medications accurately and safely, the home care aide follows the Six "Rights" of Assisting with Medications (Box 18-1).
1. Right drug
2. Right client
3. Right dose
4. Right route
5. Right time
6. Right documentation

Right Drug
The name of the drug will be listed on the medication sheet and on the medication container. Read the label, and compare with the medication sheet. Be sure you are assisting the client to take the right drug.

Right Client
Check the label on the medication container; be sure the drug is for your client (Figure 18-3). The label should have your client's first and last name on it. In some homes, two people may have the same name. Be certain you are assisting your client to take medications that are for his or her use only.

MEDICATION RECORD

Name	Delbert Sullivan							
Day		SUN	MON	TUE	WED	THUR	FRI	SAT
Date		7/11	7/12	7/13	7/14	7/15	7/16	7/17
Drug Name	Lasix (water pill)							
Dose	1 tablet							
Action	Increases urination							
Time	One (1) daily	8 a.m.	8 a.m.	8 a.m.	8 a.m.	8 a.m.	8 a.m.	8 a.m.

Special Instructions	Daily weight at 8 a.m.
	Drink plenty of fluids.
	Watch for and report any weight gain or swelling.
	Do not omit or increase dosage.
	Call doctor if unable to take medication.

Immediately Report	

Day		SUN	MON	TUE	WED	THUR	FRI	SAT
Date		7/11	7/12	7/13	7/14	7/15	7/16	7/17
Drug Name	Ferrous Sulfate (iron pill)							
Dose	1 tablet							
Action	Replaces iron in blood.							
Time	Three (3) times daily	9 a.m.	9 a.m.	9 a.m.	9 a.m.	9 a.m.	9 a.m.	9 a.m.
		1 p.m.	1 p.m.	1 p.m.	1 p.m.	1 p.m.	1 p.m.	1 p.m.
		5 p.m.	5 p.m.	5 p.m.	5 p.m.	5 p.m.	5 p.m.	5 p.m.

Special Instructions	Take between meals.
	Take with full glass of water.
	Do not take with milk or antacids.
	Will change color of stool to black.
	Do not crush tablet.
	May cause constipation.

Immediately Report	Nausea, vomiting, and diarrhea
	Abdominal pain

Fig 18-1 A sample medication sheet.

Fig 18-2 Medication reminder boxes can help clients keep track of their daily medications.

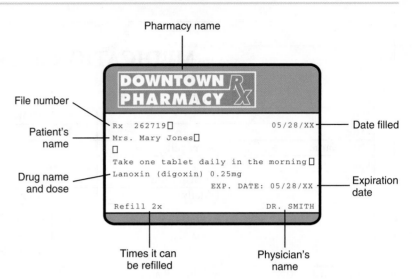

Pharmacy name

File number

Patient's name

Drug name and dose

DOWNTOWN PHARMACY Rx

Rx 262719☐   05/28/XX
Mrs. Mary Jones☐
☐
Take one tablet daily in the morning☐
Lanoxin (digoxin) 0.25mg
                        EXP. DATE: 05/28/XX

Refill 2x   DR. SMITH

Date filled

Expiration date

Times it can be refilled

Physician's name

Fig 18-3 Read the label before the client takes any medications.

BOX 18-1 | The Six "Rights" of Assisting with Medications

When assisting clients to take medications, remember the six "rights."

1. Right Drug	Read the container label. Check it against the medication list.
2. Right Client	Check the container label; be sure the drug is for the client. In some homes, two people may have the same name.
3. Right Dose	Be sure you understand how much medication your client should be taking.
4. Right Route	Be sure you know the correct route and form of the drug.
5. Right Time	Bring the drug to the client at the correct time, or remind the client about taking medications.
6. Right Documentation	Observe as the client records what was taken. If the client is not able, you record. Record what you observed.

If you have any questions or problems with the six "rights," notify your supervisor.

Right Dose

The dose is listed on the medication sheet and on each prescription container. For example: "Take one tablet daily," or "Apply ointment to left elbow twice a day." The correct amount of medication must be taken. For example, if Mrs. Jones takes two tablets from the container but should take only one tablet, you must remind her that she is to take only one tablet.

When the medication is in a liquid form, the dose may be in teaspoons, tablespoons, or milliliters. Be sure to bring the client the correct standard measuring spoon or medication cup to use when pouring the medicine.

Right Route

The method in which the medication is taken is called the *route*. This includes the following:

1. Oral medications: Solids or liquids taken by mouth, such as tablets and cough syrup
2. Sublingual medications: Placed under the tongue, where they dissolve
3. Topical medications: Applied to the skin and mucous membranes, such as ointments and eyedrops
4. Transdermal disks, patches, and gels: Medications applied to the skin
5. Metered-dose inhalers: Medication sprayed into the throat and inhaled into the lungs

6. Injections (sometimes called *parenteral medications*) may be
   a. Subcutaneous: Under the skin
   b. Intramuscular: Into the muscle
   c. Intravenous: Into the vein

Right Time

Medications must be taken at the correct time to work properly. Some are given only once a day; others may be given two, three, or four times a day. The directions on the prescription will give instructions on the time the medication is to be taken. For example, a client may have a medication that must be taken every 6 hours; this means four times during a 24-hour period. Your client's medication schedule should be in the care plan or medication sheet. Some drugs have to be taken at times when the stomach is empty, that is, 1 hour before or 2 hours after eating. Other medications need to be taken at mealtime to reduce stomach upset and help with absorption. These prescriptions usually have labels that say "take on an empty stomach" or "take with food or milk."

A client may also need to avoid certain foods or beverages when taking some medications. The prescription container may carry such special instructions as "avoid alcoholic beverages." If they are not avoided, internal bleeding or liver damage could occur. Also, mixing certain drugs with alcohol and tobacco can cause serious harm, such as depressed respirations, unconsciousness, or even death. For these reasons, clients should not take any drugs without the doctor's knowledge, including OTC medications or herbal mixtures.

Sometimes clients are confused about when to take their medications. For example, a client may say, "I can never remember. Do I take two tablets at 3 o'clock, or three tablets at 2 o'clock?" Alert your supervisor if this happens. Your client may need a "refresher" course on taking medications properly. Assist your client to take all medications at the right time.

Right Documentation

Ideally, clients should keep their own medication records. The nurse is the one who teaches the client how to do this. However, some clients may be unable to write on the medication sheet because of physical disability or vision problems. In these cases, the home care aide will record the information for the client. Always follow your agency's policy regarding documentation (recording), and ask your supervisor for help, if needed.

GUIDELINES FOR ASSISTING WITH MEDICATIONS

When assisting clients with medications, observe the following guidelines:
1. Always follow agency policy.
2. Carefully review the care plan with your supervisor before assisting client with medications. Follow the Six "Rights" of Assisting with Medications (see Box 18-1).
3. Make sure you bring the correct medication containers to the client. Read the labels carefully. There may be more than one person in the home with the same name. Compare container labels with the medication sheet to be sure you have the correct medication.
4. Know the correct dose of each medication. Check the care plan.
5. Give a glass of water (or other liquid) with oral medications as ordered.
6. Store medications as follows.
   - Separately from those of other family members, in a special location, just for client's medications
   - In a dry, cool place (not in the bathroom medicine cabinet)

- Out of reach of children and confused persons
- In original containers
- With lids tightly closed
- According to any special storage directions, such as "store in refrigerator"

7. Do not leave medications at the bedside and assume that the client will take them correctly. Remain with the client until he or she has finished taking the medications.
8. Do not remove labels from medication containers.
9. Never use any medication container that is not labeled or take medication from a container where the label cannot be read.
10. Do not use discolored or deteriorated drugs. Notify your supervisor.
11. Be sure prescriptions are refilled before medications are completely used. Remind client/family to reorder medication when only a few days' supply remains.
12. Listen to your client. If he or she questions something about a medication, STOP—do not assist with administration. Call your supervisor immediately.
13. Report to your supervisor if your client
    - Does not use the medication sheet and/or does not take the drugs correctly
    - Does not know why the drug is being taken, the dosage, or the time schedule
    - Refuses to take the medication, forgets, or omits a dose; the client should not take a double dose if one is omitted
    - Shows any side effects (e.g., vomiting, rash, breathing difficulty, itching, diarrhea)
    - Takes any medications that are not listed on the medication sheet, particularly OTC drugs
14. Check with your supervisor before discarding any unused medication.
15. Record what you have done on the client's care record. Client should record on the medication sheet. Assist as necessary.
16. Record if a medication is not taken or omitted, and why. Follow Procedures 18-1 to 18-6 for assisting clients with medications.

PROCEDURE 18-1 | Assisting With Oral Medications

Materials Needed
- Oral medications
- Teaspoon or tablespoon, if needed (use standard measuring spoon)
- Glass of water
- Straw (optional)

Procedure
1. Explain what you are going to do.
2. Check care plan and medication sheet.
3. Wash your hands.
4. Obtain materials listed above.
5. Help client to wash hands.
6. Check label on each prescription (see Figure 18-3) or on each prepoured medication for
   Right drug
   Right client
   Right dose
   Right route
   Right time
7. Loosen lid(s) on container(s) if client is unable to do so. Tell client the name of each medication (read from label).
8. Place containers where client can reach them, or hand container to client. Let client read name of medication to you. Be sure client is wearing eyeglasses if client needs them to read.
9. Assist client with oral medications.
   - Give sip of water to moisten mouth.
   - Support hand as necessary to pour medication.
   - Give a full glass of water or other cool liquid after client puts medication in mouth.
   - Remind client to lower chin while swallowing.
10. Close containers.
11. Have client record medications taken. Home care aide may record for client, if necessary.
12. Store materials in proper location.
13. Wash your hands.
14. Record what you have done. Report any unusual conditions to your supervisor.

PROCEDURE 18-2 | Assisting With Rectal Suppositories

Materials Needed
- Suppository
- Water-soluble lubricant
- Disposable glove
- Toilet tissue
- Handwashing supplies

Procedure
1. Explain what you are going to do.
2. Check care plan and medication sheet.
3. Wash your hands.
4. Obtain materials listed above.
5. Provide privacy (close door, shut drapes, pull shades).
6. Assist client into bed and in Sims' position.
7. Remove clothing to expose anal area.
8. Check label on the suppository for
    Right drug
    Right client
    Right dose
    Right route
    Right time
9. Unwrap suppository.
10. Apply water-soluble lubricant to suppository. Do not use petroleum jelly because it is not water-soluble.
11. Give glove to client to put on.
12. Hand suppository to client to insert into rectum. Guide client's hand, if necessary.
13. Observe as client inserts medication and wipes anus with toilet tissue.
14. Have client remove and discard glove into waste container.
15. Help client to wash hands.
16. Discard used materials in waste container.
17. Have client record medication taken. Home care aide may record for client, if necessary.
18. Remind client to remain on side for 15 to 20 minutes to allow suppository to melt and medication to be absorbed.
19. Wash your hands.
20. Record what you have done. Report any unusual conditions to your supervisor.

PROCEDURE 18-3 | Assisting With Eye Medications or Ointment

Materials Needed
- Eye medication or ointment
- Tissues or cotton balls
- Small hand mirror
- Disposable gloves (if necessary)

Procedure
1. Explain what you are going to do.
2. Check care plan and medication sheet.
3. Wash your hands.
4. Obtain materials listed above.
5. Help client to wash hands.
6. Check label on prescription container for
    Right drug: Be certain the preparation is for use in the eyes only
    Right client
    Right dose: Be certain the strength of the solution/ointment in the container is correct
    Right route: Which eye, or both eyes
    Right time
7. Loosen lid on container, if client is unable to do so.
8. Place container within client's reach, or hand container to him or her as necessary. Be sure client is wearing eyeglasses if client needs them to read.
9. Hold mirror so client can see to administer eye medication.
10. Remove client's eyeglasses, if worn.
11. Assist client with
    Eye medications
    - Guide client's hand to grasp lower lid.
    - Observe that client looks up and releases drops into lower lid.
    - Observe that client closes eye to distribute medication.
    - Make sure that dropper does not touch client's eye.
    Eye ointment
    - Guide client's hand to grasp lower lid.
    - Observe that client looks up and squeezes a small ribbon of ointment into the lower lid from inner corner of eye to outer corner of eye.
    - Observe that client closes eye to allow medication to melt and be distributed.
    - Make sure that tip of tube does not touch eye surface.
12. Reseal container.
13. Have client record medications taken. Home care aide may record for client, if necessary.
14. Store materials in proper location.
15. Wash your hands.
16. Record what you have done. Report any unusual conditions to your supervisor.

PROCEDURE 18-4 | Assisting With Transdermal Disks or Patches

Materials Needed
- Medicated transdermal disk or patch
- Disposable gloves (if necessary)

Procedure
1. Explain what you are going to do.
2. Check care plan and medication sheet.
3. Wash your hands.
4. Obtain materials listed above.
5. Provide privacy (close door, shut drapes, pull shades).
6. Help client to wash hands.
7. Check label on container for
   Right drug
   Right client
   Right dose
   Right route
   Right time
8. Have client remove and discard old disk or patch into waste container. Wash skin that had been covered by old disk or patch.
9. Ask client to select new site for new disk or patch (any area without hair), usually the chest or upper arm.
10. Observe as client applies new disk or patch to skin surface. Be sure that the medication is not touched with ungloved fingers. (Your skin may absorb some of the drug.)
11. Discard wrapper and other used materials.
12. Have client record medications taken. Home care aide may record for client, if necessary.
13. Store materials in proper location.
14. Wash your hands.
15. Record what you have done. Report any unusual conditions to your supervisor.

PROCEDURE 18-5 | Assisting With Medicated Gels

Materials Needed
- Tube of medicated gel
- Dosing card

Procedure
1. Explain what you are going to do.
2. Check the care plan and medication sheet.
3. Wash your hands.
4. Obtain materials listed above.
5. Provide privacy (close door, shut drapes, pull shades).
6. Help client to wash hands.
7. Check label on carton or tube for
   a. Right drug
   b. Right client
   c. Right dose
   d. Right route
   e. Right time
8. Remove dosing card from the package, and place on a flat surface so client can read it.
9. Uncap the tube.
10. Observe as client squeezes the gel to the prescribed dosage on to the dosing card.
11. Put cap back on tube.
12. Observe as client applies the gel to prescribed area (e.g., hand, wrist, knee). Client should rub entire amount of gel into the skin in the proper area. Do not touch the gel—your skin may absorb some of the drug.
13. Have client wash hands (unless the gel was applied to that area).
14. Have client record medication applied. Home care aide may record for client, if necessary.
15. Hold end of dosing card with fingertips, rinse, and dry. Store materials in proper location.
16. Wash your hands.
17. Record what you have done. Report any unusual conditions to your supervisor.

APPLICATIONS OF HEAT AND COLD

Heat and cold are applied to parts of the body to treat many types of problems, such as pain, swelling, and soreness. Applying heat or cold to the body is done only when the doctor orders such treatment. The care plan indicates the type of treatment and the number of times each day the treatment is to be given. In some states, the home care

PROCEDURE 18-6   Assisting With Metered-Dose Inhalers

Materials Needed
- Metered-dose inhaler container of prescription drugs
- Disposable gloves (if necessary)

Procedure
1. Explain what you are going to do.
2. Check care plan and medication sheet.
3. Wash your hands.
4. Obtain materials listed above.
5. Provide privacy.
6. Help client to wash hands.
7. Check label on prescription container for
   Right drug
   Right client
   Right dose
   Right route
   Right time
8. Hand metered-dose inhaler to client, who then uses it to inhale the medication (Figure 18-4).
9. Have client record medication taken. Home care aide may record for client, if necessary.
10. Clean inhaler, wearing disposable gloves, according to manufacturer's instructions, and store in proper location.
11. Remove and discard gloves. Wash your hands.
12. Record what you have done. Report any unusual conditions to your supervisor.
13. Assist client with oral hygiene as needed.

Fig 18-4 Client inhales medication (Step 8).

aide is not permitted to apply heat or cold. Be sure you know what your state (and agency) allows you to do.

There are two types of hot or cold applications: dry and moist.

1. Dry: The heat or cold does not come in direct contact with the client's skin. An example is a hot water bag or an ice bag. Dry heat or cold does not produce its effects as deeply or as quickly as moist heat or cold, but there still is risk of skin damage.
2. Moist: The heat or cold comes in direct contact with the client's skin, such as hot water soaks and cold compresses. Moist heat or cold produces the desired effects more quickly and more effectively. However, because heat or cold comes in direct contact with the skin, risk of skin damage is greater.

EFFECTS OF HEAT

Applying heat to a part of the body causes blood vessels in the area to dilate. These enlarged blood vessels help bring more blood, containing oxygen and nutrients, to the surrounding tissues. Heat applications are used to
- Provide warmth and comfort
- Help to relax sore muscles
- Relieve soreness in joints
- Increase blood circulation to the area

EFFECTS OF COLD

Applying cold to a part of the body causes blood vessels in the area to constrict. As the blood vessels become smaller, circulation to the area is reduced. The sensation of pain is usually reduced because nerve endings in the skin become less sensitive. Cold applications are used to

- Stop bleeding
- Reduce pain
- Reduce swelling
- Reduce heat in the tissues

SAFETY

Whenever heat or cold is applied to the body, there is risk of skin damage. Clients at greatest risk include the following:

- Fair-skinned individuals: Their skin is delicate, thin, and fragile and is more easily injured.
- Infants, young children, and confused adults: These clients cannot tell you when the application is too hot or too cold.
- Older adults: Their skin is thin, and reaction to heat or cold may be delayed.
- Unconscious or paralyzed individuals: These clients cannot feel the effects of heat or cold.
- Diabetic clients: Their nerve endings are not as sensitive to changes in temperature.

Check your client's skin frequently after applying heat or cold. If the client complains of pain or numbness in the area, remove the application immediately and notify your supervisor. Record the client's reaction, appearance of skin, and time the treatment was stopped (Box 18-2, Signs of Skin Injury When Applying Heat and Cold).

The following general safety rules should be used when applying heat or cold:

- Use a cooking thermometer, if available, to check the temperature of the water.
- Follow the manufacturer's directions for operating equipment safely; contact your supervisor when in doubt.
- Follow your agency's guidelines for temperature ranges for hot and cold applications.
- Cover a hot water bag, hot or cold pack, or ice bag with a towel or other covering before placing it on the client's skin.
- Check the client's skin every 10 minutes; for those at risk of skin damage, check more frequently.
- Remove the application immediately if there is any sign of skin injury (see Box 18-2).

BOX 18-2   Signs of Skin Injury When Applying Heat and Cold

HEAT APPLICATIONS
- Client complains of burning sensation or pain in area
- Skin is
  Red
  Blistering

COLD APPLICATIONS
- Client complains of burning sensation, numbness, or pain in area
- Skin is
  Red
  Pale
  Bluish

APPLYING DRY HEAT

The most common ways of applying dry heat are with a hot water bag, heating pad, or hot pack. The care plan will indicate how long dry heat should be applied and how frequently. Sometimes, the client may ask you to apply dry heat even though it is not listed in the care plan. "I feel so cold—please get the heating pad and put it on my shoulders." This may sound like a reasonable request. But remember, as a home care aide, you may apply heat only when ordered by the doctor and approved by your agency. In this case, helping the client to put on an extra sweater or placing a blanket over the shoulders may be a good substitute. Explain why you are not able to apply the heating pad.

Before applying dry heat with a heating pad or hot pack, read the manufacturer's directions and be sure you understand how to use the appliance. Do not allow the client to lie on top of the heating pad or pack because this position increases the risk for burns.

Your client may use commercially made hot packs (pads, pillows, cushions, or wraps) (Figure 18-5). These items have gel in the center of the pack. They are prepared by heating in the microwave. The gel becomes hot and radiates warmth to the rest of the pack. Read the manufacturer's directions about heating, applying, and reheating this type of hot pack. Heat the pack for the lowest time recommended by the manufacturer. Cover the pack with a towel or cover provided by the manufacturer before applying it to the client's skin. Hot wraps may have Velcro closures that can be easily wrapped around the ankle, elbow, or wrist.

See Procedure 18-7, Applying a Hot Water Bag, and Procedure 18-8, Applying a Hot or Cold Pack.

APPLYING MOIST HEAT

Moist heat is used when there is a need to provide warmth deeper in the tissues. The most common forms of moist heat are hot soaks, compresses, and sitz baths. It is very important to check the temperature of the water before the client's skin comes in contact with the water; burns can occur immediately if the water is too hot. When the client's skin is prone to burns, Vaseline or another protective substance may be used around the outer part of the skin to protect it from the heat of the hot compress. Contact your supervisor for instructions.

Fig 18-5 A commercially made hot pack. (Courtesy Southwest Technologies, Inc., Kansas City, Missouri.)

PROCEDURE 18-7   Applying a Hot Water Bag

Materials Needed
- Hot water bag
- Soft cloth or towel
- Cooking thermometer (if available)
- Pencil
- Paper

Procedure
1. Explain what you are going to do.
2. Wash your hands.
3. Obtain materials listed above.
4. Provide privacy.
5. Fill hot water bag with water. Secure with stopper. Turn bag upside down to check for leaks.
6. Remove stopper, and empty bag.
7. Run more hot water, and test with cooking thermometer; adjust water temperature to 115° to 130° F (46° to 54.4° C).
8. Fill bag one-third to one-half full.
9. Lay bag flat to remove air. Place stopper in bag while it is still flat.
10. Cover bag with soft cloth or towel, and apply to client's affected area.
11. Write on paper the time the bag was applied.
12. Refill bag when it becomes cool.
13. Check client's skin every 10 minutes for danger signs (see Box 18-2).
14. Remove bag according to time required. Write time of removal on paper.
15. Remove stopper, empty bag, and hang bag upside down to dry. Place cloth or towel in laundry container to be washed.
16. Wash your hands.
17. Record what you have done. Report any unusual conditions to your supervisor.
18. When bag is dry, blow air into it and replace stopper to prevent insides of bag from sticking together. Store in proper location.

PROCEDURE 18-8   Applying a Hot or Cold Pack

Materials Needed
- Hot or cold pack
- Soft cloth, towel, or cover
- Pencil
- Paper

Procedure
1. Explain what you are going to do.
2. Wash your hands.
3. Obtain materials listed above.
4. Provide privacy.
5. Place hot pack in microwave, and heat according to manufacturer's directions. Or, remove cold pack from freezer.
6. Cover pack with soft cloth or towel, or cover and apply to client's affected area.
7. Write on paper the time the pack was applied.
8. Check client's skin every 10 minutes for danger signs (see Box 18-2).
9. Remove pack according to time required. Write time of removal on paper.
10. Store pack according to manufacturer's directions. Place cloth, towel, or cover in laundry container to be washed.
11. Wash your hands.
12. Record what you have done. Report any unusual conditions to your supervisor.

While the client is receiving moist heat, check the skin every 10 minutes for signs of burns. Also, add water as needed to maintain the proper water temperature. See Procedure 18-9, Applying Hot Compresses, and Procedure 18-10, Applying Hot Soaks.

Sitz Bath

The sitz bath is a method of applying moist heat to the client's perineum and pelvic area. The purpose of the sitz bath is to increase the circulation of blood to the area. It also helps to promote healing, clean a wound of the rectal or perineal area, or ease discomfort after surgery or childbirth.

Equipment needed includes a plastic sitz bath that fits on the rim of the toilet bowl and a water bag with tubing and a clamp (Figure 18-7). Warm water is placed in the

PROCEDURE 18-9   Applying Hot Compresses

Materials Needed
- Basin or container
- Hot water
- Cooking thermometer (if available)
- Compresses (small towel, washcloth, or gauze squares)
- Bath towel
- Waterproof protector pad
- Disposable gloves
- Plastic wrap
- Tape
- Pencil
- Paper

Procedure
1. Explain what you are going to do.
2. Wash your hands.
3. Obtain materials listed above.
4. Provide privacy (close door, shut drapes, pull shades).
5. Place waterproof protector pad under the body part where compress is to be applied.
6. Fill basin or container one-half to two-thirds full of water at 105° to 115° F (40.5° to 46.1° C). (Check temperature with cooking thermometer.)
7. Put on gloves.
8. Place compress in the water.
9. Wring out compress, and apply to area (Figure 18-6). Note time applied.
10. Cover compress quickly with plastic wrap. Secure edges of plastic wrap with tape. Cover with bath towel.
11. Write on paper the time compress was applied.
12. Apply, according to directions, a hot water bag or rubber-protected heating pad over the plastic wrap to keep compress hot.
13. Check client's skin every 10 minutes for danger signs (see Box 18-2).
14. Change compress, if cooling occurs.
15. Remove compress according to time required.
16. Write time of removal on paper.
17. Pat area dry with towel. Discard used gauze or compress. Place used cloths or towels in laundry container to be washed.
18. Remove and discard gloves.
19. Wash your hands.
20. Clean and store materials in proper location.
21. Record what you have done. Report any unusual conditions to your supervisor.

Fig 18-6 Wring out the compress, and apply to the area (Step 9).

plastic sitz bath. The client sits in the warm water. The water bag holds additional warmer water. When the water in the sitz bath begins to cool, the tubing is unclamped and warmer water enters the sitz bath. The client may be taught how to control the flow of water. For clients who are unable to handle the clamp, the home care aide will perform this task.

Warm water increases the circulation to the perineal area. When this happens, there is less blood flow to other parts of the body. As a result, the client may become pale, weak, or feel light-headed or dizzy. It is important to check the client every 5 minutes for these signs. Also, the shoulders and legs may become cold. To avoid chilling during the procedure, cover the shoulders and knees.

Do not use a regular bathtub to give a sitz bath. Keeping the legs under hot water causes blood vessels in the legs to dilate and decreases circulation to the perineal area. See Procedure 18-11, Giving a Sitz Bath.

PROCEDURE 18-10 | Applying Hot Soaks

Materials Needed
- Basin or other container
- Hot water
- Cooking thermometer (if available)
- Waterproof protector pad
- Towel

Procedure
1. Explain what you are going to do.
2. Wash your hands.
3. Obtain materials listed above.
4. Provide privacy.
5. Assist client to comfortable position.
6. Place waterproof protector pad under the area to be soaked.
7. Fill basin or container one-half full of water 105° to 110° F (40.5° to 43.3° C). (Check temperature with cooking thermometer.)
8. Expose only the part to be soaked.
9. Place area to be soaked into the water.
10. Check water temperature and skin of area being soaked every 10 minutes. Remove from water if danger signs are noticed (see Box 18-2).
11. Remove body part from water according to time required.
12. Write time of removal on paper.
13. Pat body part dry. Assist client to replace clothing and to get comfortable.
14. Clean and store materials in proper location.
15. Put used towel in laundry container to be washed.
16. Wash your hands.
17. Record what you have done. Report any unusual conditions to your supervisor.

APPLYING DRY COLD

Ice bags and cold packs or wraps are commonly used to apply dry cold to a part of the body. Similar to hot packs, cold packs or wraps contain gel in the center of the appliance. They are prepared by placing them in the freezer section of the refrigerator until the gel is frozen. Be sure to follow the manufacturer's directions about freezing, applying, and refreezing these packs or wraps.

Inexpensive substitutes for an ice bag include a freezer bag or heavy-duty plastic bag filled with crushed ice, or a bag of frozen peas or corn. When the treatment is

Fig 18-7 A sitz bath.

PROCEDURE 18-11 Giving a Sitz Bath

Materials Needed
- Portable plastic sitz bowl
- Hot water
- Water bag and tubing
- Pitcher
- Blanket or large towel
- Cooking thermometer (if available)
- Clean dressing or sanitary pad (if needed)
- Disposable gloves (two pairs, if needed)
- Paper bag

Procedure
1. Explain what you are going to do.
2. Wash your hands.
3. Obtain materials listed above.
4. Assist client to bathroom or commode.
5. Provide privacy.
6. Put on gloves.
7. Help client to remove clothing from below waist.
8. Ask client to remove and discard dressing or sanitary pad, if worn. Assist, if needed. Observe amount and color of drainage.
9. Ask client to void before beginning the procedure.
10. Raise toilet seat. Place sitz bowl so that drainage holes are at the back of the toilet. Fill half of plastic sitz bowl with warm water, 94° to 98° F (34° to 37° C). (Check temperature with cooking thermometer.)
11. Close side clamp of bag tubing. Fill water bag with warm water, 120° F (49° C). Hang bag so that it is higher than the toilet (on towel bar, top of toilet tank, or vanity).
12. Assist client to sit in sitz bowl. If client feels cold, cover shoulders and knees with blanket or towel.
13. Place tube end of water bag in outlet at front of the bowl.
14. Instruct client to open clamp of water bag to let warmer water into the bowl when water begins to cool. Assist as needed.
15. Instruct client to call for assistance, if needed. Explain that the procedure will take 15 to 20 minutes.
16. Remove and discard gloves.
17. Wash your hands.
18. Check client's condition every 5 minutes or more frequently, if needed.
19. When time is up, clamp tubing and remove from sitz bath.
20. Wash hands. Put on second pair of gloves.
21. Assist client to slowly assume standing position.
22. Inspect perineal area; note any drainage in water. Dry area, and reapply dressing or pad, if needed.
23. Assist client to dress, as needed, and to return to chair or bed.
24. Empty and disinfect plastic bowl. Flush tubing with water, and clean end of tubing. Return equipment to proper location.
25. Remove and discard gloves.
26. Wash your hands.
27. Straighten bathroom.
28. Record on care record, noting color and amount of drainage on dressing or pad. Report any unusual conditions to your supervisor.

finished, the bag of peas or corn can be refrozen for later use. Be sure to mark the bag so that it is not used as food.

Change the cover of the ice bag, cold pack, or wrap when it becomes moist. You may need to refill the ice bag or get another bag of frozen peas when the contents begin to melt. Sometimes the client may feel chilly while receiving applications of cold; this is not unusual. A sweater or blanket may help to relieve the feeling. See Procedure 18-12, Applying an Ice Bag.

APPLYING MOIST COLD

Cold compresses are the usual way to apply moist cold. Just as moist heat is more penetrating than dry heat, moist cold is more effective than dry cold. Covering the cold compress with plastic wrap or a piece of plastic helps to retain the cold. Cold compresses become warm quickly because of the body's heat. Change the compress as soon as it becomes warm. Cold compresses are often used for areas such as the eyes. Be careful to avoid pressing on the area that is usually sensitive to the touch. Follow Procedure 18-13, Applying Cold Compresses.

PROCEDURE 18-12   Applying an Ice Bag

Materials Needed
- Ice bag
- Soft cloth or towel
- Crushed ice
- Pencil
- Paper

Procedure
1. Explain what you are going to do.
2. Wash your hands.
3. Obtain materials listed above.
4. Provide privacy (close door, shut drapes, pull shades).
5. Fill ice bag with water. Secure with stopper. Turn bag upside down to check for leaks.
6. Remove stopper, and empty bag.
7. Crush the ice, and fill the bag (one-half to two-thirds full).
8. Lay bag flat to remove air. Place stopper in bag while it is still flat.
9. Cover bag with soft cloth or towel, and apply to client's affected area.
10. Write on paper the time bag was applied.
11. Add ice as bag warms. Change towel if it becomes moist.
12. Check client's skin every 10 minutes for danger signs (see Box 18-2).
13. Remove bag according to time required. Write time of removal on paper.
14. Remove stopper, empty bag, and place bag upside down to dry. Place cloth or towel in laundry container to be washed.
15. Wash your hands.
16. Record what you have done. Report any unusual conditions to your supervisor.
17. When bag is dry, blow air into it and replace stopper to prevent insides of bag from sticking together. Store in proper location.

PROCEDURE 18-13   Applying Cold Compresses

Materials Needed
- Basin or container
- Bath towel
- Plastic wrap
- Pencil
- Compresses (small towel, washcloth, or gauze squares)
- Ice water
- Disposable gloves
- Tape
- Paper
- Waterproof protector pad

Procedure
1. Explain what you are going to do.
2. Wash your hands.
3. Obtain materials listed above.
4. Provide privacy (close door, shut drapes, pull shades).
5. Place waterproof protector pad under the body part where compress is to be applied.
6. Fill basin or container one-half to two-thirds full with ice water.
7. Put on gloves.
8. Place compress in water.
9. Wring out compress, and apply to area.
10. Cover compress quickly with plastic wrap. Secure edges of plastic wrap with tape. Cover with bath towel.
11. Write on paper the time compress was applied.
12. Check client's skin every 10 minutes for danger signs (see Box 18-2).
13. Change compress when warming occurs.
14. Remove compress according to time required.
15. Write time of removal on paper.
16. Pat area dry with towel. Discard used gauze square or compresses. Place used washcloth and towels in laundry container to be washed.
17. Remove and discard gloves.
18. Wash your hands.
19. Clean and store materials in proper location.
20. Record what you have done. Report any unusual conditions to your supervisor.

OXYGEN THERAPY

Clients who have difficulty breathing and are not receiving enough oxygen through the air may need additional amounts of oxygen. The doctor orders the amount and the method to be given, usually by nasal tube or mask. Oxygen is a drug and is part of the client's treatment or therapy.

When the client is receiving oxygen therapy in the home, the doctor may want to monitor how well the client's body is using the oxygen—the level of oxygen concentration in the blood. The pulse oximeter is a convenient measuring device (Figure 18-8). Placed on a fingertip, it measures the percentage of oxygen in the blood. It also measures the pulse. The electronic screen of the pulse oximeter shows the percentage of oxygen and the pulse. Normal ranges for oxygen are from 95% to 100%. The client's care plan will indicate at what percentage level below 95% oxygen therapy is required.

Oxygen is supplied to homes by companies that specialize in delivering and providing breathing equipment. The respiratory therapist or company representative explains the correct use of the equipment to the client and family caregiver. Care of equipment, including ways of disinfecting parts and proper maintenance, is also explained. If your client is receiving oxygen therapy, the name, address, and telephone number of the oxygen supplier should be available in case of an emergency.

TYPES OF EQUIPMENT

There are two basic types of oxygen systems that are used to deliver oxygen in the home.

1. Gas cylinders: Oxygen is stored under pressure in metal cylinders (Figure 18-9). They may be stationary, usually at the side of the bed for clients who are immobile, or portable, wheeled in a cart or worn by the client in a shoulder bag to permit easy movement.

Fig 18-8 A pulse oximeter. (From Sorrentino SA: *Mosby's textbook for long-term care nursing assistants,* ed 6, St. Louis, 2011, Mosby.)

Fig 18-9 A portable oxygen tank with carrying case. (Courtesy Invacare Corporation, Elyria, Ohio.)

Fig 18-10 An oxygen concentrator.

2. Oxygen concentrators: This equipment separates oxygen from the other gasses in the air and stores it in a tank (Figure 18-10). The concentrator runs on a continuous supply of electricity. Backup power sources or an oxygen cylinder must be available in case of an electrical failure. Portable oxygen concentrators that can operate on battery power are also available.

OXYGEN SAFETY

ONE OF THE THREE REQUIREMENTS NEEDED TO PRODUCE A FIRE IS OXYGEN. THEREFORE, THE DANGER OF FIRE AND EXPLOSION IN THE HOME IS ALWAYS PRESENT WHEN OXYGEN IS BEING USED. IT IS VERY IMPORTANT THAT EVERYONE IN THE HOME—YOU, THE CLIENT, FAMILY MEMBERS, AND VISITORS—FOLLOW THE RULES OF OXYGEN SAFETY.

The home care aide should make sure of the following:

- "No Smoking" and "Oxygen in Use" signs are placed on the front door of the client's home, apartment, or room and in the client's room where oxygen is being used.
- Fire hazards are removed (see Chapter 8).
- Client uses oxygen in areas free from the danger of fire.
- Client stays out of areas where open flames (pilot lights) and electrical equipment may cause sparks (e.g., kitchen, basement, garage).
- Cigarettes, cigars, lighters, and matches are removed from client's area.
- Client does not use alcohol or other flammable liquids (e.g., nail polish, perfume, aftershave lotion) when receiving oxygen.
- A working, fully charged fire extinguisher is available for use in case of an emergency.
- Name and telephone number of oxygen supplier are available.
- Oxygen tanks are properly secured in the floor stand provided by the supplier and are at least 6 inches from walls, drapes, and heating units.
- Oxygen tanks are stored away from sun and other heat sources.

Fig 18-11 A nasal cannula.

Fig 18-12 A face mask.

CARING FOR THE CLIENT RECEIVING OXYGEN

Nasal Cannula

In the home, the most common method of administering oxygen is by nasal cannula. It is easy to use, and the client can talk and eat while the cannula is in place (Figure 18-11). There are two prongs that project from the plastic tubing. They are inserted about ½ inch into the nostrils. The respiratory therapist adjusts the length of the prongs to make them comfortable for the client. The tubing is attached to the source of oxygen.

When caring for a client with a nasal cannula

- Place padding (cotton balls, gauze) between the strap and the ears, if needed.
- Wash and dry the area around the nostrils and ears carefully.
- Apply water-soluble lubricant around nostrils, if irritation is present.
- Do not use petroleum jelly (Vaseline) as a lubricant because it can act as a fuel to produce fire.
- Note any skin irritation around the nostrils and ears.
- Immediately notify your supervisor of any skin irritation (redness, broken skin) and its location.

Face Mask

When oxygen is needed on an occasional basis, a face mask may be used (Figure 18-12). Talking is difficult when wearing a mask, and it must be removed before eating. The mask fits snugly over the client's nose and mouth. Straps are adjusted around the head and over the ears. Some masks have small holes on both sides that allow carbon dioxide to escape during exhaling. These holes also allow air from the room to enter during inhaling.

When caring for a client with a face mask

- Place padding (cotton balls, gauze) between the strap and the ears, if needed.
- Wash and dry the face carefully.
- Note any irritation on the nose or face where the mask touches the skin.
- Immediately report signs of irritation (redness, breaks in skin) and location to your supervisor.

Oxygen dries the membranes of the mouth and respiratory system. An oxygen humidifier may be used to add moisture to the oxygen. This special container for sterile water is attached to the oxygen delivery system. When the oxygen is turned on, it bubbles through the sterile water.

Humidifiers must be cleaned and refilled on a regular basis. Your supervisor will explain how to check the water level in the humidifier and how to add more. Store the

Fig 18-13 Intravenous equipment.

sterile water supply in the refrigerator; write the date it was opened on the container and discard if not used within 2 weeks. Clean the humidifier as instructed by your supervisor or the respiratory therapist.

Clients receiving oxygen therapy need frequent mouth care. Check with your supervisor about the frequency of giving mouth care. Encourage the client to drink water and other fluids to provide added moisture to the mouth's mucous membranes.

INTRAVENOUS INFUSIONS

Intravenous (IV) infusions are used to administer medications and to supply needed fluids. IV equipment includes the following (Figure 18-13).
- Fluid container: Plastic bag with fluid
- Pole: Holds fluid container
- Tubing: Plastic tubing carries fluid from the bag to the client
- Needle or catheter: Inserted into a vein in the client's arm or hand and secured with tape
- Meter: Controls the flow of fluid (number of drops per minute)

CARING FOR THE CLIENT RECEIVING IV THERAPY

The home care aide has limited responsibilities regarding the use of IV therapy in the home. Most of the responsibilities are those of the nurse. The nurse is the person who adjusts the rate of flow of the medications and performs all procedures regarding the use and disposal of IV equipment. Your responsibility is to observe and report any problems with the equipment and to observe and report any changes in the client as follows:

Equipment
- Rate of fluid is too slow or too fast
- Fluid is leaking around the needle

- Meter is "beeping"
- Fluid in bag is low and needs to be changed

Client

- Has swelling (edema) or redness where needle is inserted
- Complains of pain or burning sensation around needle
- Feels itchy, nauseous or vomits
- Has sudden chills, headache, skin rash, or difficulty breathing
- Becomes restless and may be injured by needle or equipment
- Tries to pull needle out

After you have talked with your supervisor, be sure to record on the care record the time you called, what your supervisor told you to do, and what you did.

DRY DRESSINGS

Dressings are gauze squares that are used to cover wounds or surgical openings. They protect the area from clothing and microorganisms in the air and help to absorb any drainage from the wound. There are two types of dressings: sterile and unsterile. The home care aide does not apply or remove sterile dressings or apply dressings with ointments or other types of medication; these tasks are the responsibility of the nurse.

APPLYING AND REMOVING DRY DRESSINGS

You may be required to apply and remove unsterile dry dressings or to reinforce a dressing already in place. Dressings are reinforced when drainage is leaking from the dressing or when the dressing becomes loosened. Use standard (universal) precautions when applying and removing dressings because of the risk of bloodborne pathogens. Observe the area carefully. Note the size of the area and color of the skin around the area; also note the color, amount, and odor of drainage, if any. Record this information on the care record. Report any changes in the appearance of the area to your supervisor.

Tape is used to secure the dressing to the skin. Make sure the edges of the dressing are taped to prevent movement of the dressing (Figure 18-14). When removing tape, pull the tape toward the dressing, not away from the dressing. Injury can occur if pressure is applied when pulling tape away from the bandaged area. Inspect the skin under the tape. If reddened or broken, notify your supervisor. Do not reapply tape over irritated skin.

The dressing may stick to the skin if drainage from the wound dries. If this happens, follow the care plan or ask your supervisor what to do. Notify your supervisor if there

Fig 18-14 Tape the edges to prevent movement of the dressing.

PROCEDURE 18-14   Removing a Soiled Dressing and Applying a Clean, Dry Dressing

Materials Needed
- Gauze dressing pad
- Tape
- Scissors
- Waterproof protector pad (if needed)
- Tongs or spring-clip clothespin (if available)
- Paper or plastic bag
- Disposable gloves (two pairs)

Procedure
1. Explain what you are going to do.
2. Wash your hands.
3. Obtain materials listed above.
4. Provide privacy (close door, shut drapes, pull shades).
5. Cut length of tapes needed, and hang them on edge of table for use later.
6. Put on gloves.

REMOVING A SOILED DRESSING

7. Expose area where dressing is to be removed.
8. Place paper or plastic bag nearby.
9. Remove all tape from skin by pulling tape toward the dressing/wound.
10. Gently remove soiled dressing using tongs or clothespin to grasp the edges. If tongs or clothespin is not available, grasp the cleanest part of the dressing and remove. Inspect dressing and skin. Note color, amount of drainage, and odor. Discard into paper bag.
11. Discard soiled gloves. Wash hands. Put on clean gloves.

APPLYING A CLEAN, DRY DRESSING

12. Remove clean, dry dressing from cover, touching edge of dressing only.
13. Apply dressing to area.
14. Take strips of precut tape, and apply to secure dressing.
15. Place dressing cover in paper bag and discard.
16. Remove and discard gloves in paper or plastic bag.
17. Wash your hands.
18. Record what you have done. Report any unusual conditions to your supervisor such as
Excessive drainage
Change in color of drainage
Redness
Bleeding
Swelling
Odor

is bleeding or drainage as a result of removing the dressing. Follow Procedure 18-14, Removing a Soiled Dressing and Applying a Clean, Dry Dressing.

PROMOTING CIRCULATION

Many factors affect clients' circulation, including
- Inactivity and immobilization
- Paralysis
- Disease conditions of the heart, blood, and blood vessels
- Surgery
- Trauma
- Pregnancy

Clients with these conditions may have slow or sluggish circulation. In some cases, an abnormal blood clot, or thrombus, may form. If a thrombus, or some part of it, travels through the circulatory system, it may damage vital organs—heart, lungs, brain. A moving blood clot is called an embolus.

Moving, exercising, coughing, and deep breathing can improve circulation. Encouraging clients to do as much as possible for themselves is one method of improving circulation. Blood collects in the lower extremities, and leg exercises help the blood to return to the heart. Walking is the best exercise, but, if this is not possible, leg exercises may be ordered. The nurse or therapist will teach the leg exercises. Follow the care

BOX 18-3 **Caring for the Client Who Wears Elastic Stockings or Bandages**

- Check toes (or fingers) for
  Coldness
  Bluish skin
- Check with client to see if he or she has any complaints of
  Numbness
  Pain
  Tingling
- Remove elastic stocking (bandage), and observe skin condition.
- Report unusual observations to your supervisor.
- Record what you have done.

plan, and assist your client to perform the exercises as scheduled. Follow Procedure 14-15 (p. 262) for range-of-motion leg exercises. NEVER MASSAGE A CLIENT'S LEGS. YOU MAY DISLODGE A THROMBUS, CAUSING IT TO TRAVEL TO A VITAL ORGAN.

ELASTIC STOCKINGS

Elastic stockings, called *TEDs* or antiembolism stockings, are used to improve circulation of the legs and feet and prevent the formation of blood clots. They create pressure on the leg veins, increasing the return of blood to the heart. These stockings come in many sizes and in both knee-high and thigh-high lengths. The client's legs are measured by the nurse to determine the proper size stockings. Ideally, clients will apply their own stockings. You may or may not be permitted to apply elastic stockings; it depends on your agency's policy.

Stockings are removed three times a day to check for color and warmth of feet and toes. The client should be sitting with the legs up or lying down while stockings are off. Stockings should be reapplied before the client stands or while sitting on the side of the bed. Improper application can block circulation and damage tissues. See Box 18-3 for hints on checking the client's circulation when elastic stockings or bandages are worn. Change the stockings daily after bathing the legs. Stockings should be washed regularly. Hand-wash and air-dry according to manufacturer's instructions (see Procedure 18-15, Applying Elastic Stockings).

ELASTIC BANDAGES

Elastic bandages, sometimes called *ACE bandages,* are used for the same purpose as elastic stockings. In addition, elastic bandages are used to provide support and reduce swelling after musculoskeletal injuries. These may be applied to arms and/or legs. Ideally, clients will apply their own elastic bandages. If they require assistance, follow the care plan. Not all agencies permit home care aides to apply elastic bandages; follow agency policy.

When applying elastic bandages, follow these guidelines:
- Use bandages of proper length and width.
- Leave furthest part of limb (fingers, toes) exposed to check for proper circulation.
- Keep limb elevated while applying bandage.
- Wrap evenly with no wrinkles or folds.
- Do not wrap too tightly.

PROCEDURE 18-15   Applying Elastic Stockings

Materials Needed
- Clean elastic stockings

Procedure
1. Explain what you are going to do.
2. Wash your hands.
3. Obtain elastic stockings.
4. Provide privacy.
5. Put client in supine position.
6. Expose legs. Check to see that legs are clean and dry.
7. Turn stocking inside out by placing one hand into sock, holding toe of sock with other hand, and pulling (Figure 18-15, A).
8. Put client's toes into foot of stocking. Make sure sock is smooth (Figure 18-15, B).
9. Slide remaining portion of sock over client's foot and heel. Make sure foot fits into the toe and heel position of the sock. The sock will now be right side out (Figure 18-15, C).
10. Pull stocking up over client's calf until stocking is fully extended (Figure 18-15, D).
11. Inspect stocking to make sure there are no wrinkles or binding at the top of the stocking.
12. Make sure client is safe and comfortable.
13. Wash your hands.
14. Record what you have done. Report any unusual conditions to your supervisor.
15. Check for proper circulation regularly according to care plan.

Fig 18-15 **A,** Turn the stocking inside out (Step 7). **B,** Put client's toes into foot of the stocking (Step 8). **C,** Slide stocking over the client's foot and heel (Step 9). **D,** Pull stocking up over the calf (Step 10). (From Potter PA, Perry AG, Stockert P, Hall A: *Fundamentals of nursing,* ed. 8, St. Louis, 2013, Mosby.)

PROCEDURE 18-16 | Applying Elastic Bandages

Materials Needed

- Elastic bandages
- Fasteners (clips, safety pins, tape)

Procedure

1. Explain what you are going to do.
2. Wash your hands.
3. Obtain materials listed above.
4. Provide privacy.
5. Assist client to comfortable position: supine for legs and feet; other positions according to care plan and part to be bandaged.
6. Expose part. Check to see that it is clean and dry.
7. Hold bandage with roll up (Figure 18-16).
8. Apply one end of bandage to smallest part (e.g., wrist, ankle).
9. Wrap two turns to anchor bandage.
10. Continue wrapping in spiral turns upward (overlap previous turn by two thirds). Apply firmly but NOT TOO TIGHTLY.
11. Fasten end with clip, safety pin, or tape.
12. Wash your hands.
13. Record what you have done. Report any unusual conditions to your supervisor.
14. Check for proper circulation regularly according to care plan.

Fig 18-16 Hold bandage with roll up (Step 7).

BOX 18-4 | Infection Control When Performing Special Procedures

- Wash your hands before and after wearing gloves.
- Wear gloves when
  There is risk of contact with body fluids, including drainage from wounds
  Disposing of soiled dressings and perineal pads
  Cleaning oxygen equipment
- Wear PPE when needed.
- Dispose of soiled dressings, pads, and gloves in paper or plastic bag. Place in plastic trash bag, and discard immediately.

Wash and dry bandages according to manufacturer's instructions. Avoid heat, as it will destroy the elastic. Overstretched elastic bandages should be replaced with new ones. Follow Procedure 18-16, Applying Elastic Bandages.

INFECTION CONTROL

It is very important to use standard (universal) precautions when in contact with the client's body fluids and waste materials. To prevent the spread of possible infection, also practice medical asepsis techniques discussed in Chapter 11. Box 18-4 reviews important rules of standard (universal) precautions and medical asepsis when performing procedures discussed in this chapter.

CHAPTER SUMMARY

- Special procedures are important in the treatment of the client's condition. However, in some states, home care aides are not permitted to perform these procedures.
- Special procedures are listed in the care plan. Some procedures are done by the home care aide and some by the client, and other procedures are the responsibility of other members of the home care team.
- Home care aides assist clients to take their own medications; home care aides never administer medications of any type.
- Applications of heat and cold are used for their helpful effects. Improper use of heat and/or cold may cause a client to have a severe injury. Home care aides must follow all safety rules about applications of heat and/or cold.
- Oxygen is used for clients who have difficulty breathing and cannot get enough oxygen through the air. There is great risk of fire when oxygen is being used in the home. Home care aides must know and follow safety rules pertaining to oxygen use.
- Home care aides observe and report problems with intravenous equipment or any client complaints during IV therapy.
- Home care aides may be responsible for other treatments, including: applying clean, dry dressings and assisting clients to apply elastic stockings or bandages.
- Three important responsibilities of the home care aide in every special procedure are observing, recording, and reporting to the supervisor.
- Use standard (universal) precautions and medical asepsis rules when performing the special procedures discussed in this chapter.

STUDY QUESTIONS

1. List seven guidelines for special procedures.
2. What is the difference between administering medications and assisting with medications?
3. List 10 guidelines to follow when assisting clients to take medications.
4. What are two desired effects of hot applications? Cold applications?
5. Describe two safety rules to follow for each of the following procedures:
   a. Applying a hot water bottle
   b. Applying a hot compress
   c. Giving a sitz bath
   d. Applying an ice bag
   e. Applying a hot soak
6. List six rules of safety to follow when the client is receiving oxygen.
7. Your client is receiving an intravenous infusion. List four observations you would report to your supervisor.
8. How does the home care aide practice infection control and standard (universal) precautions when removing a soiled dressing and applying a clean, dry dressing?
9. Identify three responsibilities of the home care aide when caring for clients with elastic stockings.
10. When checking a client's extremities for proper circulation, what will you look for?
11. Identify three ways the home care aide can prevent the spread of infection when performing special procedures.

19

Caring for Older Adults

OBJECTIVES

After you read this chapter, you will be able to:

1. Define the terms *aging, young old, middle old,* and *oldest old.*
2. Identify three common myths about older adults and the realities about these myths.
3. Discuss four adjustments older adults need to make as they age.
4. Identify eight common physical changes experienced by older adults and eight ways the home care aide can assist the client to cope with them.
5. Discuss three safety factors to consider when caring for older adults.
6. Define and describe three signs of possible physical abuse, emotional abuse, and material or financial abuse.
7. Discuss five guidelines to follow when caring for older adults.
8. Discuss the problem of alcoholism in older adults.
9. Identify two warning signals of suicide in older adults.
10. Apply principles of standard (universal) precautions and infection control when caring for older adults.

KEY TERMS

Abuse Mistreating or causing harm
Baby boomers Those born between 1946 and 1964
Gerontologists Specialists in the study of aging
Informal caregivers Unpaid persons, usually family members, who care for clients on a voluntary basis

Mourning Reaction to a great personal loss
Neglect Inability or failure to provide needed care
Stereotype Generalization about a form of behavior in an individual or a group

HOW OLD IS OLD?

Aging is the process of growing old that begins at birth and continues until death. Aging is inevitable. The rate at which aging takes place differs with each person, but it increases and becomes more noticeable during the later years.

The term *old* has a very personal meaning for each of us. If you are 22 years old, then age 35 may seem very "old" to you. At age 75, a person may consider

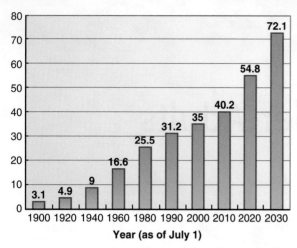

Fig 19-1 Number of persons 65 years of age and older from 1900 to 2030 (in millions). Note: Increments in years are uneven. (From A Profile of Older Americans: 2010. Administration on Aging, U.S. Department of Health and Human Services.)

Fig 19-2 Most older adults remain in their homes and continue with daily routines, such as shopping.

"old" to be anyone 5 years older than himself. And a 95-year-old may consider herself to be "old."

No one really knows what causes aging to occur. Much research is being done in this area, and **gerontologists** have many theories. These include the following:

- Cells wear out
- Each person has a personal "time clock" that controls aging
- The genes determine the rate of aging

This is the first time there have been so many older adults. Because of this, we are able to learn more and more about the aging process. For example, certain conditions, such as Alzheimer's disease, have been recognized as disease processes, not a part of the normal aging process. As research continues, the secrets to the aging process may be uncovered.

Although 65 is the usual age for retirement and Social Security benefits, gerontologists classify the older adult population according to the following groups:

- Young old age   65 to 74 years
- Middle old age   75 to 84 years
- Oldest old age   85 to 100+ years

FACTS ABOUT OLDER ADULTS

At the beginning of the twentieth century, 1 of every 25 people was 65 and older, only about 4% of the population. Today, Russ' observation that there are "a lot of older people" is correct. More than 12.9% of the total U.S. population is older than 65 years of age, about one in every eight Americans. In fact, the fastest growing group is 85 years of age and older.

The number of older adults will continue to grow rapidly as the population of "**baby boomers**" begins to turn 65, the largest group ever in the United States to head toward retirement. By 2030, there will be about 72.1 million older adults, more than twice the number in 2000 (Figure 19-1).

Most older adults are well and live at home. They continue with daily routines, like shopping, and they pursue recreational activities (Figures 19-2 and 19-3). In fact, 20% of older adults are employed. This percentage may continue to rise as economic

Fig 19-3 Many older adults enjoy the popular sport of golf.

BOX 19-1 **Facts about Older Adults**

- There are 39.6 million adults 65 years of age and older living in the United States. This represents 12.9% of the total population.
- A 65-year-old man can expect to live to be 82.5 years old. A 65-year-old woman can expect to live to be 84.9 years old.
- There are more older women than men: 22.7 million older women to 16.8 million older men (135 women to every 100 men).
- Older men (77%) are much more likely to be married than are older women (42%).
- About 30% of older adults live alone: 8.3 million women and 4.0 million men.
- Only 4.1% of older adults are living in institutions.
- About 14.8% of the white population is 65 years of age and older. Other groups are represented as follows:

African Americans	8.3%
Asians and Pacific Islanders	3.4%
Hispanics	7.0%
American Indians or Native Alaskans	1.0%

- About 8.9% of older Americans live below the poverty level. The highest poverty rates (44.6%) are for older Hispanic women living alone.
- The educational level of older adults is increasing. More than 78.3% have completed high school, and 21.7% are college graduates.
- A child born in 2007 can expect to live 77.9 years, about 30 years longer than a child born in 1900.

---

conditions force many older adults to postpone retirement and continue full or part-time employment. Only 4.1% are in institutions, and these are usually the oldest old. See Box 19-1 for more facts about the older population.

MYTHS AND REALITIES

In the United States, the focus is on youth. Television commercials sell creams and lotions to reduce wrinkles; give smooth, young skin; and erase the effects of aging. We get the idea that to be young is "okay" and to be old is dull, boring, not "cool." Older adults are portrayed as grouchy, forgetful, rigid, helpless, worthless, useless,

Fig 19-4 A home care aide takes time to share the past with a client.

TABLE 19-1	Myths and Realities of Aging
THE MYTH	**THE REALITY**
Older adults cannot learn new things or adjust to changes.	It may take longer, but older adults can learn new routines and new skills. They can adjust to changes with help and support from others.
Incontinence is a sign of aging.	Incontinence is a sign of an abnormal condition that requires medical treatment.
Most older adults are sick and are in nursing homes.	Only about 4.1% of older adults are in nursing homes and other institutions.
Mental confusion is a normal part of growing old.	Mental confusion is an abnormal condition that must be reported to your supervisor.
Older adults are no longer concerned about looking attractive.	The need to look attractive does not change as the aging process continues.
Forgetfulness is a sure sign of illness.	Forgetfulness is not necessarily a sign of illness or disease.

unproductive, stupid, and slow. Society has created an unfair and untruthful **stereotype** of the older population.

There is no typical older adult. Each is a unique individual who will age at his or her own rate and in his or her own way. For example, if Mr. Felder was a happy, pleasant person in his younger years, chances are that he will have the same personality as he becomes an older adult. Grouchy, complaining Mr. Green will be even better at complaining when he gets older. After all, he has had years of practice. Grandma Bennett likes to sit in the rocker on her porch and watch the flowers grow, but her 76-year-old sister runs in the marathon each year and says she does not have time to waste "watching the roses bloom."

As people age from young old to oldest old, they usually become more frail and have more chronic illnesses. They experience an increasing loss of strength and mobility. There is a big difference between the 70-year-old and the 90-year-old. Although there are exceptions, the oldest old require more help with performing activities of daily living and caring for and maintaining their homes.

Many older adults enjoy reminiscing about the "old days" and the "old times." Listen to them; it is a wonderful opportunity to learn about their history and culture (Figure 19-4). Sometimes, you may hear the same story over and over and over again. Be patient; those older adults who have memory problems will forget what they have told you and repeat it frequently. This can be trying for the listener, but smile, be patient, and listen again. Review Chapter 3 to sharpen your communication skills. Table 19-1 lists some myths and realities about aging.

AGEISM

Ageism is a form of discrimination practiced against older adults. Younger generations may "look down" on older adults and treat them as mindless, stupid, and worthless. Ageism puts older adults into categories such as senile, rigid in thought and behavior, and old fashioned in morality and skills. It allows younger persons to see older people as different from themselves. They no longer identify older people as human beings. Ageism may take many forms.

- Being denied a job because of age
- Discrimination in housing
- "Rip-offs" in home repairs and maintenance
- Treating older adults as if they are not able to think or make decisions for themselves

Our cultural background and personal experiences with older persons influence our views of aging. In some cultures, older adults are revered and respected. They are always cared for at home and would never be sent to a nursing home. In other cases, older adults live far away from children and grandchildren, so younger persons may have little or no experience with their elders. This may lead to a stereotyped view of older adults. Also, ageism protects younger persons from thinking about the future— and the issues of their own illness, aging, and death.

ADJUSTING TO GROWING OLDER

As a person grows older, many changes occur. These changes are not only physical but also social and emotional. The older person must face these changes and learn how to adjust to them in order for meaningful aging to occur (Box 19-2).

RETIREMENT AND REDUCED INCOME

The usual age for retirement is 65 years of age. With downsizing and restructuring of government and industry, some people retire at an earlier age, some as early as 50 years

---

BOX 19-2 Adjusting to Growing Older

- Adjusting to retirement and reduced income
- Finding a meaning in life
- Maintaining satisfactory living arrangements
- Finding satisfaction within the family
- Facing the reality of death
- Accepting oneself as an aging person
- Adjusting to decreasing health and physical strength

Fig 19-5 Part-time employment fills social and financial needs.

of age. The change from working outside of the home to not going to work requires a lot of adjustment. Many people associate employment with a feeling of worth and not working with a feeling of uselessness. Some view retirement as a permanent vacation and are delighted to do nothing. Others cannot sit still and are easily bored. Whatever the case, the income may be reduced or, at best, remains the same. Budgeting, wise use of credit and credit cards, and careful shopping are now a necessary way of life. Social Security checks may not be enough to live on, and some pensions are barely enough. Health care costs are so high, especially medications, that the older adult may be forced to choose between food and medicine.

Many older adults continue employment because of the increased cost of living forces them to keep working. Others find part-time jobs to keep pace with the necessities of life. For both groups, retirement becomes a dream, not a reality. However, there are healthy older adults who choose to be employed as long as they are able.

If one is wealthy, there is no problem with finances. But for most people, the money they have now has to last for a lifetime. As a result, most older adults are cautious and very careful about their money. Notify your supervisor if your client is having financial problems. There are community agencies to help older adults with everything from financial counseling to food stamps or other government assistance programs.

MEANINGFUL LIFE

Older adults find meaning in life in many ways. Most will continue to do what they have always done: participate in the same clubs, church activities, social groups, and volunteer activities and enjoy their children and grandchildren. Others need to fill the gap created by retirement. This is done by finding part-time or full-time employment (Figure 19-5), beginning a new career, developing new hobbies or interests, participating in volunteer activities (Figure 19-6), continuing one's education, and joining senior citizens' clubs.

Many older adults enroll in courses offered at community senior centers, local community colleges, or adult evening programs at area high schools. These courses include information about a variety of interests, such as learning to operate one's personal computer or other electronic devices. Through the personal computer, e-mail, and

Fig 19-6 Volunteer service provides meaningful activity and the chance for socializing.

Fig 19-7 This older adult uses the computer to keep in touch with family and friends.

social networks, older adults keep in touch with children, grandchildren, other relatives, and friends living near and far away (Figure 19-7).

Loneliness is a common experience for older adults. Advancing age and the inability to drive or use public transportation isolate them from the community. They are lonely because they have outlived many of their own generation, and they continue to experience what seems to them an ongoing, never-ending series of losses. They feel these losses very deeply. After a lifetime of human contact, they may now be alone without the loving touch of another human being. They need the nonverbal communication of hand-holding, a gentle touch, or hug. Sometimes, the home care aide is the only person visiting the client, providing personal care, and meeting the need for human contact. Remember to give older clients a smile, a comforting touch (Figure 19-8), and a hug (if appropriate to their culture).

Pets provide companionship and love, especially for the person who is alone. Animals enjoy hugs and kisses; humans enjoy giving this love to their pets (Figure 19-9). These animals may become the older adult's "family." Be kind to your client's animals. If you are afraid of the pet, are allergic to its hair, or dislike dogs or cats, ask the client to secure the animal where you will not have contact with it. Tell your client that you cannot be around animals because of health reasons. If you are very allergic to animals, inform your supervisor.

SATISFACTORY LIVING ARRANGEMENTS

Most older adults stay in the home where they have always lived. Others may live with one of their children. Some older adults live in assisted living facilities, senior citizen apartments, retirement communities, group homes, single-room occupancy

Fig 19-8 Touch is an important means of communicating.

Fig 19-9 Pets are like family members.

hotels, or adult foster homes. Still others may live in a Continuing Care Retirement Community (CCRC). They "buy into" the community, live in an apartment, and then move to the community nursing home when necessary and remain a resident of the CCRC until death. Clients in all of these living facilities will use the services of a home care aide.

SATISFACTION WITHIN THE FAMILY

With retirement, married couples spend a great deal of time together. Some partners may not have had so much togetherness since their honeymoon. It is a time of adjustments and getting to know each other again.

Older adults have the opportunity to build adult relationships with their grown children and resolve any problems of the past. For most elders, grandchildren are a special delight. Some older adults provide child care for their grandchildren while the children's parents work. Some grandparents raise their grandchildren because the children's parents are sick, deceased, unemployed, divorced, or in prison. In other cases, older adults have no families, may be abandoned or ignored by family members, or outlive relatives. There may be no opportunity for satisfaction within the family.

REALITY OF DEATH

Older adulthood is the final stage of life; the next step is death. Older adults are very aware of the reality of death. They have lost friends, relatives, and perhaps a spouse or partner. Preparing a will, purchasing a burial site, preplanning with a funeral director, and making advance decisions about care and treatment all remind the older adult of what is to come.

The death of a spouse or partner causes deep sadness and grief. Mourning has many physical, social, and emotional effects. It will take the survivor several years to recover from the death. Even then, life is changed forever, and many adjustments must be made to living on one's own.

SELF-ACCEPTANCE

We all need to accept ourselves just as we are (Figure 19-10). Some older adults have difficulty facing the fact that they are "older adults." They do not like the changes

Fig 19-10 Accepting the physical changes of aging is a task of older adults.

caused by the aging process. They long for their youth and the "good old days." But most older adults adjust to the changes in their lives and learn to accept things as they are.

Exercise, proper diet, and rest are important factors in feeling good and staying healthy. Grooming, hygiene, and cleanliness are important factors in looking and feeling good. An interest in life, getting out, reading, and being a part of the community help to promote a positive attitude and emotional well-being. All of these things help a person with self-image and self-acceptance.

DECREASING HEALTH AND PHYSICAL STRENGTH

Some older adults may ignore problems with seeing, hearing, and walking, saying that they are "just a part of old age." These difficulties can interfere with daily living. They can also lead to medical problems and increasing dependence. For example, a person who cannot see to read the medication labels may take the wrong drug at the wrong time. As a result, he or she may become confused, may fall, or may need to be hospitalized.

As aging progresses, most people do not have the strength they formerly had. It takes longer to do the tasks they used to do, and these jobs are very tiring. Many of the oldest old are unable to perform household duties or activities of daily living because chronic illness interferes with mobility. These older adults require assistance with home maintenance and personal care, such as bathing and grooming. It is hard for the independent-minded older adult to accept help with such personal activities. They may become frustrated and angry with their slowness and dependency. Be patient; give them time and assistance as needed.

Older adults cherish their independence and will do almost anything to remain living "at home." They have a basic need to make their own decisions and choices about their care and future.

PHYSICAL SIGNS OF AGING

Although the aging process begins at birth, the physical signs of this process do not become noticeable until later in life. Aging affects all the body systems but at different rates of speed. Physical changes begin gradually and may not be obvious right away. For example, hair begins to lose its color very gradually—a few hairs at a time—until there are many gray hairs. The ability to perform strenuous physical activity without rest periods also decreases gradually as we age. But there are always exceptions: the 80-year-old woman who does not have one gray hair, or the 85-year-old man who runs in the marathon race.

The changes that occur are influenced by many factors: heredity, health practices and lifestyle (e.g., rest, sleep, exercise, eating habits, smoking, alcohol use, illegal drug use), stresses of life, and one's occupation.

The following are a few of the signs of aging.

- Wrinkling of the skin: Loss of fatty tissue and elastic quality of the skin
- Thinning and graying of hair: Glandular changes and loss of color of the hair
- Decrease in physical strength and endurance: Changes in the skeletomuscular, circulatory, and respiratory systems
- Difficulty in adjusting to shadows, glare, or dim lights: Changes in the eye
- Increase in time needed to react to emergency situations: Changes in the nervous system

The material that follows explains (1) the basic changes in each body system, (2) common situations experienced by the client, and (3) ways that the home care aide can assist the client to cope with these normal changes.

CHANGES IN THE SKELETOMUSCULAR SYSTEM

"I used to be 5'4"—now I'm only 5 feet tall! And I just don't seem to have as much energy as I had when I was younger."

Perhaps the change that is most noticeable in this body system is that older adults are just not as tall as they used to be. As aging occurs, there is a shortening of the spinal column. This is a very gradual process. In some people, the upper spine becomes curved and the head bends forward. Bones lose calcium, causing them to become weak and brittle—a disease called osteoporosis (Box 19-3). So, these older adults are more prone to fractures. When fractures occur, healing takes longer, too.

BOX 19-3   Osteoporosis

What is it? Thinning and weakness of the bones from loss of calcium

Who has it? 10 million Americans are estimated to have the disease—8 million are women. 35% of all women over 65 years of age have it. Another 34 million Americans have low bone density.

Who gets it? Anyone can, but mostly women who are
- Postmenopausal
- Smokers
- Alcohol consumers
- Physically inactive

What happens? Fractures of the hip, spine, and wrist are complications of osteoporosis. Women are most at risk for hip fractures—more than 75% of all hip fractures occur in older women.

Prevention Men and women of all ages are encouraged to have recommended amounts of calcium-rich foods in the diet and to be physically active.

Treatment is different for each person, but may include
- Change in lifestyle to eliminate smoking and reduce alcohol intake
- Increased activity, if possible, especially weight-bearing exercise, such as daily walking
- Adequate amounts of calcium in the daily diet (see Chapter 10 for good sources of calcium)
- Calcium and vitamin D supplements and prescription medications as prescribed by a doctor

BOX 19-4   Skeletomuscular System

Common Situations	Suggestions for Helping the Client
Stiffness in joints and muscles	Assist client to put joints through range of motion during activities of daily living.
	Help client to change position at least every 2 hours.
Difficulty removing and recapping jars, toothpaste tubes, medication containers, or opening cereal boxes	Remove caps or lids on containers, or open boxes, as needed.
	Encourage client to use assistive devices such as rubber bands around edges of lids.
Difficulty handling heavy cups, mugs, and glassware	When possible, use lightweight plasticware with handles. Fill cups ½ full to reduce weight and prevent spills.
Takes more time to perform activities	Assist client when needed, but do not perform activity for client.
	Allow extra time for activities; do not rush client.
Tires easily	Allow for rest periods between activities to avoid exhaustion.
	Schedule hygiene activities at a time when energy levels are highest, if possible.

Changes also occur in the joints and muscles. Generally, there is a decrease in the strength and flexibility of the muscles. Joints stiffen, especially after a period of sleep or rest. Lack of exercise, including walking, contributes to further muscle weakness and joint stiffness. Box 19-4 lists suggestions for helping clients with common situations resulting from changes in the skeletomuscular system.

CHANGES IN THE INTEGUMENTARY SYSTEM

"My skin used to be very oily. Now, it's so dry and flaky."

Most of the changes that occur in this system do not produce major physical problems. Rather, they are outward signs of the aging process. There is a redistribution of fatty tissue under the skin. These fatty deposits are gradually lost from the face, arms, and legs; they may seem to "reappear" in the abdomen and hips. Loss of fatty tissue, especially in the arms and legs, and changes in metabolism may cause the older person to complain of being cold, even when it is warm outside.

Glands do not produce as much oil to lubricate the skin naturally. So, the skin becomes dry and flaky. The elbows, hip bones, and shoulder blades become more visible because of the lack of fatty tissue covering the bones. Also, the skin loses its elastic quality, and blood vessels near the surface of the skin are more visible, especially in the hands and arms.

The fingernails become ridged and brittle, while the toenails tend to become hard and thick. They can be very difficult to cut.

Prolonged exposure to the sun's damaging rays hastens the aging of the skin, especially of the face. Wrinkles and crow's feet around the eyes are the results of repeated use of facial muscles over a long period of time. Box 19-5 lists suggestions for helping clients with common situations resulting from changes in the integumentary system.

CHANGES IN THE CIRCULATORY AND RESPIRATORY SYSTEMS

"My hands and feet are cold all the time, even in the summer."

Generally, these two body systems become less effective as the body ages. The muscles of the heart and blood vessels gradually begin to lose their strength and

---

BOX 19-5 Integumentary System

Common Situations	Suggestions for Helping the Client
Dry, flaky skin	Use soap sparingly.
	Do not give daily tub bath or shower unless care plan indicates.
	Apply moisturizing creams or lotions to skin *after* bathing.
	Do not put oils in bathtub due to risk of falls.
	Avoid alcohol-based products, as they tend to dry skin.
Brittle fingernails	File, as needed. Apply lotion to soften nails.
Thick, hard toenails	Do not cut or file toenails. Notify your supervisor; a podiatrist may need to be contacted.

BOX 19-6 Normal Range of Vital Signs for Clients 85 Years of Age and Older

Temperature

Oral	95° to 97° F (35° to 36.1° C)
Rectal	95.2° to 98.6° F (35.1° to 37° C)
Axillary	94° to 96° F (34.4° to 35.5° C)
Tympanic	95° to 97° F (35° to 36.1° C)
Pulse	70 to 76
Respirations	20 to 22 (more shallow than a younger adult)
Blood Pressure	$\frac{120}{80}$

---

efficiency in transporting blood to all parts of the body. The process of returning blood through the veins to the heart also becomes less efficient. The openings of the blood vessels narrow due to the deposits of calcium, cholesterol, and other fatty substances.

The number of alveoli decreases, and each one becomes less elastic, so the exchange of oxygen and carbon dioxide is less efficient. Secretions of the mucous membrane that lines the entire respiratory tract tend to thicken. They can be difficult to expel. See Box 19-6 for normal vital signs of clients 85 years of age and older.

The body's resistance to infection and disease is lowered because the immune system does not function as efficiently as before. Therefore, older adults are at greater risk for infection. It is very important for the home care aide to observe, record, and report beginning signs of infection immediately so that treatment can begin promptly.

Box 19-7 lists suggestions for helping clients with common situations resulting from changes in the circulatory and respiratory systems.

CHANGES IN THE DIGESTIVE SYSTEM

"Food just doesn't taste the same anymore."

Many older clients' concerns result from changes in the digestive system. The number of taste buds in the tongue are reduced, especially those that affect the sweet and salty tastes. The sense of thirst is decreased. Lack of teeth or poorly fitting dentures prevent many older clients from eating the foods they once enjoyed. Salivary glands secrete less saliva. Gastric juices produced by the stomach are reduced, and food remains in the stomach longer. As a result, clients complain of bloating and indigestion. Muscles of the large intestine do not work as well, and peristalsis is decreased. The nerve

BOX 19-7   Circulatory and Respiratory Systems

Common Situations	Suggestions for Helping the Client
Complains of being cold, especially in hands and feet	Assist client to put on sweater, socks, gloves; use an extra blanket in bed. Dress by layering.
	Place thermostat on higher setting. Caution client not to use hot water bottles or heating pads to keep warm.
	Encourage client to avoid crossing legs when sitting.
	Avoid use of constricting clothing: tight socks and wristbands, knee-high stockings, round garters.
Rapid heart beat when stressed; takes longer to return to "normal" heart rate	Pace activities to avoid rushing.
	Allow plenty of time to perform care procedures.
	Try to reduce stressful situations.
Shortness of breath with increased activity	Provide frequent rest periods when assisting client with activities of daily living.

BOX 19-8   Digestive System

Commons Situations	Suggestions for Helping the Client
Dry mouth	Encourage client to drink fluids: 2 quarts (2000 milliliters) daily. Offer small amounts of fluids frequently.
	Offer fluids to moisten the mouth before assisting client to take oral medications.
	Offer frequent mouth care.
Loss of teeth	Provide soft foods (pureed, chopped meats, fruits, and vegetables) according to care plan (see Chapter 10).
Gas, bloating, indigestion, heartburn	Report and record on care record if these complaints are new to the client.
	Encourage client to eat slowly and chew food thoroughly.
	Have client maintain a sitting position for $\frac{1}{2}$ hour after eating.
	Avoid serving gas-forming, fatty, and highly seasoned foods (see Chapter 10).
	Offer six to eight small meals daily.
Constipation	Encourage client to eat foods high in fiber, and offer fluids frequently.
	Allow plenty of time in bathroom for bowel movement; do not rush.

sensation that signals the need to defecate may also be dulled. These factors, coupled with a decreased fluid intake and a diet low in fiber, make constipation a real problem for many older adults. Box 19-8 lists suggestions for helping clients with common situations resulting from changes in the digestive system.

CHANGES IN THE NERVOUS SYSTEM AND SENSES

"I can remember exactly what I did on my 10th birthday. But, what did I do yesterday?"

Perhaps the best way to describe the normal aging nervous system is that it is slower—slower to receive and send messages to other parts of the body. This slowness is due to loss of nerve cells, which begin to decline at around 25 years of age. Memory loss for recent events is a common concern for many older adults. Forgetting the home

BOX 19-9   Nervous System and Senses

Commons Situations	Suggestions for Helping the Client
Forgetfulness	Encourage client to jot down reminders on pad.
Short-term memory loss, such as names of persons who visited yesterday	Provide clues to client to refresh memory.
Difficulty adjusting to depths (going up and down steps and stairs)	Encourage client to use hand rails, if available; provide support as needed. Do not rush; allow plenty of time.
Trouble getting to sleep	Avoid caffeine after evening meal (e.g., coffee, tea, chocolate). Avoid alcohol at night. Give back rub. Give warm milk before bedtime, if allowed. Encourage physical activity during the day.
Unsteady balance when changing position suddenly	Encourage client to change position slowly, such as turning around. Count to 10 after client rises from a sitting position, then proceed to assist the client to walk. Provide support when walking. Do not rush client.
Difficulty adjusting to sudden changes in light or darkness	Encourage client to wait a few minutes until the eyes can adjust to the darkness or light. Use a night light.
Changes in ability to see and hear	See Chapter 3 for communicating with the visually- and hearing-impaired client.

care aide's name or where their eyeglasses are can be embarrassing or frustrating for the older adult. But they are not necessarily signs of illness. One's intelligence does not lessen as aging continues. The ability to learn continues. It may just take longer to learn and remember new information. Adjusting to stress and change in one's life becomes more difficult and takes longer for the older adult.

The sensory organs also become slower in receiving and sending impulses to the brain. The most common of all complaints involving the senses is the decreased ability to hear. This is a very gradual process, hardly noticed, until sounds used in normal conversation become more difficult to hear. Normal changes in the eye result in a decreased amount of tears, decreased side vision, and decreased ability to see certain colors (blues and greens are more difficult to see than reds and yellows).

Other sensory changes include reduced sense of smell, reduced taste buds, and reduced sense of touch in the fingers and toes.

Many older adults say that their patterns of sleep have changed. Before, they could sleep all night without waking. Now, sleep is disrupted by frequent trips to the bathroom or wakefulness. Lack of physical activity, anxiety, and long naps during the day can cause nighttime insomnia. Box 19-9 lists suggestions for helping clients with common situations resulting from changes in the nervous system and senses.

CHANGES IN URINARY AND REPRODUCTIVE SYSTEMS

"When I have the urge to go to the bathroom, I have to go fast! I can't hold my water very well."

| BOX 19-10 | Urinary and Reproductive Systems |

Common Situations	Suggestions for Helping the Client
Urgent need to void; difficulty holding urine	Clothing should be easy to remove: elastic waistband on slacks (no buttons, zippers). *DO NOT* reduce fluids during the day. May need to help client to bathroom every 2 hours or less.
Interrupted sleep due to nighttime voiding	Avoid drinks with caffeine after evening meal (coffee, teas, colas). Avoid salty and spicy foods for last meal of day. Avoid alcohol, particularly beer, in the evening. Place commode at bedside. Put on night light. Make sure passage to bathroom is uncluttered, if commode is not used at bedside.
Dryness of genital area	Avoid hot tub baths.

This comment is usually due to the weakness of the bladder muscles or to medications that increase urinary output. Some older adults can only hold half as much urine at one time as they could when they were younger. As a result, frequent trips to the bathroom are common. Other older adults retain large quantities of urine because the bladder muscles become stretched and have difficulty contracting. In these situations, the client may complain of leaking. This usually means that the bladder is overfilled.

Urinary incontinence is not part of the normal aging process. There can be many causes for urinary incontinence. It is an abnormal condition that should be reported to your supervisor immediately (see Chapter 15).

As the male reproductive system ages, the prostate gland usually increases in size. This is not a problem unless the gland causes the urethra to constrict and interferes with the normal flow of urine from the bladder. The testes continue to manufacture sperm for much of the older man's life.

In the female, fatty tissue in the breasts and external genitals is reduced. Mucous secretions of the vagina also are reduced. These are due to ovarian hormone changes that occurred during menopause.

Older adults do not lose their interest as sexual beings. The need to continue satisfying sexual relationships is a normal part of aging. Sexual activity may need to be modified because of physical changes. Frail older adults, for example, may find that cuddling, kissing, hugging, and hand-holding can be satisfying types of sexual expression and pleasure. For others, the use of vaginal lubricants to replace the lack of mucous secretions may need to be used, or it may take longer to achieve an erection. However, these changes do not reduce the amount of sexual pleasure. Respect the client's need for privacy. Box 19-10 lists suggestions for helping clients with common situations resulting from changes in the urinary and reproductive systems.

NUTRITION

The ChooseMyPlate Food Guide can be individualized to meet the nutritional needs of all persons including older adults. Additional information is available from the home care agency's dietitian or from the ChooseMyPlate.gov Internet website. Older adults usually do not drink enough fluids because the sense of thirst is reduced. Other reasons for not drinking fluids include:

- Fear of not being able to get to the bathroom in time due to problems with mobility
- Difficulty removing clothing quickly enough resulting in soiled garments and embarrassment
- Pain that results from walking or transferring from wheelchair to commode

It is very important for older adults to drink plenty of fluids (2 quarts or 2000 milliliters) including water and other fluids each day. So, encourage clients to use the commode or toilet, before the urge to void is felt, about every 2 hours or less.

SAFETY AND THE OLDER ADULT

Because of the physical changes that take place, older adults are at great risk for injury due to accidents. Nursing research indicates that some older adults are at even greater risk because of advanced age, side effects of medications, and severe disability (Box 19-11). Each year, hospital emergency rooms treat older adults for injuries, such as burns and falls, which are associated with products they live with and use every day. Burns, caused by faulty cooking practices, are the most common fire-related injury. Seventy-five percent of all falls occur either inside the house or outside, but nearby. About 87% of all fractures in older adults are due to falls. And, falls are the leading cause of death due to injury in older adults.

Tripping over something on the floor or uneven pavement outdoors can contribute to falls. The older adult's strength is not sufficient to correct one's balance, and so the fall occurs. Participating in classes to increase physical strength and practicing Tai Chi to improve balance are highly recommended for older adults.

The home care aide must be alert to potential safety hazards in the home and remove them, if possible. When they cannot be removed, inform a family member, if available; record and report the hazard to your supervisor.

See Box 19-12 for making the home safer for older adults.

BOX 19-11 Older Clients at Greater Risk for Accidents

Clients Who Are	Clients Who Have	Clients Who Use
Women	Poor eyesight	Canes or walkers incorrectly
85 Years and older	Unsteady gait	Prescription medications, especially blood pressure medications and sedatives
Living alone	Problems with balance	Over-the-counter medications
Frail	Muscle weakness	Alcohol or abuse alcohol or other addictive substances

---

BOX 19-12 Safety and the Older Adult

- See Chapter 8 to review home safety practices.
- Confine pets at night or if client may fall over animals.
- Close cabinet and closet doors and drawers after use.
- Keep client areas well lighted; use night lights.
- Encourage clients to use brighter light bulbs, especially in bathrooms, stairways, and other frequently used areas.
- Encourage client to have grab bars installed near toilet and in bathing area.

BOX 19-13	Watch for Sudden or Gradual Changes

C   Communicating with others
H   Hydration
A   Activities of daily living (ability to function); appearance
N   Nutrition, nervous system (memory loss, muscle weakness)
G   Gait, gastrointestinal problems
E   Environment, emotions
S   Sensory problems (seeing, hearing, tasting, balance, smelling, feeling) and vital signs

ILLNESS IN THE LATER YEARS

Although older adults make up 12.9% of the total population, they occupy more than 50% of acute care hospital beds. More than 70% of available health care services (including home care) are used by older adults. Each year, the average older adult has more than 30 prescriptions filled; the average adult fills about a dozen prescriptions each year. While the prescription may be filled, only about half of the people take their medications as directed. Skipping a dose or not taking the medication at all are some of the common errors made by older adults. Also, they have five times more adverse reactions to medications than younger persons.

Illness can occur very quickly in the older adult because of the many physical changes due to aging (Box 19-13). Beginning signs of illness may be ignored or not reported to the doctor. There are several reasons for not reporting symptoms; these include the following:

- Communication barriers (language, deafness, culture)
- Fear of hospital or nursing home admission
- Cost of treatment
- Fear of outcome

Most commonly, however, the older adult fails to recognize that minor symptoms can quickly develop into a serious medical condition. Prompt treatment can often prevent serious illness and hospitalization.

Some important symptoms to recognize and report are:
- Sudden confusion and agitation
- Urinary incontinence and/or retention
- Eating changes, particularly anorexia
- Energy and activity changes
- Frequent and recurrent falls
- Decreased fluid intake

IF THESE SYMPTOMS ARE NEW, NOT A PART OF THE CLIENT'S HISTORY, REPORT THEM TO YOUR SUPERVISOR IMMEDIATELY. DO NOT ASSUME THAT THESE SYMPTOMS ARE "JUST A PART OF GETTING OLD." THEY MAY BE SYMPTOMS OF DRUG REACTION, INFECTION, OR ANOTHER SERIOUS MEDICAL PROBLEM THAT REQUIRES TREATMENT.

Caring for the older adult can be rewarding and challenging. Some general principles for caring for older adults are listed in Box 19-14.

INFECTION CONTROL

Physical changes of aging combined with the older client's existing illness place him or her at great risk for infection. Be alert for signs of infection, including

---

BOX 19-14   Caring for Older Clients: General Principles

- Allow plenty of time for self-care activities of daily living.
- Encourage client to assume as much responsibility for care as possible.
- Help client only when needed; avoid "doing for" clients when they can "do" for themselves.
- Pace activities to avoid rushing the client; rushing can result in frustration for both client and home care aide.
- Offer fluids frequently, even though the client says he or she is not thirsty.
- Encourage physical activity according to the care plan.

- Be aware of possible safety hazards in client's environment; eliminate them, if possible.
- Respect client's routine; make changes only when necessary.
- Be alert for gradual or sudden changes in client's physical, mental, or emotional condition; record and report them to your supervisor.
- Listen to client when he or she is reminiscing, even when the story is repeated several times. Be patient, and use the communication skills discussed in Chapter 3.
- Practice standard (universal) precautions because of the great risk for infection.

- Elevation of temperature, pulse, and respirations
- Cold or flulike symptoms

Other signs of infection are found in Box 11-2 (p. 171). If your client has any of these symptoms, notify your supervisor immediately. Review the Boxes in Chapter 11 for a quick refresher in the principles of infection control and medical asepsis.

WHO ARE THE CAREGIVERS?

According to national statistics, 80% of all home care services are provided by family caregivers. And, almost one third of the U.S. adult population plays the role of caregiver—about 65.7 million people. This includes 31% of all households. Seven in ten caregivers provide care to someone older than 50 years of age.

The majority of informal caregivers of older adults are family members who provide as little as 20 hours a week or as much as 24 hours each day of the week. Although there is no typical informal caregiver, most are women: wives or adult daughters. The typical female caregiver is

- Age 48
- Working outside of the home
- Caring for her own family
- Coping with her own stresses and health problems
- Caring for a family member who is 69 years old
- Spending 17 years caring for her own children and 18 years caring for an aging parent(s)

About 70% of older adults in the community live with a caregiver. Sometimes an older adult becomes the caregiver. More and more people older than 65 years of age are providing care to both children (grandchildren) and other older adults. This shift to an older population of caregivers requires that help from others (family, friends, neighbors, and social service programs) is needed to support them in their caregiving.

Your client may be cared for by an elderly partner, or a 90-year-old person may be the caregiver for a 70-year-old "child." Adult children, in-laws, or grandchildren may also be caregivers. Sometimes, it is elderly siblings, younger nieces or nephews, neighbors, or friends who provide the care.

Home care aides are assigned to give client care, but they also provide assistance to caregivers in the following ways:

- Offering emotional support by listening to concerns, problems, and questions
- Assuming some of the responsibility for physical care of the client (according to the care plan)
- Enabling them to get out of the house for a few hours
- Encouraging the use of agency resources to deal with problem situations

Very often, the care given by the home care aide (if only for a few hours a week) helps the caregiver to feel restored and able to continue with his or her responsibilities.

ELDER NEGLECT AND ABUSE

Television and radio programs, magazines, and newspapers have brought cases of abuse and neglect of older adults to the public's attention. It is estimated that one in every seven older adults has been a victim of physical, emotional, or financial abuse usually by someone on whom they depend for care and protection. Unfortunately, many victims of elder abuse are too embarrassed, too trusting, or afraid to seek help. And so, only about one in five cases of neglect or abuse are reported each year.

SOME DEFINITIONS

Neglect is the inability or failure to provide needed care. For example, the older adult, living alone, is unable to care for himself or herself, and no one is assuming responsibility for the care. Or, the caregiver fails to provide adequate food or clothing, leaves the client alone for long periods of time, or withholds needed medications or other necessary items.

Abuse is mistreating or causing harm. There are four types.

1. *Physical:* Producing physical injury and pain by hitting, kicking, biting, burning, pushing, punching, or by other means, including sexual abuse. Confining a person against his or her will is also considered physical abuse.
2. *Emotional:* Threatening or insulting language that produces fear in the person being abused. The types of behavior considered to be emotional abuse vary according to state laws.
3. *Financial or Material:* Stealing money, Social Security checks or other checks, valuables, or possessions or misusing the client's money or possessions.
4. *Abandonment:* Desertion of an elder by those responsible for their care and custody.

THE ABUSED

Research shows that those who are at the greatest risk of being abused are older adults who have physical or mental conditions. They may live with another person or may live alone. Isolation and loneliness are key factors in financial or material abuse. The older adult may seek friendship and companionship from a stranger and trusts the person, who later becomes the abuser.

THE ABUSERS

Most of the abuse of the older adult is usually committed by a family member—the spouse, adult daughter, or other family member or friend who is assuming responsibility as caregiver. The stress of months and years of continuous caregiving can take its toll on both older adult and caregiver. While it is difficult to understand why this happens, the following are some possible reasons:

- The caregiver takes out the frustration and stress of caregiving on the "victim," the person needing care.
- There is history of violence in the family as a way of handling problems.
- Alcohol or drug abuse by family members may cause physical or mental conditions leading to abuse.
- The abuser is "paying back" the older adult for being abused in the past.

Employed caregivers, unfortunately, account for about 4% of elder abuse. Reasons for abuse may be similar to that of the family caregiver. Frustration and the stress of caregiving are factors leading to elder abuse by the employed.

SIGNS OF NEGLECT AND ABUSE

The following are signs of possible client neglect or abuse.

Neglect

- Dirty hair, body, and clothing
- Urine or feces in the bed, on clothing, or in the client's area
- Weight loss, dehydration, or malnutrition
- Missing assistive devices (e.g., eyeglasses, hearing aids, dentures, canes, walkers)

Physical Abuse

- Bruises, cuts, sores, or burns on the skin
- Bruises, cuts, or burns in the genital area
- Unusual vaginal discharge
- Frequent "falls," fractures, sprains
- Patchy hair loss

Emotional Abuse

- Changes in behavior (e.g., withdrawn, cries a lot, is very quiet)
- Behaves in a fearful manner, especially when abuser is present
- Does not want to be left alone with caregiver or family members
- Is yelled at, threatened, humiliated, or belittled by caregiver

Material or Financial Abuse

- Mentions that money, checks, or valuables are being stolen
- Tells of being forced to sign over property or other financial documents
- Tells of being forced to sign checks or pay outrageous prices for services or products
- Unpaid utility bills
- Lack of food or medication
- Unanswered mail or unpaid bills

WHAT THE HOME CARE AIDE CAN DO

Your agency has rules to follow if you suspect that your client is being neglected or abused. It is very important to record your observations and report this information to your supervisor immediately. Record exactly what your client has told you. Do not assume. For example, record the following: "The client said, 'My granddaughter calls me nasty names—I just feel terrible when she does it. She tells me that if I don't turn over my Social Security check to her, she won't give me anything to eat.'" Do not record that the client's granddaughter is abusing the client emotionally and financially. This may or may not be correct. State the facts as clearly as possible so that your agency can investigate the situation further and take the most appropriate steps to protect your client. Elder abuse or neglect is a very serious matter. Many states have laws that require that signs of abuse or neglect be reported to the appropriate authorities. This will be done by your agency as necessary.

ALCOHOLISM

Alcoholism is a serious and often unrecognized problem in older adults. It is estimated that more than 2.5 million older Americans have some drinking problem. It is the number one addiction among older adults. Widowers 75 years of age and older have the highest rate of alcoholism in the country. As a person ages, problems with alcohol may develop. The body's tolerance for alcohol decreases with age, so what was considered moderate drinking in middle age may be problem drinking in old age. Furthermore, the effects of alcohol may be increased by the many medications taken by older adults.

A minority of older adults find comfort in excessive alcohol consumption due to life changes (loss of spouse or loved one), loneliness, boredom, lack of sleep, or physical pain. However, the majority of older alcoholics have had a history of long-term alcohol abuse, some starting in adolescence or young adulthood.

Now that the Baby Boomer generation is reaching older adulthood, it is believed that the number of older adults with alcohol and substance abuse problems will be many times greater than those seeking professional help. For many older adults, addiction to alcohol and other substances is a deeply shameful condition that hinders them from seeking the help they need.

Many problems occur as a result of alcohol abuse.
- Reduced self-control
- Anger, hostility, nastiness, and aggression
- Verbal, physical, and/or emotional abuse of family, friends, and caregivers
- Avoiding others
- Social isolation
- Falls
- Confusion, loss of memory, blackouts
- Malnutrition and weight loss

Alcoholism may be suspected when these problems occur. However, there often are other causes for these symptoms. Evidence of a drinking problem may be found in the home. Many empty alcohol containers and a large stock of alcoholic beverages may indicate a drinking problem. IF YOU SUSPECT THAT YOUR CLIENT HAS A PROBLEM WITH ALCOHOL, NOTIFY YOUR SUPERVISOR. IT IS NOT YOUR JOB TO DIAGNOSE OR TREAT ALCOHOLISM. YOU CANNOT MAKE SOMEONE STOP DRINKING. Specialized medical treatment is needed. If your client or family member asks you what to do about problem drinking, refer them to your supervisor. Home care agencies know of many community resources for assistance with this problem.

SUICIDE

Charlie's daughter, Angela, has been concerned that, when her father visits her second-floor apartment, he has difficulty walking up even a few steps without having to stop to catch his breath. Also, his appetite has been very poor since the death of his wife about 6 months earlier. When Angela finally got him to see a doctor for a physical examination, oxygen therapy was ordered to help him to breathe more easily. The respiratory therapist visits to instruct Charlie about exercises to help increase his lung capacity. Russ Larson has been assigned to give personal care.

At first, Charlie rarely talked while Russ gave him care. Russ tried various topics—sports, world news, local news, and so on—but Charlie was just not interested. Then, Russ remembered that many older adults like to reminisce about their past. "What was it like to live in this area in the 40s, Charlie?" Russ said. Then, Russ listened carefully. Over a period of several visits, he learned that Charlie, age 83, had been a coal miner for 45 years. He married his high school sweetheart, Lucy, and had two children. "Those were good years—we didn't have much money, but we managed. When I was forced to retire from the mines, I didn't know what to do to spend the time. I'd go to the local bar with my friends and drink too much. The smoking doesn't help, either. I know it's not good for my breathing but it's my only vice, that and the six-pack of beer each night with a few shots of whiskey! Don't tell Angela! Since Lucy died, I just don't have the 'get up and go' like I did. Lucy used to get me out of the house to go shopping or visit friends, but now she's gone," says Charlie, with tears in his eyes. "She was such a good cook. My cooking is pretty bad. I don't have much of an appetite. Eating alone is no fun. I'd rather drink my beer and munch on the pretzels."

Today, while Russ was helping him to shower, Charlie said, "You know, Russ, life's not worth living anymore. It takes all my strength just to breathe—I'm a mess. Sometimes I feel like taking one more breath and calling it quits. It's not worth living this way without my Lucy." Russ replies, "Oh, Charlie, don't feel that way. Things will get better; don't worry. You have a wonderful daughter who loves you." Charlie gets angry and says, "Russ, you just don't understand what it's like. Leave me alone!"

Russ is upset by what Charlie said and records this conversation in the care record. Then he calls Mrs. Quick, his supervisor. Mrs. Quick meets with Russ to discuss how he might have responded to Charlie in a more supportive way. She says that Charlie may be expressing behaviors that are symptoms of depression (see Chapter 21). Mrs. Quick thanked Russ for contacting her and scheduled a visit to talk to Charlie before calling his doctor.

Older adults have the highest suicide rate of any age group in the United States. Each year as many as 10,000 older adults will die from suicide. There are many theories about the reasons for suicide. These include changes in brain chemistry; emotional illness, particularly depression; and physical problems, such as heart disease, chronic pain, and loss of a body part or function. Other factors associated with suicide in older adults are as follows:

- A pattern of successive losses with little time in between for grieving and recovery
- Alcohol and/or drug dependence
- Retirement
- Social isolation and lack of a support system
- Prolonged illness

BOX 19-15 Warning Signs of Suicide in Older Adults

STATEMENTS SUCH AS

"I'm going to kill myself."
"I just want to end it all."
"My family would be better off without me."
"There's no point in going on."

PUTTING LIFE IN ORDER, SUCH AS

Giving valuables away
Making or changing a will
Finalizing funeral or burial plans

SELF-NEGLECT, SUCH AS

Not eating
Not drinking
Refusing to take medications or taking too
   much medicine
Hiding medications to take later in large
   quantities
Overeating, not sticking to prescribed diet

Unlike younger persons, older adults do not make suicide attempts or gestures. Elders who attempt suicide are almost always successful on the first attempt. Methods range from guns to drugs and other poisonous substances. Some people just quietly refuse to eat or drink or take their medications.

Home care aides should be alert for warning signs of suicide (Box 19-15). Pay attention to these signs, take them seriously, and report them to your supervisor immediately. There are many things that can be done to improve the quality of life for older adults. Depression can usually be treated with good results.

CHAPTER SUMMARY

- Aging begins at birth and becomes more noticeable in the later years.
- Each person ages at his or her own rate and in his or her own way.
- Only 4.1% of older adults live in institutions.
- Ageism is a form of discrimination practiced against older adults.
- The normal aging process causes many social, emotional, and physical changes. There are many adjustments to be made during this period, including
    Adjusting to retirement and reduced income
    Finding meaning in life
    Finding satisfaction within the family
    Facing the reality of death
    Accepting oneself as an aging person
    Adjusting to decreasing health and physical strength
- Aging causes many changes in the body systems. Home care aides help clients to cope with these changes.

- Older adults are at greater risk for injuries from falls and other accidents. Safety is an important factor to remember when caring for older adults.
- Older adults may not report the beginning signs of illness because they are not aware of the possible serious medical problems that may develop.
- Most older adults are cared for at home by an informal caregiver.
- Elder abuse and neglect are serious problems that must be reported to your supervisor.
- Alcoholism is often unrecognized in older adults.
- Older adults have the highest rate of suicide in the United States.
- It is important to practice infection control and medical asepsis to protect the older client.

STUDY QUESTIONS

1. Define aging, young old, middle old, and oldest old.
2. List three myths about older adults and the reality about each myth.
3. Discuss four adjustments older adults need to make for meaningful aging to occur.
4. List eight common physical changes experienced by older adults. Discuss what the home care aide can do to assist the client to cope with each change.
5. Define physical abuse, emotional abuse, financial abuse, and neglect. Give an example of each.
6. Why are older adults at risk for accidents? Describe three safety factors to be considered when caring for older adults.
7. List five guidelines to follow when caring for older adults.
8. Why is alcoholism often unrecognized in the older adult?
9. Describe two warning signs of suicide in the older adult.
10. List five signs of infection in older adults.

20

Caring for Mothers, Infants, and Children

OBJECTIVES

After you read this chapter, you will be able to:

1. Describe four normal changes that occur in the mother following the birth of the infant.
2. Discuss the responsibilities of the home care aide in caring for mothers of newborns.
3. Identify seven abnormal conditions of the mother that must be reported to the supervisor.
4. Discuss safety factors to be considered when caring for infants.
5. Identify five signs of infant illness that must be reported to the supervisor.
6. List four signs of stress in children.
7. Discuss the difference between discipline and punishment.
8. Identify five ways the home care aide can form positive relationships with children.
9. Recognize five common signs of child abuse.
10. Perform the procedures listed in this chapter.
11. List five ways the home care aide can prevent infection when caring for mothers, infants, and children.

KEY TERMS

Areola Colored, circular area surrounding the nipple

Bond Emotional attachment between infant and parents, especially the mother

Cesarean birth Surgical procedure in which the baby is delivered through an incision in the abdomen

Discipline System of rules that governs the way we act

Fontanel(s) Space covered by tough membranes between bones of the infant's skull (soft spot[s])

Full term Completion of 37 to 40 weeks of pregnancy

Gestation Period of time between conception and birth

Hemorrhoids Enlarged veins in the rectum or anus

Lochia Discharge from the vagina after childbirth

Postpartum period First 6 weeks after the birth of the baby

Prognosis Educated guess about the probable outcome of an illness

Respite care Short-term care provided so that main caregivers in the family can have a break from their responsibilities

Rooting reflex Normal reaction infants have that makes them begin to suck when their cheeks are stroked

Caring for mothers, their infants, and children is both demanding and satisfying for the home care aide because of the variety of clients being served. Many are well, such as the mother and her newborn infant. Other clients, such as children or teenagers, may be recovering from illnesses. Some clients, while not ill, have disabilities that require special care, such as cerebral palsy. The age of the client may range from a 2-day-old newborn to a mother who may be older than 40 years of age. A review of normal growth and development patterns (Chapter 4) will help you to understand each client's needs.

Being *flexible* and *patient* are two important abilities that will be frequently used during visits to these clients. Mothers are usually returning home with their newborns to an established household. This household may include the partner, other children, and relatives. Routines and patterns of behavior may be well established. Caring for your client means taking into consideration the family's existing routines; being flexible, when possible, so that you can reinforce these routines; and practicing patience when the schedule does not go as planned.

CARING FOR MOTHERS

Many years ago, the pregnant woman was admitted to the hospital to have her baby and returned home a week later. Seven or more days in the hospital was not unusual after a normal delivery. Gradually, the length of stay has been shortened. Today, healthy mothers and newborns return home from medical centers or birthing centers within 1 or 2 days. As a result, home care services are in great demand to provide care for mothers and their newborns during this important period following childbirth. The home care aide's responsibilities may include assisting the mother in her own physical care and helping her to care for the newborn. Other duties may include supervising an older child or children and performing housekeeping tasks, according to the care plan. Providing emotional support, encouragement, and practicing positive listening skills are also important aspects of client care.

THE POSTPARTUM PERIOD

The first 6 weeks following the birth of the baby is called the postpartum period. This is a time when the reproductive organs gradually return to their nonpregnant state. Just as hormones influenced the physical condition and emotions during pregnancy and childbirth, they continue to influence the changes that take place during the postpartum period. Important changes include the following:
- *Uterus:* Immediately after childbirth, the uterus (about 7 inches long and 2 lb in weight) contracts. This prevents excessive bleeding from taking place. The uterine muscles continue to contract, causing the uterus to become smaller as muscles tighten. By the end of the postpartum period, the uterus has reached a size similar to its nonpregnant state (about 3 inches long and 2 oz in weight).
- Lochia: Vaginal drainage after childbirth is dark red and may contain some clots of blood for 2 to 3 days. It has a fleshy odor. Gradually, the lochia changes in color as follows:
  - Pinkish-brownish: Days 4 to 10
  - Creamy: Days 11 to 21
  - The amount of lochia gradually decreases until no drainage is present and total healing has taken place.

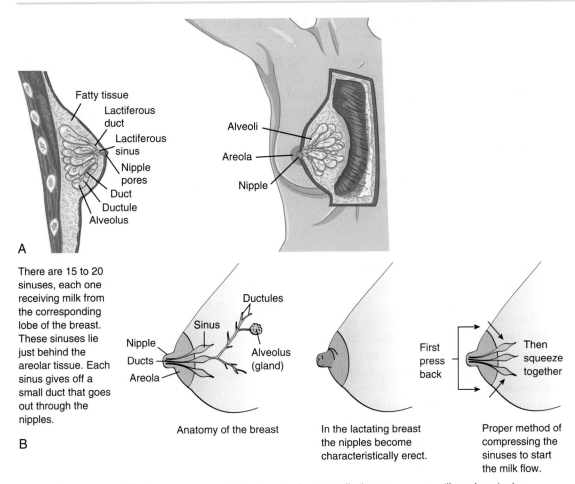

There are 15 to 20 sinuses, each one receiving milk from the corresponding lobe of the breast. These sinuses lie just behind the areolar tissue. Each sinus gives off a small duct that goes out through the nipples.

Fig 20-1 **A,** Milk ducts transport milk to the nipples. **B,** Milk ducts transport milk to the nipples.

- *Perineum:* Sometimes the perineum is torn during the birth process. The repair by the doctor is commonly called "stitches." Hemorrhoids may be visible in the anal area. These may have been present during pregnancy or appear after delivery because of the pressure experienced during labor and delivery.
- *Breasts:* At the third day after childbirth, the breasts become swollen and tender because of milk "coming in." Hormones are responsible for stimulating the glands in the breast to produce milk. Milk ducts transport the milk to openings in the nipple. Each nipple contains 15 to 20 openings (Figure 20-1). As the infant sucks the nipple, milk flow is stimulated. Usually, milk will continue to be produced as long as the infant sucks at the breast.
- *Weight Loss:* Losing the weight gained during pregnancy is usually an important goal that the mother wants to accomplish. About 18 to 20 lb are lost during the first 10 days after giving birth. Getting rid of the remaining weight takes a longer time. Eating a normal, nutritious diet, along with exercise, helps to take weight off slowly. Under normal conditions, it takes 6 to 8 weeks for the mother to return to her prepregnancy weight (provided there has been a weight gain of 20 to 30 lb).
- *Other Changes:* Some mothers have had a cesarean birth. This means that an abdominal incision has been made, and the baby has been delivered through the abdomen rather than through the vagina. In addition to the changes listed above, these mothers also have abdominal sutures or staples and a dressing covering the incision. Healing of the incision takes place gradually. See Chapter 22, p. 439, The Postoperative Client.

CARING FOR THE PHYSICAL NEEDS OF THE MOTHER

The mother will be instructed about caring for herself before she leaves the hospital, medical center, or birthing center. She is taught to notice signs that she should report immediately to the doctor, perform perineal care, observe the color of lochia, attend to daily hygiene needs, and care for her breasts. If the mother has had a cesarean birth, care of the incision and other precautions are also included. The amount of exercise, rest, and sleep should be discussed. Your role, as the home care aide, is to help the mother perform these activities according to the care plan.

Care of the mother includes the following six areas as discussed over the next few pages.

PROMOTE REST/SLEEP

The process of delivering an infant takes lots of energy. After the delivery, the mother is usually exhausted. Many changes have taken place, both physically and emotionally. The first-time mother needs to learn how to care for her infant and herself. The mother who has other children needs to learn how to schedule time for rest periods between caring for herself and the other children. Encourage the mother to rest or sleep when the infant is sleeping. If another child or children are at home, your role may be to supervise and care for them while the mother takes a much needed rest.

Friends and relatives of the family are usually eager to see the newborn and mother, but their visits should not interfere with the mother's need for rest and sleep. Be careful that these visits do not tire the mother.

OBSERVE LOCHIA

ORR

The color and amount of lochia are indications of the healing process within the uterus. Therefore, it is very important to observe and record this information on the care record. Check the pad each time it is changed. Always put on gloves before handling the pad. Observe the color (red, pinkish-brownish, creamy). Is it normal for the number of days following delivery? If not, report this to your supervisor. Notify your supervisor immediately if these conditions are present.

- Bright red discharge appears after pinkish-brownish or creamy lochia has been present
- Lochia has a foul odor
- Large number of blood clots
- More than one pad per hour is saturated for 2 to 3 hours in a row or two or more pads used within 1 hour
- Discharge makes client itch

The soiled pad should be removed by the mother and placed in a plastic or paper bag. It is your responsibility to put it in the trash.

ASSIST WITH PERSONAL HYGIENE

ORR

The mother gives herself perineal care after changing pads, after urinating, and after a bowel movement. If you are responsible for this procedure, follow the instructions given in Procedure 14-8 in Chapter 14. Observe the condition of the perineum for any signs of infection, such as swelling, redness, or unusual odor or drainage. Also, observe any change in the condition of hemorrhoids, if present. Box 20-1 lists additional information to be reported to your supervisor.

Remove and apply perineal pads from front to back so that any organisms from the anal area do not come in contact with the perineum or vagina. Clients with perineal

> **BOX 20-1**   **Changes in the Mother to Be Reported to Your Supervisor**
>
> - Change in color, odor, and amount of lochia
> - Bright red bleeding
> - Large number of clots
> - Two or more pads saturated within 1 hour
> - More than one pad per hour for 2 to 3 hours
> - Fever of more than 101° F (38.4° C) oral, chills, elevated pulse rate, poor appetite
> - Swelling, redness, unusual odor in perineum
> - Scant urination, painful urination
> - Redness, swelling, unusual odor around abdominal incision (cesarean birth)
> - Changes in behavior (e.g., withdrawn, uninterested in surroundings, suspicious, constant crying)
> - Pain, tenderness, or swelling in calf muscle of leg
> - Chest pain

sutures may find that a sitz bath helps to relieve the discomfort. It is ordered by the doctor. If the care plan indicates the need for this treatment, follow Procedure 18-11 in Chapter 18.

Assist your client to shower or take a sponge bath. Tub baths are usually not allowed until lochia is no longer present and the perineum is healed.

OBSERVE BLADDER AND BOWEL ELIMINATION

It is important that the urinary and digestive systems are working properly after childbirth. Make sure that the mother drinks plenty of fluids. This is particularly important if she is breast-feeding. Constipation may be a problem, especially for mothers who have hemorrhoids. A diet high in fiber and fluids with plenty of fruits and vegetables provides the bulk and fluid needed to soften the stool for easy elimination. Commercial stool softeners may be recommended by the doctor.

ENCOURAGE PROPER DIET

The period after the birth of an infant is a time when the mother is regaining energy and repairing body tissues. Therefore, eating well-balanced meals is very important. A diet that includes all the requirements of the MyPlate Food Guide is essential. Some mothers who are very anxious to lose the weight gained during pregnancy may go on a "crash diet." This is not the time to diet because the mother's body needs to repair itself after childbirth. Notify your supervisor if your client's eating habits show signs of improper food intake.

Nutrition for Breast-Feeding Mothers

The nutritional needs of breast-feeding mothers do not change very much from the needs during pregnancy. However, the need for fluids increases to produce enough milk for the baby. Mothers should be encouraged to drink fluids each time they nurse their babies. The doctor orders the type of diet needed and the amount of fluids. For teenage mothers, an additional serving from the dairy group is usually needed (see Chapter 10, p. 147, Figure 10-3).

The kinds of food and other substances that the mother takes into her body are secreted into her milk. This includes alcohol, any medication, caffeine, chocolate, garlic, and other seasonings. Nicotine, from cigarette smoke, is also transmitted in breast milk. Studies have shown that the positive effects of breast milk in providing infants with protection

---

BOX 20-2   Signs of Breast or Nipple Infection

- Painful breasts: red, hard, or hot to the touch
- Cracked skin around the nipples
- Open sores around the nipples
- Cracked nipples
- Bruised nipples
- Bleeding nipples
- Elevated oral temperature: 101° F (38.4° C) or higher
  REPORT ANY OF THESE SIGNS TO YOUR SUPERVISOR IMMEDIATELY.

---

from disease are decreased when the mother smokes. Mothers who are breast-feeding should avoid the use of alcohol, caffeine, and herbal preparations; stop smoking; and check with the doctor about using prescription and over-the-counter drugs.

If the mother notices a connection between a certain food she has eaten and the infant's reaction (fussiness, diarrhea, gas), she may consider avoiding that food. At a later time, the mother may want to try the food again because the food may not have been the real problem.

ASSIST WITH BREAST CARE

Before leaving the hospital, all mothers are taught how to care for their breasts. This care is very important for those who breast-feed and bottle-feed. Proper care of the breasts helps to prevent infection.

Clear water is used to clean the breasts, usually once a day. Soap is not used because it has a drying effect on the nipples. Breasts should be supported by wearing a well-fitting bra. It is important that the nipples and breasts are free of any signs of infection or injury (Box 20-2).

For breast-feeding mothers, absorbent breast pads help to keep the breasts dry between feedings, once the milk is flowing. To prevent growth of organisms that produce infection, the pads need to be changed frequently. After each feeding, the nipples should be exposed to the air to dry thoroughly. Frequent washing of the nipples tends to remove the natural protective body oils. Therefore, washing the breasts and nipples once a day is usually sufficient.

THE "BABY BLUES"

The body's hormones not only cause physical changes after childbirth but also influence the mother's emotions. It is not unusual for the mother to have periods of feeling sad, or bouts of crying, for no real reason. This is called the "baby blues." Coping with all the body changes and the new responsibilities of parenthood may cause these feelings. It is important to reassure the mother that the "blues" is not a sign of serious emotional problems but a normal reaction to the many changes in her life. Listen to what she has to say, and provide positive feedback. As the mother's body returns to the prepregnancy state and the family learns new skills in caring for the newborn, the periods of feeling blue decrease.

Some observations to report include:

- Poor bonding between mother and baby
- Neglecting the infant
- Mother's comments about harming the infant and/or other children
- Any dangerous situation

These could be signs of serious emotional problems.

OTHER SITUATIONS

Most babies are born healthy and at **full term**. Bringing baby home is a joyful time for the family. However, these two statements may not apply to all of your clients. You may experience the following situations:

The mother returns home without the newborn because

- The baby was born earlier than expected and remains in the hospital for expert care
- The baby died (before, during, or after birth)
- The baby is being placed for adoption
- The baby has severe physical or mental disorders
- The mother or father (or both) did not want this pregnancy, and the baby may not be welcomed
- The mother or father (or both) wanted one baby but, instead, had twins, triplets, or more

These situations may be ones where the usual joys of childbirth are replaced with sorrow, sadness, frustration, or even anger. Your supervisor will advise you about handling these difficult situations. PROVIDING EMOTIONAL SUPPORT TO THE MOTHER AND OTHER FAMILY MEMBERS IS AN IMPORTANT PART OF THE PLAN OF CARE. Listen to what your client is saying. Use your listening skills as discussed in Chapter 3.

CARING FOR INFANTS

It is true that newborn infants require a lot of care and attention. They are completely helpless and dependent on adults for their care. Even though they may sleep most of the time, it seems that their need for care is almost endless. Consider that the normal newborn's daily needs include the following:

- Changing diapers 6 to 12 times
- Feeding every 2 to 4 hours
- Burping
- Bathing
- Changing clothing after feeding and at bedtime
- Snuggling and loving
- Protecting from harm and injury

A newborn infant changes the whole family's routines. The mother is often exhausted after having the baby and needs short-term assistance with infant care. This help may be provided by the home care aide. Duties and responsibilities are listed on the care plan. Mother and aide establish a daily routine that can be followed when the aide is no longer in the home.

THE NORMAL INFANT

APPEARANCE

Length and Weight

The weight of the average newborn infant is about 7½ lb (3400 g). During the first few days of life, 10% of this weight may be lost, but it is quickly regained. At birth, babies are about 18 to 21 inches (46.4 to 54.4 cm) long.

Head: The head appears large, and it may be bruised or swollen from the trip through the birth canal. The neck is very weak and must be supported when the baby is lifted or carried (Box 20-3). There are two soft spots, known as **fontanels**, in the infant's skull. The large anterior fontanel, toward the front of the skull, is closed (becomes hard) by the end of the second year of life. The posterior fontanel, at the back of the skull, is closed after 2 months. These areas of soft bone allow for molding of the head during delivery and for brain growth after birth.

The baby may have lots of thick hair, no hair, or just a fuzzy growth on the scalp. There is no average when it comes to infant's hair. Newborns usually have cloudy blue

---

BOX 20-3 Holding an Infant

There are several methods for holding infants.
1. Lift baby by placing one hand under the head and neck for support (Figure 20-2, *A*). Place other hand under infant's body. Raise infant's head up to your shoulder. Continue to support head and neck (Figure 20-2, *B*).
2. Lift up baby, supporting head and neck in bend of your elbow. Trunk rests on forearm. This is called the "football hold." Infant may be held facing up (Figure 20-2, *C*) or facing down (Figure 20-2, *D*).
3. Lay baby on his or her tummy across your lap with head turned toward the side (Figure 20-2, *E*).

Fig 20-2 Holding an infant.

eyes and may have a whitish discharge from the eye for a few days. True eye color appears at around 6 weeks of age.

Skin

The newborn's skin may appear reddish. Newborns chill quickly, and their hands and feet become bluish and cold. This is normal. Keep the baby dressed and wrapped as appropriate to the climate and the culture. Infants with black skin tend to be very pale at birth, but the skin darkens as they get older. Fingernails and toenails grow quickly. They may be cut by the parent while the infant sleeps or with help when the child is awake.

Umbilical Cord

The stump of the umbilical cord remains in place for about 2 weeks before it dries up and falls off. It may be cleaned with an alcohol wipe according to the care plan. Keep the cord dry. It should not come in contact with stool, feces, or soiled diapers. Fold the diaper down so it does not touch the cord. Likewise, fold the shirt up so it will not touch the cord. Until the cord falls off, babies are given sponge baths. See Procedure 20-1, Bathing an Infant: Sponge Bath; Procedure 20-2, Bathing an Infant: Tub Bath; and Procedure 20-3, Dressing an Infant.

Genitalia

Female genitalia appear large, and there may be some mucus or blood-tinged drainage from the vagina. This is normal and comes from exposure to the mother's hormones before birth.

When the male infant's scrotum becomes cold, the testes may move up in the sac in an effort to be warm. Sometimes one testicle appears to be higher than another. This is normal. In about 3% of male infants, the testicles may be undescended. They may descend during the first 3 months of life. If not, the physician will recommend treatment at the proper age. If the infant has been circumcised, follow instructions for care of the area.

PROCEDURE 20-1   Bathing an Infant: Sponge Bath

Materials Needed

- Basin, bowl, or bathinette with water comfortably warm to the elbow
- Washcloth
- Towels (two)
- Hooded bath towel (optional) or receiving blanket
- Sterile cotton balls
- Rubbing alcohol or alcohol wipes for cleaning umbilical cord stump
- Vaseline or other dressing, if needed for circumcision (according to care plan)
- Mild soap
- Disposable gloves (for diaper change)
- Wastebasket
- Clean clothing
- Toilet paper or tissues

Procedure

1. Wash your hands.
2. Obtain materials listed above.
3. Place all materials in easy reach. Spread hooded towel or receiving blanket on flat surface (e.g., kitchen table, crib, changing table) near where you will bathe baby.
4. Place baby on receiving blanket or hooded towel next to basin of warm water. Always keep one hand on baby. **Never leave baby unattended. If you have forgotten something, take baby with you to get it.**
5. Begin with the head.
   a. Wet a cotton ball with plain water, and gently clean eye by wiping from inner corner to outer corner. Discard cotton ball. Use a new one to clean other eye.

Continued

PROCEDURE 20-1 | Bathing an Infant: Sponge Bath—cont'd

b. Wet washcloth and sponge face, ears, and folds in neck. Pat dry. Do not use cotton swabs to clean nostrils or ears. You may damage delicate tissues.

c. Pick up baby, holding in the football hold, facing upright. Hold head over basin. With free hand, wet washcloth and wring out over baby's scalp. Put a small amount of soap on the palm of your hand. Rub gently on to the infant's scalp (Figure 20-3). Rinse by wringing wet washcloth over head. Dry gently. Cover head with hooded towel or receiving blanket.

6. Remove shirt. Wash chest, upper abdomen, arms, and hands. Pat dry. Turn baby; wash and dry back.

7. Put on clean shirt.

8. Clean umbilical cord with alcohol (according to care plan).

9. Remove lower clothing. Wash legs and feet. Dry.

10. Put on gloves.

11. Remove diaper. Wipe any feces away with tissue, and clean perineal area. Discard diaper, or set aside for laundry. Wash perineum.

a. Girls: Wash from front to back. Rinse thoroughly. Gently pat dry.

b. Boys: Wash entire scrotum. Care for circumcision according to care plan.

12. Put on dry diaper.

13. Remove and discard gloves.

14. Finish dressing baby. Wrap in receiving blanket.

15. Place baby in a safe and comfortable position.

16. Clean materials, and return to proper location.

17. Record what you have done. Report any unusual observations to your supervisor.

Fig 20-3 Gently rub small amount of soap onto infant's scalp (Step 5c).

PROCEDURE 20-2 | Bathing an Infant: Tub Bath

Materials Needed

- Baby bathtub or bathinette with water comfortably warm to the elbow
- Washcloth
- Towel
- Hooded towel or receiving blanket
- Mild soap
- Clean clothing
- Toilet paper or tissues
- Disposable gloves (for diaper change)
- Wastebasket

Procedure

1. Wash your hands.

2. Obtain materials listed above.

3. Place all materials in easy reach. Spread hooded towel or receiving blanket on flat surface (e.g., kitchen table, crib, changing table) near where you will bathe baby.

4. Place baby on receiving blanket or hooded towel next to basin of warm water. Always keep one hand on baby. **Never leave baby unattended. If you have forgotten something, take baby with you to get it.**

5. Begin with the head.

a. Wet a cotton ball with plain water, and gently clean eye by wiping from inner corner to outer corner. Discard cotton ball. Use a new one to clean other eye.

b. Wet washcloth and sponge face, ears, and folds in neck. Pat dry. Do not use cotton swabs to clean nostrils or ears. You may damage delicate tissues.

c. Pick up baby, holding in the football hold, facing upright. Hold head over basin. With free hand, wet washcloth and wring out over baby's scalp. Put a small amount of soap on the palm of your hand. Rub gently onto the infant's scalp. Rinse by wringing wet washcloth over head (see Figure 20-3). Dry gently. Cover head with hooded towel or receiving blanket.

6. Lay baby back on flat surface.

PROCEDURE 20-2   Bathing an Infant: Tub Bath—cont'd

7. Remove shirt.
8. Put on gloves.
9. Remove diaper. Wipe any feces away with tissue and clean perineal area. Discard diaper or set aside for laundry.
10. Remove and discard gloves.
11. Hold infant.
    a. Place left hand under baby's shoulders. Your thumb should be over the baby's left shoulder. Your hand is holding the upper left arm.
    b. Use your right hand to support the baby's buttocks. Slide your hand under the thigh. Hold left thigh with your right hand (Figure 20-4).
12. Lower baby into water, feet first.
13. Wash front of infant's body, using your right hand.

14. Change your hold.
    a. Use right hand to support baby in a sitting forward position.
    b. Support and hold fingers around baby's upper arm and your hand under the infant's chin, as in lap position for burping (Figure 20-5).
15. Wash baby's back.
16. Return to previous position.
17. Wash genital area.
18. Lift baby out of water and onto towel.
19. Wrap in towel, covering head.
20. Pat baby dry.
21. Put on dry diaper.
22. Finish dressing baby. Wrap in receiving blanket.
23. Place baby in safe and comfortable position.
24. Clean materials, and return to proper location.
25. Record what you have done. Report any unusual observations to your supervisor.

Fig 20-4 Hold left thigh with right hand (Step 11b).

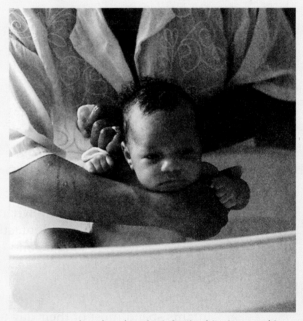

Fig 20-5 Place hand under infant's chin (Step 14b).

OUTPUT

Stools

For the first 3 or 4 days, the bowel movements are dark and tarry. These are called *meconium stools*. As the baby takes breast milk, the stools become pasty and mustard colored. Formula-fed infants have stools that are somewhat solid and brownish-yellow in color.

Voiding

Infants seem to urinate constantly. They have small bladders and void about every 2 hours. In fact, infants seem to eliminate at the same time they feed. Diaper changing

PROCEDURE 20-3 | Dressing an Infant

Materials Needed
- Shirt
- Sleeper
- Booties (optional)
- Receiving blanket
- Other garments according to climate

Procedure
1. Apply shirt.
   a. Stretch neck of shirt, and pull over baby's head (Figure 20-6).
   b. Place your hand inside sleeve, and reach up through sleeve to grasp baby's hand and pull through (Figure 20-7).
   c. Repeat on other side.
   d. Pull shirt down over chest. If umbilical stump is still present, fold bottom of shirt up to avoid rubbing.
2. Apply one-piece sleeper.
   a. Unfasten all snaps on sleeper.
   b. Lay garment on flat surface.
   c. Place baby on garment.
   d. Insert feet into lower portion of sleeper.
   e. Reach through sleeves (as for shirts) to put on upper portion of sleeper.
   f. Snap up garment.
3. Apply booties.
   a. Roll bootie over your hand, inside out.
   b. Grasp infant's toes, and turn bootie up and over foot with other hand.

Fig 20-6 Stretch neck of shirt and pull over baby's head (Step 1a).

Fig 20-7 Reach through sleeve to grasp baby's hand (Step 1b).

is a constant responsibility when caring for a newborn. Soiled and wet diapers can cause skin breakdown and infection. See Procedure 20-4, Changing a Diaper, and Box 20-4 for laundering diapers and other garments.

ACTIVITY

Sleeping
Infants spend most of their day sleeping. They wake up to be fed and changed. They are not yet able to turn over and to change positions. Pediatricians recommend that babies be placed on their backs when lying down, not on the abdomen or side. Placing healthy babies on their backs to sleep has been shown to reduce the risk of "crib deaths" or SIDS (sudden infant death syndrome). This sudden, unexplained death of an infant younger than 1 year of age strikes 2500 babies each year in the United States.

Do not use soft, fluffy covers, pillows, and blankets, because they can block the child's nose and mouth, causing suffocation. Not every baby will have a crib to sleep in. Some may sleep in a playpen, bureau drawer, laundry basket, and so on. Some safety rules for infants are in Box 20-5.

Crying
Infants cry because they are hungry, soiled, or uncomfortable. Crying is the only way that an infant can communicate its needs. Do not worry about spoiling a newborn baby.

PROCEDURE 20-4   Changing a Diaper

Materials Needed

- Clean diaper: Cloth or disposable
- Diaper pail or waste basket
- Diaper pins (for cloth diapers)
- Protective plastic pants (for use with cloth diapers)
- Baby wipes (optional)
- Washcloth (used for diaper changing only)
- Basin of warm water
- Soap
- Disposable gloves

Procedure

1. Wash your hands.
2. Obtain materials listed above.
3. Put on gloves.
4. Place baby on changing surface near materials. Be sure to protect baby from rolling off surface.
5. Open soiled diaper.
6. Wipe genital area with front of diaper (if dry). Wipe from front to back.
7. Roll diaper so that urine and feces are inside. Set aside for later disposal.
8. Wash the perineal area with soap and water, or use baby wipes. Rinse and dry thoroughly.
9. Give cord/circumcision care according to care plan.
10. Raise baby's legs. Place clean diaper in place. Cloth diapers may be folded to better fit baby.
    a. Girls: Extra fold in back
    b. Boys: Extra fold in front
11. Pin or fasten diaper in place. Keep diaper below umbilical stump. Be careful not to stick baby with diaper pin. Have your finger under the diaper when you insert pin.
12. Apply plastic pants (if cloth diaper is used).
13. Place baby in a safe and comfortable position.
14. Rinse (or dump) feces from diaper into toilet. Flush. Rinse cloth diaper with cold water, and place in diaper pail for laundering (see Box 20-4). Discard disposable diaper in garbage.
15. Remove and discard gloves.
16. Wash your hands.
17. Record what you have done. Report any unusual observations to your supervisor.

BOX 20-4   Baby Laundry

DIAPERS

Keep diapers separate from all other home laundry. Wash diapers daily or every other day.

1. Rinse dirty cloth diaper in cold water after changing baby.
2. Soak in hot water with $\frac{1}{2}$ cup bleach (4 oz, 120 mL) to 1 gallon (4 L) of water while waiting to be washed.
3. Wash in hot water using detergent and bleach according to label directions. Fabric softener is not recommended. It may irritate the infant's skin.
4. Rinse thoroughly in cold water. Dry.

OTHER BABY CLOTHING

1. If stained with formula or breast milk, rinse in cool water and pretreat with nonchlorine bleach or detergent according to label instructions.
2. Wash in warm water in a separate load.
3. Rinse thoroughly in warm water. Dry.

Crying means that the child needs attention. Never let an infant cry for a prolonged period of time. Change, feed, burp, gently rock, sing to the child—whatever is appropriate. Prompt and loving attention helps the infant **bond** with the primary caregiver. An occasional smile may be observed, but real social smiling occurs during the second month of life.

When a baby's cries cannot be quieted by feeding, burping, changing, loving, rocking, singing, or other usual means, there may be a problem. The baby may be ill.

BOX 20-5   Infant Safety

1. Do not place infants on
   - Water beds
   - Soft, stuffed bedding, such as fluffy quilts
   - Pillows of any type
2. Do not place infants on abdomen in crib or playpen. Position infants on their backs.
3. Keep sides on cribs raised at all times.
4. Hold baby on changing table. If changing table has a belt, use it to secure baby. A good rule to follow when changing or bathing an infant is: **"One hand on the baby at all times."**
5. Do not leave infants unattended on any surface (e.g., bed, sofa, table) where they could roll off.
6. Do not place anything in the infant's immediate surroundings that could cause choking or suffocation, such as stuffed toys, pillows, clothing, propped bottle, crib bumper pads, or plastic bags of any type.
7. Do not bathe infants in kitchen or bathroom sinks. Burns may be caused by hot water dripping on the baby. Older infants may touch hot faucets and be burned.
8. Do not bathe infants in the bathroom tub until they are able to sit up alone. Because of danger of drowning, NEVER EVER leave an infant alone in bath water.
9. Do not place anything around the infant's neck (necklace, cord, pacifier, or string).

BOX 20-6   Signs of Infant Illness

Notify supervisor if the newborn infant
- Has a rectal temperature of 100.4° F (38° C)
- Becomes unusually quiet or limp
- Develops skin rash or diaper rash
- Vomits (not the usual baby "spit up") or loses appetite
- Develops diarrhea
- May have fallen, been dropped, or bumped
- Shows sign of possible injury, such as swelling or bruising
- Develops a yellow coloring of the skin or whites of the eyes
- Cries constantly and is not comforted by any of the usual methods
  Call 9-1-1 or emergency medical services if baby has any trouble breathing or if baby stops breathing.

Notify your supervisor about a baby that cries constantly and cannot be comforted. Other signs of infant illness are listed in Box 20-6.

Eating

Newborn infants eat every 2 to 4 hours. They may be breast-fed or bottle-fed. Breast-feeding is started almost immediately after birth. The first milk is called *colostrum*. It is a clear fluid that contains special substances to protect the baby from infection. True milk "comes in" about 3 days after delivery. Infants who get enough milk will gain weight, appear satisfied after feeding, and produce at least six wet diapers and several fairly liquid, mustard-colored stools each day. For information on assisting a mother with breast-feeding, see Procedure 20-5.

The bottle-fed baby will drink a formula suggested by the pediatrician. Formula comes in a variety of forms: as a powder, which is added to sterile water; as a liquid, which is diluted with sterile water; and in disposable, single-feeding containers.

PROCEDURE 20-5   **Assisting Mother to Breast-Feed**

1. Wash your hands.
2. Have mother wash hands. Nipples are washed with plain water (if called for in care plan) in a circular motion from nipple outward (Figure 20-8).
3. Help the mother to a comfortable position.
   - In a chair with feet up on a stool
   - In bed with pillows behind back and head for support; adjust pillows until mother is comfortable
4. Change baby's diaper, if needed.
5. Bring baby to mother.
6. Have mother touch infant's cheek on side nearest the breast. This stimulates the **rooting reflex** and causes the newborn to turn toward the nipple.
7. Mother holds back breast tissue so the baby can "latch on" to the entire nipple and most of the **areola**. The infant's lips should cover this area. Baby's tongue should be under the nipple (Figure 20-9).
8. Baby should nurse for about 10 minutes on each breast. Sucking will be more vigorous on the first breast, and baby will empty that one faster. If baby falls asleep during feeding, mother can remove him or her from the breast. Awaken baby by washing face, changing diaper, or tapping feet. Put baby back to breast.

9. Remind mother how to remove baby from the breast: by inserting her finger into the corner of the baby's mouth to break the suction.
10. Mother burps the baby before moving baby to the other breast.
11. When feeding is over, change diaper.
12. Place baby on back.
13. Mother may massage a little milk/colostrum on nipples after feeding. Breasts may be air-dried. Nipples should be kept dry. Breast pads may be used as needed and changed when wet.
14. Assist mother with dressing, if necessary. A nursing bra may be worn.
15. Record what you have done. Report any unusual observations to your supervisor.

Fig 20-8 Cleanse breast in circular motion from nipple outward (Step 2).

Fig 20-9 Baby "latches on" to entire nipple and most of areola (Step 7).

PROCEDURE 20-6 | Preparing Formula From Powder

Materials Needed
- Clean bottles and nipples
- Powdered formula and scoop
- Funnel or measuring cup
- Long-handled spoon
- Water

Procedure
1. Wash your hands.
2. Obtain materials listed above.

3. Boil water and allow to cool (Figure 20-10, *A*).
4. Pour cooled water into bottle (Figure 20-10, *B*).
5. Add powdered formula using scoop, according to label instructions (Figure 20-10, *C*).
6. Shake well to mix (Figure 20-10, *D*).
7. Cap, seal, and store bottles in the refrigerator until needed.

Fig 20-10 **A,** Boil water and allow it to cool (Step 3). **B,** Pour cooled water into bottles (Step 4). **C,** Add proper amount of powder to bottles (Step 5). **D,** Shake well to mix (Step 6).

Formula preparation is discussed in Procedures 20-6, 20-7, and 20-8. Formula is given at room temperature. Cold formula may be warmed by placing the bottle in a container of warm water. **NEVER WARM A BOTTLE OF INFANT'S FORMULA IN A MICROWAVE.** The formula may become too hot and burn the infant's mouth. The newborn will take about 2 to 3 oz (60 to 90 mL) at each feeding. With growth, the infant will drink more formula at a feeding and will need to eat less often. Do not prop a bottle in a baby's mouth because the baby may suffocate. See Procedure 20-9, Assisting Mother to Bottle-Feed.

Infants swallow a lot of air when they are feeding. Babies need to be burped to help get rid of the air, or gas. Some babies are very "gassy"; others are not. For ways to burp a baby, see Box 20-7. Be sure to use a cloth or diaper to protect your clothing when

PROCEDURE 20-7 — Preparing Formula Using Concentrated Formula

Materials Needed
- Clean bottles and nipples
- Canned concentrated formula
- Water funnel or measuring cup

Procedure
1. Wash your hands.
2. Obtain materials listed above.
3. Boil water and allow to cool (Figure 20-11, A).

4. Wash can lid with hot soapy water. Rinse. Open can.
5. Pour appropriate amount of water into bottle (Figure 20-11, B).
6. Add appropriate amount of formula through funnel into bottle (Figure 20-11, C).
7. Shake well to mix (Figure 20-11, D).
8. Cap, seal, and store bottles in the refrigerator until needed.

Fig 20-11 **A,** Boil water and allow it to cool (Step 3). **B,** Pour cooled water into bottles (Step 5). **C,** Add proper amount of concentrate to bottles (Step 6). **D,** Shake well to mix (Step 7).

PROCEDURE 20-8 — Preparing Formula From Ready-to-Use Supply

Materials Needed
- Clean bottles and nipples
- Funnel or measuring cup

Procedure
1. Wash your hands.
2. Obtain materials listed above.

3. Wash can lid with hot soapy water. Rinse. Open can.
4. Pour formula into bottle using funnel.
5. Cap, seal, and store formula in refrigerator until needed.

PROCEDURE 20-9 | Assisting Mother to Bottle-Feed

Materials Needed
- Bottle of formula
- "Spit-up" cloth

Procedure
1. Wash your hands.
2. Obtain materials listed above.
3. Warm bottle (if cold) by placing in a pan of warm water until it is about room temperature.
4. Have mother wash her hands.
5. Help the mother to a comfortable position.
6. Change baby's diaper, if necessary.
7. Bring bottle and baby to mother.
8. Bottle should be tilted so that neck of the bottle and nipple are always covered with formula (Figure 20-12). Never prop the bottle.
9. Have mother burp the baby halfway during the feeding and at the end.
10. Feeding is discontinued when baby is no longer eating.
11. Change diaper.

Fig 20-12 Tilt bottle so that neck of bottle and nipple are covered with formula (Step 8).

12. Place baby on back.
13. Wash your hands.
14. Record what you have done and the amount of formula taken. Report any unusual observations to your supervisor.

BOX 20-7 | Burping an Infant

There are several methods for burping an infant.
1. Place diaper or "spit-up" pad over your shoulder. Hold the baby up to your shoulder. Remember to support head and neck. Gently pat or rub infant's back until burp is heard (Figure 20-13, *A*).
2. Sit infant in your lap. Support with hand under infant's chin. Hold "spit-up" pad in this hand. Rub or pat back until burp is heard (Figure 20-13, *B*).
3. Lay baby across your lap with head a little higher than rest of body. Place "spit-up" pad under infant's head. Rub or pat back until burp is heard (Figure 20-13, *C*).

A   B   C

Fig 20-13 Burping an infant.

burping a baby. Some infants will "spit up" part of the feeding along with the burp. This may happen when the baby has eaten too fast or too much. After feeding, place the infant on his or her back. There is no evidence that placing an infant on the back causes choking.

Some pediatricians will add one or two bottles of sterile water to the feeding routine if the baby seems thirsty.

THE PREMATURE INFANT

The premature infant is any baby born before 37 weeks' gestation. They have a low birth weight, and their organs are not fully developed. There is great variety in the condition and prognosis for each infant. With specialized care given in intensive care premature nurseries, some of these infants do well, but it takes them a while to "catch up" to full-term babies.

WORKING WITH CHILDREN

Home care aides will have some experiences with children throughout their careers. There may be children or grandchildren in the home of a client, or at some time you may be assigned to care for a sick or disabled child.

Whatever the case, you will need some understanding of children to work with them. Begin by reviewing the material on normal growth and development in Chapter 4. Additional information follows. Always consult with your supervisor regarding questions and concerns when working with children.

Lily Chiang has had a difficult pregnancy, and for the past 6 weeks, Betty Randolph visited three times a week to give her personal care. Lily's 4-year-old daughter, Elizabeth, likes to talk to Betty about what she's doing at the nursery school. "She's a very bright child, and I am preparing her for the time when I bring the twins home. Elizabeth can't wait to hold them and help me take care of them," said Lily.

Two weeks ago, Lily was admitted to the medical center because of high blood pressure and swelling in her hands and feet. Elizabeth was very upset! Visiting her mother in the hospital didn't make her feel better. Last week, Lily delivered identical twin boys. Because of their low birth weights, the boys didn't come home with Lily.

While Betty was helping Lily to shower, Lily started to cry. "I don't know how I'm going to take care of the babies and, at the same time, give Elizabeth the attention she needs. Since I came home, Elizabeth clings to me. I can't even go into the next room without her following me. I tell her, 'You're no baby; why are you doing this?' I'm worried, Betty, something must be wrong with her—she even wets her pants and she's been toilet trained for such a long time. If my husband knew about this, he would be very angry with her. I'm afraid I have three babies, not two, to care for. Elizabeth used to be so independent; what happened to her?"

Betty replied, "Elizabeth has a lot of adjusting to do—two new brothers who will come home soon. When you went to the hospital, perhaps she was afraid that you wouldn't come back. Now, she follows you to make sure you don't do it again! There are many changes in her life now, and she needs a lot of love from all of us as she adjusts to them. As she gets used to her new role as big sister, Elizabeth will give up her 'baby ways.' I've seen this happen over the many years I've worked in home care. But perhaps you'd like to talk to my supervisor about your concerns and ways you can help Elizabeth."

"Yes, Betty, but just talking to you makes me feel better," says Lily.

NEED FOR SERVICE

Home care agencies may provide care for children in many situations including the following:
- Respite care for developmentally disabled children
- When a parent requires supervision and assistance, for example, a teenage mother with a sick or disabled infant
- When ordered by the court in cases of real or suspected child abuse
- In group homes for children and mothers
- When a child is recovering from an illness
- When a parent is ill and unable to provide child care
- When a parent has died, and the family needs temporary assistance until satisfactory child care plans can be made

INDICATIONS OF STRESS IN CHILDREN

Reactions of families to illness are covered in Chapter 7. However, children react deeply to any threat to their security. When a primary caregiver (parents or other) is ill or absent from the home, children and adolescents may display signs of fear and anxiety. This is shown in a variety of behaviors, including the following:
- Nightmares and fear of going to bed or going to sleep
- Being afraid of the dark
- Crying and sobbing
- Hiding and withdrawing from others
- Aggressive acting out, may be directed toward the sick or disabled person or sibling (hitting, punching, swearing, cursing)
- Regression in toilet training, a return to soiling and wetting (this is more common in toddlers and preschoolers)
- Jealousy and anger toward a sick or disabled sibling
- Trying to be "perfect," to please everyone
- Playing one parent (or another important adult) against another
- Testing the limits of rules, regulations, and routines in a family/household

Often children are unable to verbally express their fears, anxieties, and other feelings. The younger the child, the more difficulty he or she will have in asking questions and in telling "how they are feeling." Teenagers may keep their feelings to themselves and be unable to verbally communicate their emotions. Anxiety and fear are often communicated through some of the behaviors listed above.

DISCIPLINE VERSUS PUNISHMENT

DISCIPLINE

When supervising or caring for children, you probably will have the opportunity to reinforce the rules of acceptable behavior in the home. This system of rules that governs the way we act is known as discipline. Discipline is a positive way of teaching responsible behavior. It sets limits and provides guidelines so that children can learn how to behave in an appropriate way when the parent or caregiver is not present. Discipline should be
- Known: The child knows the rules and what will happen if a rule is broken.
- Consistent: Each time a rule is broken, the consequence is the same.

Recognizing the child's attempts to comply with the rules of the household and praising these efforts help to encourage acceptable behavior.

Your role as the home care aide in disciplining the child is to
- Know the rules of acceptable behavior in each family situation.
- Ask the family member to clarify the rules, if you are unsure.
- Reinforce the existing rules.
- Be consistent when using discipline.
- Praise the child's efforts to comply with the rules.

ORR

Sometimes, you may be in a home where there are very few rules of discipline. Or, you are not able to follow the existing rules because they appear to be too harsh or too loose. In such cases, contact your supervisor for assistance in handling these situations. New rules may need to be set up. Do not set up new rules of discipline without the help of your supervisor.

PUNISHMENT

ORR

Punishment is a harsh response that occurs when the discipline or rule is broken. Punishing a child for failing to follow the rules of the household is not a responsibility of the home care aide. If a family member tells you to do so, explain that it is not your agency's policy to carry out punishment. Ask the family member to contact your supervisor if they have further questions. Record this information on the care record, and notify your supervisor concerning the situation.

ROLE OF THE HOME CARE AIDE

The goal is to provide a stable, secure, and safe atmosphere for the family. This is very important for sick children and for those who are experiencing stress because of illness of a family member. Recognizing each family member's needs (Chapter 4) and the family's reaction to illness (Chapter 7) can help the home care aide to provide personalized care to meet these needs and concerns. Although the home care aide's responsibilities will be different in each family situation, the following are usually included:
- Opening and maintaining lines of communication among all family members
- Providing a safe, secure, and stable environment
- Developing positive relationships with all family members
- Maintaining the existing rules of behavior
- Maintaining the daily routines as much as possible
- Being alert to situations that may add stress or that may result in harm to the family (Box 20-8)
- Reporting situations that threaten the well-being of the family
- Practicing standard (universal) precautions to prevent infection (Box 20-9)

BOX 20-8   **Changes or Events in the Home**

Report the following to your supervisor immediately.
- Violent behavior of family member (physical or verbal)
- Presence of firearms
- Frequent visits by "strangers"
- Suspected drug abuse
- Excessive drinking
- Electricity, heat, or water turned off resulting from failure to pay bills
- Severe shortage of food or clothing
- Failure of child (children) to go to school
- Illness of child
- Sudden departure of caregiver
- Unexpected return of family member

BOX 20-9   Infection Control

WHEN CARING FOR

New Mothers

- Wash hands before and after giving personal care.
- Wear gloves when handling breast or vaginal pads.
- Apply vaginal pad from front to back.
- Change breast pads when wet.
- Always use standard (universal) precautions.

Infants

- Wash hands before and after giving personal care.
- Wear gloves when changing diapers.
- Dispose of or launder soiled diapers properly.
- Keep area around baby's cord clean and dry.
- Always use standard (universal) precautions.

WHEN PREPARING FORMULA

- Wash hands before and after preparing formula.
- Follow each procedure carefully to avoid contamination of bottles, nipples, and/or formula.

GUIDELINES FOR CARING FOR CHILDREN IN THE HOME

The following guidelines should be used when interacting with children.

Communication
- Use listening skills: maintain eye contact, concentrate on what is being said.
- Watch for nonverbal communication cues: frown, lack of eye contact, smile, hands on hips.
- Answer questions simply, honestly, and clearly.
- Provide nonverbal communication: a hug, touch on shoulder or arm (according to acceptable custom and culture) to comfort child.
- Offer praise for something well done.
- Give encouragement when the child attempts to improve behavior, even though there is only slight progress.
- Use positive suggestions such as "Let's do …," rather than negative words; avoid "Don't do …" and "No."

Rest, Sleep, Play, and Exercise
- Reinforce the rituals of bedtime and naptime.
- Recognize the individual child's need for sleep; it varies with age.
- Supervise playtime; encourage active exercise, if allowed.
- Avoid taking sides when disagreement occurs.
- Avoid playing one child against another.
- Ignore tattling, if used to get attention.
- Treat each child as an individual of worth.
- Do not give more attention to one child and ignore others.

Mealtime
- Prepare foods that the child will eat.
- Do not force the child to eat.

CHILD ABUSE AND NEGLECT

The home should be a place where children can be secure, happy, and safe. However, each year, more than 5.5 million children are victims of physical, emotional, or sexual abuse or neglect, usually in their own homes according to the American Academy of Pediatrics. Most abusers are known and trusted by the child; this includes family members, relatives, friends of the family, and babysitters.

CAUSES OF ABUSE AND NEGLECT

The causes of child abuse and neglect are very complex. The following factors place some people at greater risk for becoming child abusers.
* Being raised by abusive parents
* Being a substance abuser (alcohol, drugs)

BOX 20-10   Child Abuse and Neglect

Type	Signs

PHYSICAL
 Injury not caused by an accident
	• Unexplained bodily injury
	    Bruises or welts
	    Burns
	    Cuts or sores
	 • Patterns on skin that suggest objects used
	    Belt
	    Cord
	    Cigarette
	    Iron
	 • Human bites

SEXUAL Using child for sex: this includes rape, incest, fondling genitals	• Bruises, bleeding, irritation of genitals, anus, mouth, or throat • Difficulty walking or sitting • Stained, torn, and bloody underwear • Discharge from vagina or penis • Painful urination
EMOTIONAL Behavior that hurts the child's feelings and damages sense of self-worth	*Abuser* • Constantly belittles or criticizes child • Uses insulting language • Ignores child; gives no love, support, or guidance • Screams at child • Uses threatening language
NEGLECT Failure to provide child with basic needs of food, clothing, shelter, medical care, or proper supervision	• Weight loss • Dirty clothes, hair, body • Urine and feces in bed • Child left unsupervised in home • Child wanders outside home unsupervised • Child always hungry • No food in refrigerator

- Being a single or adolescent parent
- Being isolated, with no one to rely on or to assist with child care
- Living in poverty

According to Prevent Child Abuse America, there are several types of child abuse: physical, sexual, emotional, and neglect. Box 20-10 defines each type of abuse and gives some signs. It is common for more than one type of abuse to occur. For example, physical and emotional abuse often occur together.

REPORTING CHILD ABUSE

ORR

The same rules apply to reporting child abuse as reporting elder abuse (Chapter 19). Follow your agency's policies and procedures when you suspect or observe child abuse in the client's home. Be sure to notify your supervisor immediately. Include the following information when reporting and recording on the care record.

- The name of the abused
- The date and time the abuse occurred, if known
- How the abuse occurred, if known
- When you discovered the abuse (date, time)
- What you
  Observed
  Heard
  Were told
- Where you
  Observed it
  Heard it
  Were told about it

YOUR AGENCY WILL TAKE STEPS TO PROTECT THE CHILD FROM FURTHER HARM. IT IS YOUR AGENCY'S RESPONSIBILITY TO NOTIFY THE APPROPRIATE LOCAL AND STATE AGENCIES.

CHAPTER SUMMARY

- Mothers experience many changes during the postpartum period.
- The home care aide's responsibilities in caring for new mothers include
  Promoting rest and sleep
  Observing lochia
  Assisting with personal hygiene
  Observing elimination
  Encouraging proper diet
  Assisting with breast care
- Home care aides should be aware of abnormal findings to report to the supervisor.
- Infants are completely dependent on adults for their basic human needs. Always protect the infant from harm and injury.

- Signs of infant illness include
  Elevated temperature
  Unusually quiet or limp
  Skin or diaper rash
  Vomiting and/or diarrhea
  Yellow coloring of skin or whites of eyes
  Constant crying
- Children react to stress in the home in a variety of ways. Often, this is expressed through nonverbal communication.
- Discipline is a system of rules that governs the way we act. It is not the responsibility of a home care aide to punish a child who does not follow the rules of the household.

CHAPTER SUMMARY—cont'd

- The home care aide forms a positive relationship with children by using the following guidelines:
  Use positive suggestions.
  Answer questions simply and honestly.
  Offer praise for something well done.
  Reinforce rituals of bedtime.
  Treat each child as an individual of worth.

- Child abuse is a serious problem that must be reported to your agency. Suspicions of abuse must also be reported.
- The home care aide practices medical asepsis and infection control when caring for mothers, infants, and children.

STUDY QUESTIONS

1. Describe the changes that occur in the new mother's
   a. Breasts
   b. Uterus
   c. Vaginal discharge
   d. Weight
   e. Emotions
2. List six responsibilities of the home care aide when caring for a new mother.
3. List seven abnormal conditions of the mother to be reported to your supervisor.
4. List five ways to keep infants safe in the home.
5. Which of the following conditions of the infant would you report to your supervisor?
   a. Blue hands and feet
   b. Whites of eyes are yellow
   c. Spits up with burping
   d. No hair on the head
   e. Limp body and very quiet
   f. Skin rash

6. What is the difference between discipline and punishment?
7. List four signs of stress in children.
8. You are caring for Grandma Fink, a 93-year-old woman who lives with her granddaughter and three great grandchildren. They are 2, 4, and 6 years old. List four guidelines to follow when forming a positive relationship with each of Mrs. Fink's great grandchildren.
9. List two signs of child abuse in the following categories:
   a. Physical
   b. Sexual
   c. Emotional
   d. Neglect
10. List two ways to prevent spread of infection when
    a. Changing an infant's diaper
    b. Preparing an infant's formula
    c. Assisting with breast-feeding

21

Caring for Clients With Mental Illness

OBJECTIVES

After you read this chapter, you will be able to:

1. List five characteristics of a well-adjusted individual.
2. Define mental illness, and list three effects on a person's life.
3. Define and describe three defense mechanisms.
4. Describe five abnormal behavior patterns that are common in mental illness.
5. Discuss the role of the home care aide in caring for clients with mental illness.
6. Discuss the problem of substance abuse and how it may affect the abuser and family members.
7. Discuss ways the home care aide can prevent infection in clients with mental illness.

KEY TERMS

Defense mechanisms Unconscious reactions that protect a person from real or perceived threats

Disoriented Unable to give correct information about time, place, or identity of persons or objects, or to perform activities correctly

Impulse(s) Sudden, uncontrollable urge(s)

Mental illness Brain disorder that affects thoughts, emotions, and behavior

Normal Conforming to a standard or following the rule

Psychotherapy Method of treating mental disorders, primarily by "talk therapy"

Often we say that a person with mental health is one who exhibits normal behavior. The dictionary defines normal as: "conforming to a standard," that is, according to the rule. So "normal" people are pretty much alike in the way they dress (warm clothing for cold weather, lighter clothing in hot or warm climates), in their behavior, and in their communication. Of course, there are great variations within the definitions of normal (Figure 21-1). Adolescents follow the "latest" dress code for their age group. Often adults may comment and complain about the bizarre appearance of some teenagers. Most are perfectly normal and are following the rule for their group.

Fig 21-1 Adolescents have their own "dress code."

BOX 21-1	Life Stresses	

Predictable	**Unpredictable**
• Parenthood	• Illness and/or disability
• Marriage	• Hospitalization
• Death/bereavement	• Loss of home/job
• Children leave home	• Accident
• Retirement	• Death of a child
• Education/testing	• Divorce
• Employment or job change	• Separation
• Responsibility for aging persons	• Natural disaster
	• Murder
	• Suicide

But there are other signs of mental health that are much broader than what we say and how we look. These have to do with a person's ability to cope with day-to-day living.

MENTAL HEALTH

WHAT IS MENTAL HEALTH?

What is mental health? Basically, it is a person's overall state of mind. It is how one feels emotionally rather than physically. People with good mental health are usually able to face and handle the stresses that come in everyday life (Box 21-1). They can control their thoughts, emotions, and behavior as they do their usual day-to-day routines.

Each person responds to life's stresses differently, however. Some people can handle more stress than others, and some situations will be more serious than others. Generally, however, people who are mentally healthy share certain characteristics. They seem to be content with their life situations and are well adjusted; they are "normal." Some characteristics of a well-adjusted person include the following:

- Giving and receiving love and affection
- Knowing one's needs and how to meet them
- Controlling one's desires and impulses until they can be appropriately fulfilled
- Learning from experience and letting go of the past
- Having a system of values and beliefs that guide behavior (a sense of right and wrong appropriate for the individual's culture)
- Viewing oneself and one's limitations realistically
- Expressing and controlling emotions in an appropriate way
- Being in contact with reality
- Adapting to changes in situations of daily life

FACTORS THAT INFLUENCE ONE'S MENTAL HEALTH

Many factors can also affect a person's overall mental health.
- Having a strong emotional support system of family and friends (and/or community agencies)—people who can be turned to when problems arise (Figure 21-2)
- Physical health, disabilities, or physical limitations
- Alcohol or drug use
- Family history of mental illness

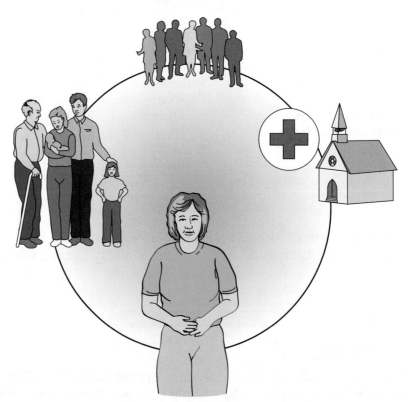

Fig 21-2 A strong support system is needed for mental health.

> **BOX 21-2**   **Warning Signs of Mental Illness**
>
> - Noticeable personality change
> - Confused behavior or thinking
> - Depression that will not go away
> - Excessive fear, anxiety, worry
> - Withdrawal from others
> - Thinking or talking about suicide
> - Violent thoughts or behavior
> - Severe change in eating and/or sleeping patterns
> - Increased use of drugs or alcohol
> - Inability to cope with daily life

MENTAL ILLNESS

WHAT IS MENTAL ILLNESS?

Mental illness can be defined as a brain disorder that affects thoughts, emotions, and behavior. People who are mentally ill have difficulties doing the normal activities of daily living (ADL). They may develop strange behaviors or lose touch with reality. A person who is mentally ill may show some of the following behaviors:

- Unable to carry on the normal daily activities: cannot sleep; does not get out of bed, dress, or prepare and eat meals
- Unable to function socially: withdraws from others; may have violent thoughts/behavior; may get into trouble with the law
- Becomes excessively worried, anxious, or fearful
- Loses touch with reality: may not recognize self or friends or family; does not know seasons, date; unable to tell correct time
- Relieves personal discomfort or troubles with increased use of drugs and/or alcohol
- Uses defense mechanisms all the time as a way to cope with stressful or unpleasant situations

Mental illness is considered an illness like any other and may be accompanied by physical symptoms as well. Clients may have headaches or other pains, anorexia, or a rapid heartbeat and may sweat heavily. Sometimes these physical symptoms mask (hide) the emotional symptoms, and this can make mental illness hard to diagnose. See Box 21-2 for warning signs of mental illness.

Mental illness can affect the quality of life of adults and children alike. Serious mental illness keeps people from leading normal lives. It can make it difficult to meet one's basic human needs, both physical and psychological. See Chapter 4 for information on understanding your client's needs.

Defense Mechanisms

Defense mechanisms are unconscious reactions that protect a person from real or perceived threats. They help block out some of the uncomfortable and threatening feelings. This makes the situation a little easier to cope with. We all use defense mechanisms from time to time to cope with pressures and stresses of everyday life. This is normal. However, many people with mental illness use defense mechanisms constantly to postpone dealing with unpleasant feelings and thoughts.

One defense mechanism that has been discussed throughout the text is denial, which can be a normal reaction to illness. When denial becomes a pattern of behavior, it can delay, postpone, or even block treatment and may lead to serious results, even death. Some other more common defense mechanisms include the following:

- *Rationalization:* Giving socially acceptable reasons to explain and justify one's unacceptable behavior, impulses, or feelings. For example, your friend says, "I had to buy that dress because it was such a great bargain," although she is 2 months behind in her rent.
- *Projection:* Assigning characteristics to others when they are actually his or her own, such as blaming others for problems rather than taking the responsibility. For example, a student fails a test and says, "That test wasn't fair. The instructor did not teach us the information that was in the test."
- *Repression:* Blocking out painful, unacceptable thoughts, experiences, and/or impulses from our conscious mind. For example, a person who was sexually abused as a child cannot remember the abuse as an adult.
- *Regression:* Returning to behavior, thoughts, or feelings used at an earlier stage of development. By acting less than one's age, the person can handle the stressful situation, or get others to take care of it. For example, an adult who is ill may show childlike behaviors and enjoy the care and attention given.

Remember that we all use defense mechanisms from time to time to help us cope with problems and painful situations. However, many mentally ill people use defense mechanisms all the time as a way of coping with life.

CAUSES OF MENTAL ILLNESS

Although the exact causes of mental illness are unknown, we do know that there are many factors that play a role in its development, including the following:
- Biochemical imbalances in the brain
- Heredity
- Chronic severe stress
- Isolation
- Alcohol and drug abuse
- Family and interpersonal relationships
- Accidents
- Untreated sexually transmitted disease
- Diseases that impair circulation to the brain

Other long-term diseases, such as Alzheimer's disease or AIDS, do affect behavior because they affect the physical structure of the brain. However, they are classified as physical illnesses.

MYTHS AND REALITIES

There are many myths and realities about mental illness, including the following:

Myths	Realities
Mentally ill persons never get well.	With treatment, people recover from mental illness. Others may develop a chronic illness that lasts for a lifetime.
Mentally ill persons are dangerous to themselves and others.	Mentally ill persons rarely harm themselves or others.
Mentally ill persons are unable to work.	If the mental illness is not severe, work is possible. In some cases, a change to a less stressful job is necessary.
Mentally ill persons can turn symptoms on and off at will.	Mentally ill persons cannot turn symptoms "on and off." Their behaviors are part of the illness and cannot be controlled.

MENTAL ILLNESS TREATMENT AND CARE

In the past, mentally ill persons were confined to large psychiatric hospitals that focused primarily on meeting the patient's physical needs. Private psychiatric hospitals offered care, but only the very wealthy could afford them. Today, treatment for mental disorders is available to anyone who seeks it. Besides hospitals, treatment is offered at community mental health centers, outpatient clinics, halfway houses, and group homes. At times, mentally ill persons may have behaviors that are harmful to themselves and/or others. Local "crisis centers" provide temporary help in such emergencies. The center provides a safe place for the person to stay while his or her condition is evaluated. The stay is short term, perhaps overnight. The next step in treatment may be the hospital or other community mental health facility as listed above.

There are several health care professionals who specialize in treating mental disorders (Box 21-3). The treatments for mental illness include psychotherapy (Figure 21-3), behavior therapy, and medication.

BOX 21-3   **Mental Health Practitioners**

1. Psychiatrist: A physician who specializes in diagnosing and treating chemical dependencies, emotional problems, and mental illnesses.
2. Psychologist: A person who holds a doctoral degree (PhD) and specializes in evaluating and treating emotional illnesses.
3. Psychiatric social worker: A person with a master's degree in social work (MSW) and specialized training in treating emotional illnesses.
4. Psychiatric nurse practitioner: A registered nurse with a master's degree in psychiatric nursing who specializes in treating emotional illnesses.

SOME PSYCHIATRIC THERAPIES

1. Psychotherapy: Method of treating mental disorders primarily by "talk therapy." This may be in an individual or a group therapy session.
2. Behavioral therapy: Attempts to solve emotional problems by changing behaviors. For example, the anxious person may learn special relaxation and breathing techniques to cope during periods of anxiety.
3. Drug therapy: Use of medications to relieve symptoms (anxiety and depression) that occur in mentally ill persons. Some drugs used to treat severe mental illness may affect behavior patterns. Drugs are used in combination with other psychotherapies.

Fig 21-3 Group therapy is one way that people can learn to cope with their conditions.

CARE OF THE MENTALLY ILL CLIENT

Clients who are mentally ill may be unable to control their thoughts, emotions, and behavior. Their strange behavior may make friends, relatives, and neighbors avoid them. Family members may be ashamed of their loved one's illness. This may leave your client feeling lonely and isolated from the world around them. Your caring attitude can go a long way to provide support and acceptance for the client and family. See Box 21-4 for guidelines when caring for the mentally ill client.

Your client may be recovering from a severe illness that required a stay in the hospital. Or, your client may suffer from a chronic illness that can be treated at home. Either way, you will have several responsibilities as part of the mental health care team.

- Follow the care plan as closely as possible to provide a consistent routine of daily activities.
- Assist the client to meet basic human needs, such as bathing, dressing, activity, nutrition, and toileting.
- Observe client's progress or condition, and report significant changes in appearance, behavior, and communication.
- Assist client to follow medication schedule, if part of the care plan.

ABNORMAL BEHAVIOR PATTERNS

Because mental illness affects the way a person thinks and behaves, your client may act quite strangely. However, the behavior is a sign of the illness and cannot be controlled. The following describes some of the more common abnormal behavior patterns that mentally ill clients may have.

BOX 21-4   Guidelines When Caring for the Mentally Ill Client

- Inform client about time of day, day of week, month, place, or person, as needed.
- Provide a safe, secure environment.
- Present reality; do not go along with client's delusions or hallucinations.
- Accept the person, not the behavior.
- Promote behavior appropriate to age and condition.
- Recognize substance abuse as a disease and not a lack of willpower or moral failure.
- Record and report changes to your supervisor.
  Increase or decrease in abnormal behavior
  Increase or decrease in performing ADL
  Ease or difficulty in making decisions
  Increase or decrease in ability to communicate
  Change in personal appearance and grooming
  Any signs of infection
- Recognize that mental illness affects everyone close to the client; listen carefully to them—offer support.
- Assist with management of the home.
- Avoid giving advice.
- Understand your feelings and how they affect your actions.
- Have an even disposition and a positive outlook.
- Follow guidelines for listening, communicating (Chapter 3), and accurate recording (Chapter 6).

Confusion

A mental state in which the client is **disoriented** about time, place, or person and may be unable to have an orderly train of thought.

Behaviors

- Time: Cannot give correct information about
  Time of day
  Day of the week
  Month
  Season, including special holidays (e.g., Thanksgiving day, Kwanza)
  Year
- Place: Cannot give correct information about
  Where they are (e.g., at home, at the doctor's office, at a relative's home)
  Where (e.g., town, city, state) or with whom they live
  Location of bathroom, bedroom, or other parts of the home
- Person: Cannot recognize
  Family members, friends, or significant others
  Cannot remember recent events
  May mistake one person for another; may confuse person's name
- Objects and activities
  Forgets names of commonly used objects (e.g., cup, plate, spoon)
  Uses incorrect name for commonly used objects
  Acts bewildered
  Wanders about the home; appears lost, especially in the evening or night
  Cannot remember how to perform ADL
  Cannot clearly think through a situation or problem

Your Role

- Communicate correct information about time, place, person, object, or activity.
- Provide clues in surroundings that will help to inform the client about time of day (clock), month, and season (calendar) (Figure 21-4).
- Explain events or procedures in simple, short sentences.
- Keep a set routine; avoid making changes.
- Encourage client to perform familiar, simple tasks and assist as needed (e.g., washing hands and face, brushing teeth).

Fig 21-4 Clocks and calendars help to inform the client about time, month, and season.

BOX 21-5 **Providing a Safe, Secure Environment for Clients**

- Place the following items out of sight and reach.
  Matches and lighters
  Sharp objects (e.g., scissors, knives, razors, breakable objects)
  Personal care items (e.g., nail polish remover, perfumes, after-shave lotion, mouthwash)
  Car and house keys
- Store the following in locked cabinets.
  Prescription and over-the-counter medications
  Laundry and household cleaning agents
  Gardening materials and fertilizers
- Keep the environment as calm as possible.
  Reduce noise
  Turn down television and radio
  Play soft, soothing music
  Work quietly
  Speak in a calm manner
  Reduce clutter
- Be sure guns, rifles, and so on, are stored in locked cabinets.
- Put bells on doors to signal that the client is trying to leave the area.
- Place a protective gate at entrances to steps and stairs.
- Follow guidelines listed in Chapter 8.

ORR

- Provide a safe, secure environment; remove potentially harmful objects (Box 21-5).
- Record and report any changes in behavior to your supervisor.
  More information on caring for the confused client is found in Chapter 22.

Anxiety and Panic

Anxiety is an uneasy, fearful feeling about real or imagined threats to a person's well-being. Panic is a sudden feeling of extreme fear. A person may be "frozen with fear" (paralyzed) or become completely hysterical. Panic attacks come without warning and may last for minutes to hours. Their frequency varies, depending on the severity of the condition.

Behaviors (Vary According to the Severity of the Condition)

- Worries constantly about everything, even small things, with no real reason
- Speaks abnormally and may be difficult to understand
- Speaks of impending doom or danger
- Difficulty sleeping; fatigued
- Paces back and forth, very restless
- Neglects personal grooming and hygiene, or is overly concerned about cleanliness or appearance
- Frequently complains of physical discomfort
- Poor appetite
- Difficulty concentrating on tasks or activities

Your Role

- Encourage routine periods of rest and activity as appropriate.
- Encourage client to do ADL, and assist when necessary.
- Be a good listener.
- Provide a safe, secure environment (see Box 21-5).
- Speak in a calm tone of voice, and use short sentences.
- Avoid discussions about client's physical complaints.
- Offer foods that are easy to eat (sandwiches, finger foods) when client is pacing.

- Encourage client to make decisions, but limit choices to make it easier.
- Offer reassurance using nonverbal behavior (sit quietly with client, touch shoulder or hand, if appropriate and culturally acceptable).
- Stay with client during panic attacks.
- Explain procedures you will perform, as needed.
- Perform tasks according to client's care plan.
- Record and report any changes in behavior to your supervisor.

Delusions and Hallucinations

Delusions are false beliefs that a mentally ill person believes to be true. For example, the client may believe that the world is going to blow up at any minute. *Hallucinations* are sensory perceptions (things seen, heard, felt, smelled) that are not actually there. For example, the client may "see," "hear," or "feel" bugs that are not there.

Alma, an employee of the A and B Community Home Care Agency, has been visiting Mrs. Morgan, an 80-year-old widow, twice a week to help with personal care. Mrs. Morgan lives with her son, Fred, an elementary school teacher.

Alma doesn't see Fred often. Usually, he's at school when she visits, but today he comes to the door to let her into the home. She's surprised to see him. He looks upset. "Hello, Fred, haven't seen you for quite a while," says Alma. He says nothing, but motions her to sit down in the hall chair. Then, he whispers, "I can't work today because the Evil One told me that I'm a very bad person and shouldn't be near any children. So, I called the school and told them I couldn't teach anymore." Alma says, "Tell me about the Evil One." Fred replies, "Come, see him. He's in the kitchen." They walk to the kitchen, but no one is there. "I don't see anyone, Fred," says Alma, but Fred insists that the Evil One is there. He keeps repeating, "See him? See him?" and becomes very upset. Alma calmly asks Fred to come with her and sit in the living room. "I need to call my supervisor about this."

Mrs. Morgan tells Alma, "He's had this problem before—I don't think that he's been taking his medicine."

Alma calls her supervisor to report what has happened and what Mrs. Morgan has said. Later, her supervisor visits the home to assess the situation.

Behaviors
- Is suspicious of others and thinks they want to do him or her harm
- Looks around a lot to see who is watching
- Believes that he or she is a king, queen, president of the United States, or other well-known person
- Mumbles to self
- Talks about unseen objects, such as animals or space ships
- Smiles, nods, and appears to be communicating to an unseen person

Your Role
- Provide a safe, secure environment (see Box 21-5).
- Leave a light on in the bedroom at night if added feeling of security is desired.
- Do not go along with the client's delusions or hallucinations or pretend to see, hear, or feel what the client is seeing, hearing, or feeling.
- Do not argue with the client about what he or she claims to see, hear, or feel.
- Give the client correct information regarding time, place, or person, as needed.
- Perform tasks according to client's care plan.
- Describe the delusions or hallucinations in the care record, and report any changes in behavior to your supervisor.

Depression

Clients with this disorder, sometimes called *clinical depression,* have feelings of extreme sadness and hopelessness. Depression can also be accompanied by symptoms of physical illness, such as headaches and stomach upset. It is an illness that, for most people, can be treated effectively.

Behaviors

- Feels very unhappy, sad most of the time
- Cries a lot
- Shows no interest in almost all ordinary activities (e.g., job, family, hobbies, relatives, sex)
- May overeat or show no interest in food at all
- May be constipated
- Gains or loses large amounts of weight rapidly
- Experiences changes in sleep patterns, such as cannot sleep or sleeps all the time
- Has no energy, feels exhausted all the time
- Feels worthless, angry, and irritable
- Cannot concentrate, remember things, or make decisions
- Speaks about committing suicide or actually attempts suicide

Your Role

- Encourage routine periods of rest and activity, as appropriate.
- Encourage the client to perform ADL and assist when necessary.
- Be a good listener; do not try to "cheer up" the client.
- Provide a safe, secure environment (see Box 21-5).
- Give information, explanations, and directions to the client in terms that he or she can understand.
- Follow the care plan to be sure that basic needs for food, fluids, and toileting are met.
- Assist the client to take medications, as required.
- 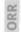 Be alert for signs of suicide (see Box 19-15), and report these immediately to your supervisor.
- Record and report any changes in behavior or problems with medications to your supervisor.

Aggression

This is the use of violent or abusive behavior to cope with anxiety.

Behaviors

- Is irritable and angry
- Paces back and forth, sometimes with fists clenched
- Appears hostile and agitated
- Expresses rage and threats of physical abuse
- Punches, kicks, or throws things in the environment
- Is suspicious of others
- May have delusions or hallucinations

Your Role

- Assist the client to take medications as required.
- Observe the client for any signs of increasing aggression, and report them to your supervisor immediately.
- Encourage the client to perform ADL (assist as directed in care plan, if your safety is not at risk).
- Do not try to give physical comfort, such as touching or hugging. The client may try to hit or kick you.
- Be a good listener; this may be calming to an angry client.
- Provide a calm, safe, secure environment (see Box 21-5).

- Speak in a calm tone of voice, and make eye contact.
- Remain calm, and try to control your facial expressions; do not show anger or fear.
- Do not wake the client by touching. The client may lash out; softly call out to the person by name.
- Do not turn your back on an aggressive client or put yourself in a position where the client could hurt you. Do not let the client get between you and an exit.
- If the client is threatening you or does hit you, leave the home and call for help.
- Contact your supervisor immediately if you have been forced to leave the client alone.

Suspicion (Paranoia)

Thoughts of persecution (that others are "out to get" him or her), secretiveness, and inability to maintain contact with reality are common behaviors with this disorder.

Behaviors

- Secretive; fearful of others
- Cannot maintain contact with reality
- Worries that someone or something is listening in on personal thoughts and watching his or her every move
- Believes that someone or something is trying to control him or her, such as the "government" through the television or telephone or by computer
- Cannot relate to others
- Refuses to eat or drink, for fear that the food has been poisoned
- May become aggressive under stressful situations
- Cannot perform personal care or ADL

Your Role

- Do not ask the client to make decisions; this may cause confusion and increase stress levels.
- Serve foods and fluids in packages that have not been opened or that could not be easily tampered with, such as
  Hard-cooked eggs that do not have cracked shells
  Juice, water, or soda in individual cans, bottles, or other single-serving containers
  Fruit cups, puddings, and yogurts in single-serving containers
  Meals that are packaged or ready to eat (client may be suspicious of the use of a microwave oven for food preparation and may believe the microwave can control or hear client's thoughts)
- Do not go along with the client's delusions or hallucinations.
- Do not argue with the client about what he or she claims to see, hear, or feel; gently change topics.
- Assist the client to take medications, as required.
- Record and report any changes in behavior or problems with medications to your supervisor immediately.

Overactivity (Mania)

This is a mood disorder in which the client may show extreme happiness or excitement accompanied by restlessness and overactivity.

Behaviors

- Extreme feelings of confidence or power, the ability to do anything, even fly
- Irritable and restless; unable to sit still and relax
- Speaks quickly in urgent tones, jumps from one topic to the next, and may be difficult to understand
- Is too busy or preoccupied with thoughts to eat, drink, or perform ADL
- May wear bright clothes, lots of makeup and jewelry

Your Role
- Provide a safe, secure environment (see Box 21-5).
- Reduce noise levels, and play soft, calming music.
- Offer foods that are easy to eat (sandwiches, finger foods) when client is pacing.
- Encourage routine periods for rest, activity, toileting, and grooming.
- Do not argue with client; this will increase irritability and may cause aggression.
- Assist the client to take medications, as required.
- Record and report any changes in behavior, especially an increase in aggression or signs of depression, to your supervisor immediately.

Sexual Acting Out

The client has an inability to control sexual desires and acts out sexual urges and fantasies to relieve the anxiety.

Behaviors
- Removes clothing, and insists on being nude in inappropriate settings
- Frequently fondles, touches self
- Masturbates frequently regardless of setting
- Makes frequent sexually suggestive remarks or is sexually aggressive to others

Your Role
- Try to keep client dressed; use layers of loose, comfortable clothing appropriate to the climate.
- Keep a robe nearby for client to use in case client undresses.
- Redress the client as often as necessary.
- Try to occupy the client with activities (e.g., hobbies, writing, video games) that will keep his or her hands busy and help to release the stress and anxiety.
- Provide privacy for the client who needs to masturbate.
- Observe the client for signs of injury and infection that may occur with continuous masturbation. These include
  Vaginal drainage
  Red and irritated perineal area
  Foul odor from perineal area
  Drainage from penis
  Red and irritated skin on penis
- Record and report to your supervisor any sexual advances made by your client.
- Try not to judge the client; remember that this is part of your client's mental illness.
- Maintain a professional attitude, because the client may mistake your friendliness for acceptance of sexual advances.
- Do not accept or ignore suggestive remarks or sexual advances; tell your client in a firm tone of voice that the behavior is not acceptable and that you do not want to be spoken to or touched in that manner. Do not scold or yell.

SUBSTANCE ABUSE

Substance abuse is the misuse of chemical substances (usually alcohol or drugs) that leads to an emotional and/or physical dependence. It is a serious problem that affects millions of Americans and their families. Unfortunately, health care workers may become substance abusers, because they often have easy access to their clients' prescription medications.

Substance abuse can alter a person's mood, consciousness, and thinking. It can cause physical changes that lead to illness, and even death. As a person becomes addicted, the body gets used to having the drugs or alcohol in the system. Then the body begins to need more and more of the substance to get the desired feeling. Soon the body becomes dependent on the substance to function. If the person tries to stop taking the substance, severe physical and mental distress will occur. Drug and alcohol addictions are very hard to overcome, but, with proper treatment, it can be done.

COMMONLY ABUSED SUBSTANCES

The most commonly abused substances are alcohol and drugs.

Alcohol

Alcohol is a legal drug that can be obtained by anyone of legal drinking age, according to state law. Alcohol abuse is a disease of about 10% of women and 30% of men in the United States. Of the over 14 million (1 in 13 adults) who have problems with drinking alcohol, about 8 million are alcoholics. Alcoholism is not only a problem of older adults; it is a serious problem for adolescents, even young children. Alcohol abuse can lead to other substance abuse, too. Reasons for alcohol abuse include to help one sleep, to reduce anxiety, to lift one's spirits, or to make socializing easier. See Chapter 19 for some of the signs and problems caused by alcohol abuse in older adults.

Prescription Medications

Medications are prescribed by the doctor to treat illness and the client's symptoms, such as pain, sleeplessness, or anxiety. Some clients continue to use these medications after the initial prescription has expired. This may be done by changing doctors frequently to get new prescriptions, changing the drug store where the prescription is filled, or obtaining prescription drugs illegally.

Illicit (Illegal) Drugs

There are many illegal drugs used in the United States. The illicit drug market tries to increase its financial profits by coming up with new drugs with exciting names to catch the interest of drug users and "hook" their victims.

SIGNS OF SUBSTANCE ABUSE

The following is a partial list of signs of substance abuse:

Physical

- Changes in appearance, such as weight loss or gain, lack of attention to personal hygiene and clean clothing
- Changes in eating habits or sleep patterns
- Wears sunglasses to hide dilated or constricted pupils of eyes
- Wears long-sleeved shirts to hide needle marks on arms
- Slurred speech; difficulty with balance
- Unusual odor to breath; unusual smell on clothing

Work or School Habits

- Difficulty concentrating on tasks to be done
- Changes in work habits, such as being late for work, calling in sick frequently, cannot perform work efficiently
- Changes in school habits, such as poor grades, lack of interest in school activities, frequently late or absent
- Disinterested in activities at work or school

Other
- Changes in personality or mood swings
- Not interested in family activities, events
- Sudden appearance of "new" friends
- Presence of large amounts of pills, alcohol, beer (may be out of sight)
- Presence of supplies such as syringes, needles, pipes, or other drug supplies

YOUR ROLE

WHEN YOU SUSPECT SUBSTANCE ABUSE

ORR If you suspect that a coworker, client, or client's family member may be a substance abuser, notify your supervisor. Do not discuss your suspicions with anyone other than your supervisor. This information should be kept confidential. Be sure to report accurately what you observed or heard that led you to suspect substance abuse. This is a serious responsibility, and accurate reporting is necessary so that further investigation can be made. Do not attempt to give advice to the suspected substance abuser. Your agency has resources available to handle the situation and help the abuser with this serious problem.

WHEN YOU SUSPECT A SUBSTANCE ABUSER IS IN YOUR CLIENT'S HOME

ORR Some substance abusers may have bizarre behavior and can cause harm to themselves and others. Safety for yourself and your client should be your first concern. If you believe that you are in immediate physical danger, get out of the home and notify your supervisor. He or she will advise you concerning the next steps to take. If you or your client are not in any present danger, follow the directions above for reporting possible substance abuse.

WHEN YOUR CLIENT IS PRESENTLY BEING TREATED FOR SUBSTANCE ABUSE

ORR Be observant for any signs that your client is returning to previous habits of abuse. Record and report your observations to your supervisor immediately so that additional help can be provided to assist your client to recover. Follow the care plan carefully. Your role includes providing support and encouragement to your client and family members during this difficult time. Recovering from substance abuse is hard work. It is important that your behavior and communication show a positive concern during this period of recovery.

INFECTION CONTROL

CLIENTS WITH MENTAL ILLNESS MAY BE UNABLE TO PERFORM THE ADL THAT WE "JUST DO" AND TAKE FOR GRANTED. THINGS LIKE GETTING OUT OF BED, PERSONAL HYGIENE, AND MEAL PREPARATION MAY BE JUST "TOO MUCH" FOR THEM. BECAUSE OF INACTIVITY, POOR HYGIENE, AND POOR NUTRITION, THEY MAY BE AT RISK FOR INFECTION. Others may be unable to communicate the symptoms of physical illness or infection. A client who is a substance abuser may concentrate only on getting the next "fix" of the substance; health, nutrition, and hydration are not important to the abuser.

ORR When caring for those with mental illness, you need to be alert for symptoms of infection. Observe the client's behavior, appearance, and conversation for any signs of illness. Is the client drinking large quantities of fluids? Voiding frequently? Having diarrhea? See Box 11-2, p. 171, to review signs and symptoms of infection. Notify your supervisor of any abnormal observations.

Remember to practice standard (universal) precautions at all times to protect yourself and your client.

CHAPTER SUMMARY

- Persons with good mental health are usually able to cope with and adjust to the predictable and unpredictable stresses of living in an acceptable way. Well-adjusted individuals are able to
    - Give and accept love and affection
    - Adapt and adjust to change
    - Deal with problems in a realistic way
    - Accept responsibility for their own decisions, feelings, and actions
    - Know their needs and how to meet them
- Mental illness is defined as a brain disorder that affects thoughts, emotions, and behavior.
- Mental illness is an illness like any other and may be accompanied by physical symptoms.
- Serious mental illness keeps people from leading normal lives.
- Defense mechanisms are behaviors that help people cope with anxiety. They protect the person from real or perceived threats. Examples of defense mechanisms are denial, rationalization, regression, repression, and projection.
- Many people with mental illness use defense mechanisms constantly to postpone dealing with unpleasant feelings and thoughts.

- Abnormal behavior patterns seen in persons who are mentally ill include confusion, anxiety and panic, delusions and hallucinations, depression, aggression, suspicion (paranoia), overactivity (mania), and sexual acting out.
- The home care aide's role includes
    - Following the care plan carefully
    - Providing daily assistance to help the client meet basic human needs
    - Observing the client's progress, and reporting significant changes in appearance, behavior, and communication
    - Assisting the client to follow the medication schedule
    - Providing emotional support and acceptance for the client and family
- Substance abuse is a serious problem that affects millions of Americans and their families. If you suspect that a coworker, client, or client's family member may be a substance abuser, notify your supervisor.
- Clients with mental illness should be observed for signs of infection. Always practice standard (universal) precautions even if the client has no sign of physical illness.

STUDY QUESTIONS

1. List five characteristics of a well-adjusted individual.
2. Define mental illness. List three ways that it affects a person's life.
3. List three defense mechanisms, and define each.
4. Describe five abnormal behavior patterns that are common in mental illness.
5. List four responsibilities of the home care aide when caring for clients with mental illness.
6. What is meant by substance abuse? What is your first responsibility when you suspect that there is a substance abuser in the home?
7. Your client's diagnosis is clinical depression. However, you notice that she is coughing, breathing rapidly, and making "wheezing sounds" when she breathes. What would you do?

22

Caring for Clients With Illnesses Requiring Home Care

OBJECTIVES

After you read this chapter, you will be able to:

1. Describe the role of the home care aide when caring for clients who have the following conditions:
   - Cardiovascular diseases
   - Cancer
   - Stroke
   - Chronic obstructive pulmonary disease (COPD)
   - Diabetes
   - Alzheimer's disease
   - Multiple sclerosis
   - Parkinson's disease
   - Arthritis
   - Fractures
   - AIDS
   - Amputation/Prosthesis

2. Discuss the role of the home care aide when caring for clients who are recovering from surgery.
3. Identify three purposes of support groups in helping clients and family members to cope with the illness.
4. Discuss the role of the home care aide in providing emotional support for clients and family members who are coping with illnesses identified in this chapter.
5. Apply principles of standard (universal) precautions and infection control when caring for clients.

KEY TERMS

Aphasia Absence of speech

Edema Abnormal amount of fluid in the tissues (swelling)

Exacerbation(s) Return of symptoms of illness or disease following a remission

Hemianopsia Blindness or defective vision in one half of the field of vision

Hemiplegia Paralysis of one side of the body

Incentive spirometer Instrument that is used to encourage the client to breathe deeply and correctly

Malignant Becomes progressively worse and causes death; for example, cancer

Perception Ability to recognize sensations through the senses

Pursed lips Lips positioned for whistling

Remission(s) Partial or complete disappearance of symptoms of illness or disease

Tremors Purposeless, continuous, quick movements of skeletal muscles, especially in the hands

Wound Physical injury causing a break in the skin during surgery or an accident

The illnesses described in this chapter have been selected because they are typical of the types of clients you may care for. It is not possible to describe all the illnesses that people have. However, if you are not familiar with your client's illness, be sure to ask for help from your supervisor. DO NOT CARE FOR A CLIENT WHEN YOU DO NOT KNOW YOUR RESPONSIBILITIES; IT CAN BE DANGEROUS FOR YOUR CLIENT AND FOR YOU.

For some clients, you will observe that their condition is improving with each visit that you make; this can be very satisfying for you and your client. For others, who have chronic illnesses, you may see little or no improvement. But remember, your care allows them to remain at home, in familiar surroundings, rather than in an institution. Many clients will experience pain. This is an important symptom that needs to be recorded and reported to your supervisor. Pain is discussed in Chapter 6, pp. 78–82. You will also care for those clients who are at or approaching the last stage of living. Basic principles of care for these clients are discussed in the Chapter 23.

When reading this chapter, you will be referred to material already covered in the book. It is important to refresh your memory by reading this information again.

CARDIOVASCULAR DISEASES

DEFINITION

Cardiovascular diseases affect the normal functioning of the heart and blood vessels. A very common disorder found among home care clients is congestive heart failure. It is due to the gradual weakening of the heart's ability to adequately pump blood to all parts of the body.

THE FACTS

Cardiovascular disease is the leading cause of death in the United States. More than 2500 Americans die of cardiovascular disease each day, an average of one death every 33 seconds.

SYMPTOMS

Clients who have congestive heart failure may have the following symptoms:
- **Edema,** especially in the feet and ankles; may also have a feeling of tightness in the fingers
- Cough due to fluid in the lungs; may or may not cough up sputum
- Difficulty breathing with or without activity and when lying flat; needs two or more pillows to sleep
- Constantly tired
- Chest pain caused by lack of blood supply to the heart muscle
- Anxiety due to chest pains; may have symptoms of depression as disease progresses

YOUR ROLE

Communicating
- Use the techniques listed in Chapter 21 for clients who are anxious.
- Clients may not want to talk a lot; it takes much energy, especially when breathing is difficult.

Maintaining a Safe Environment
- Use precautions learned for clients receiving oxygen; the client may use oxygen only when needed or all the time.

- Dispose of used tissues according to standard (universal) precautions.
- Take precautions to reduce client's risk of infection; those with congestive heart failure are at great risk for infections.

Performing Activities of Daily Living (ADL)

- Follow the guidelines in Box 22-1.
- Follow the activity schedule; some clients may be severely limited in activity.
- Keep the client's legs and feet elevated when sitting in a chair; support the area from knees to feet (Figure 22-1, *A* and *B*).
- Raise the head of bed to Fowler's position, if hospital bed is used, so client can breathe more easily; if regular bed is used, provide pillows or a backrest.
- Assist the client to bathroom or commode; client may be receiving medications to increase urinary output.

Maintaining Good Nutrition

- Follow the care plan's directions for special diet restrictions; client may be on a sodium-restricted diet to help reduce the amount of fluids in the tissues; see Chapter 10 for a review of foods to avoid.

BOX 22-1   ADL for Clients with Low Energy Levels

- Do not rush the client; allow extra time to perform activities.
- Encourage self-care and assist the client, as needed.
- Provide rest periods during bathing and dressing or when you notice the client is tiring during a procedure.
- Encourage the client to wear nonconstricting clothing that is easy to put on and take off (elastic waist bands, suspenders [not belts] for men, slip-on shoes). No bras, girdles, socks, or stockings with elastic bands. Avoid tight neck bands. Use a shawl rather than a sweater or jacket.
- Use techniques that will save the client's energy when performing ADL (chair in bathroom for bathing, toilet articles within easy reach); place underwear inside slacks and put on together.
- Schedule activities requiring a lot of energy (bath) for time of day when energy reserves are high, if possible.

A   B

Fig 22-1 **A,** Incorrect position. The legs and feet are not properly elevated, and there is no support under the knees. **B,** Correct position. The legs and feet are properly elevated, and the knees are fully supported.

- Follow the guidelines listed in Box 10-13 on p. 161 for ways to conserve the client's energy when eating.
- Encourage fluids as indicated in the care plan.

Assisting with Special Procedures

The care plan may include the following procedures:
- Apply elastic stockings (see Chapter 18, Procedure 18-15).
- Measure and record intake and output (see Chapter 15, Procedure 15-3).
- Weigh daily or when listed; weigh at the same time of day; client wears similar type of clothing.
- Assist the client to take oral medications.
- Assist the client to take medications to relieve chest pain.
- Take vital signs according to the care plan.

ORR   Observe, Record, and Report
- Shallow, rapid respirations
- Coughing up blood-tinged, frothy sputum
- Wheezing or "rattling" breathing
- Cyanosis (bluish color) of lips, nail beds, and skin
- Sweating
- Weak, rapid pulse
- Small amount of voiding
- Amount of weight gain or loss from previous time client was weighed
- Confusion and restlessness

CANCER

DEFINITION

Cancer is a term used to describe more than 100 diseases that result from the uncontrolled growth and spread of malignant cells. They may travel from the original site to other locations in the body.

THE FACTS

Cancer is the second leading cause of death in the United States. The American Cancer Society estimates that half of all men and women in the United States will develop cancer in their lifetime. While the risk of developing cancer can come at any age, the incidence of cancer increases as we grow older. The earlier the cancer is discovered, the greater the chance for successful treatment and recovery.

Winston Campbell has been receiving chemotherapy for a malignant brain tumor. A combination of new medications that his oncologist has ordered has caused bouts of diarrhea. However, he is beginning to feel better now. The doctor changed one of his medications, and that helped to relieve his symptoms. Alex is relieved, too. "We were both exhausted. Now, things are calmer, for the present, anyway." Today, after Betty helped him to shower, Winston said, "Where is Tort (the cat)? I've been too sick lately to play with her. I've missed her. Please bring her to me, Betty. Just petting her will make me feel better." Betty knows that playing with Tort is important to Winston and that the doctor has OK'd this activity. She reminds Winston to wash his hands thoroughly after playing with Tort. She also washes her hands carefully after touching the cat.

SYMPTOMS

There are no typical symptoms shown by clients with cancer. Symptoms depend on where the cancer is located, how much of the body is affected, and the type of treatment the client has received or is currently receiving.

You may care for a client who is receiving treatment to help destroy cancer cells and prevent them from spreading. Two methods are radiation (the use of x-rays) and chemotherapy (the use of strong chemicals in the form of medication). Unfortunately, these methods can also destroy healthy cells. Both types of treatments are usually given in hospitals or medical centers by health professionals. Clients return home after each treatment. However, some intravenous chemotherapy is given in the home. Your client may show the following side effects of radiation or chemotherapy:

- Tiredness, exhaustion
- Nausea and/or vomiting
- Anorexia
- Loss of taste or smell
- Skin irritation or burns in the area receiving radiation
- Loss of hair
- Sores in the mouth, around the lips and tongue
- Bleeding gums
- Upper respiratory infections: Client's immune system is not functioning well
- Diarrhea
  Other symptoms may include the following.
- Pain
- Constipation caused by medications given to relieve pain

YOUR ROLE

The information that follows is only a partial list of ways to assist the client with cancer. Be sure to review the care plan thoroughly before beginning care. It is important to know when the client has received the last treatment or the last medication for pain so that you can better understand the client's needs.

Communicating
- Listen to what the client tells you.
- Use nonverbal communication; it is just as important as verbal; show that you care by a touch of the hand and your presence; when a person is in pain, a lot of talking may not be welcome.
- Do not say anything that is untrue, such as, "I know you will get better; please do not worry."
- Encourage the client to tell you when he or she begins to be tired so that you can adjust the care routine, as needed.

Maintaining a Safe Environment
- Discourage visits from persons with colds or other infections; clients are at high risk for infections (Box 22-2).
- Practice standard (universal) precautions and infection control when handling body fluids and waste.
- Encourage client to wash hands frequently.

BOX 22-2   Preventing Infection

- Use standard (universal) precautions to protect your client and yourself.
- Dispose of body wastes properly.
- Discourage visitors who have colds or other infections.
- Use disinfectants properly.
- Keep the client's area clean and free of dust.
- Prepare and store foods properly.
- Wash your hands before and after giving client care.
- Wash your hands before and after handling food.
- Wash your hands after touching pets.
- Wash your hands before and after gloving.
- Observe the client's skin for redness or skin breakdown.

Performing ADL
- Practice techniques to conserve client's energy described in Box 22-1.
- Provide frequent oral hygiene according to the care plan; use a very soft bristled toothbrush or foam swab to avoid further injury to mouth and gums. Be gentle; avoid alcohol-based mouthwashes; use normal saline.
- Do not remove colored lines on skin that indicate the site for radiation treatments; do not wash skin within these lines.

Maintaining Good Nutrition
- Encourage fluids that the client can drink.
- Prepare foods that the client likes and can eat and swallow.
- Avoid foods with strong odors and high acid content, which can irritate mouth tissues.
- Prepare frequent small meals; they are usually better tolerated.

Assisting with Special Procedures
- Observe the skin at the site of intravenous infusion
- Notify your supervisor of any problems with equipment or changes in client's condition. See Chapter 18, Intravenous Infusions, p. 338.

Helping the Client to Cope with Pain
- Encourage the client to take medication before the pain becomes severe: bring medication to the client on time, according to the care plan; some pain medications cause constipation; record bowel movements accurately.
- Use techniques listed in the care plan to help the client to tolerate pain (e.g., back rub, warm or cool applications to area, playing soothing music).
- Attend to the client's request for spiritual aids, such as prayer or spiritual readings.
- ORR Record the type, location, and frequency of pain (see Chapter 6) on the care record, according to agency procedure.
- Assist the client with recording pain information (Figure 22-2), if requested.
- Accept the client's changed behavior due to pain; do not judge this behavior.

ORR Observe, Record, and Report
- White or yellow patches or sores in the mouth
- Other signs of infection
- Problems or changes in
  Swallowing, eating, or drinking
  Bowel habits: constipation or diarrhea

Client's Daily Pain Journal

Name: _Sol Weinstein_

Date: _Tuesday, October 10_

Location of Pain: _Lower back_

Medication(s): _Morphine sulfate 30mg. by mouth every four hours_

Pain Scale

0	1	2	3	4	5
No Pain	Mild Pain	Moderate Pain	Severe Pain	Very Severe Pain	Worst Possible Pain

TIME	LEVEL OF PAIN 0 1 2 3 4 5	MED TAKEN	ACTIVITIES AND COMMENTS
1:00 AM	3	✓	Awake and restless
2:00	1		Awake to bathroom
3:00			
4:00			
5:00	2	✓	Awake
6:00			
7:00	1		Resting in bed
8:00	1		Breakfast in kitchen
9:00	1	✓	Shower and dress
10:00	1		Read paper, watch T.V.
11:00			
12:00 noon			
1:00 PM			
2:00			
3:00			
4:00			
5:00			
6:00			
7:00			
8:00			
9:00			
10:00			
11:00			
12:00			

Directions: 1. Using a Pain Scale, select the number that most closely describes your level of pain and record.
2. Record medication taken.
3. Describe activity and any comments in column provided.

Fig 22-2 The client pain record. (Modified from Gentiva Health Services, Melville, New York.)

- Changes in type or frequency of pain
- Bruising or bleeding
- Pain that is not relieved with medication
- Changes in appearance of skin at radiation site (e.g., redness) and infusion site

CEREBROVASCULAR ACCIDENT

DEFINITION

A cerebrovascular accident (CVA) is an injury to the brain caused by lack of blood to the tissues.

THE FACTS

CVA, also known as a *stroke* or *brain attack,* is the third leading cause of death and the leading cause of adult disability in the United States. Each year, about 795,000 Americans have a new or recurrent stroke: that is one stroke every 40 seconds, according to the American Stroke Association.

SYMPTOMS

This is a very serious illness. The sooner the person receives medical care, the better the chances of survival. However, some people will not survive. Of those who do, many will be treated in a rehabilitation center before coming home. Symptoms depend on the extent of the brain injury and the area involved. Symptoms may include problems with the following:

- *Communication:* Due to difficulty receiving, understanding, and expressing speech and language. Aphasia is caused by injury to the speech center of the brain. Short attention span is also caused by brain damage. Clients may have slurred speech and problems finding the "right" word they want to say. This is very frustrating, and clients may cry or become angry because they are unable to clearly express their needs and feelings. Sometimes, they will not understand what you are asking or telling them.
- *Safety:* Due to poor balance, hemiplegia, and hemianopsia. The client is at great risk for falls.
- *ADL:* Due to limited mobility, weakness, and perception problems. There may be severe problems with performing ADL, and clients usually require a great deal of assistance with grooming and hygiene.
- *Mobility:* Due to hemiplegia and enforced bed rest.
- *Pain in affected shoulder and/or arm:* Due to weight of paralyzed arm pulling on joints.
- Elimination: Due to incontinence, urinary retention, and constipation.
- Nutrition: Due to difficulty in swallowing, self-feeding, and perception problems.
- Depression: Due to effects of serious illness, problems with mobility, and prolonged rehabilitation. Clients may have low self-esteem because of the many losses they have experienced and the need to depend on others for so much care. EMOTIONS CHANGE SO QUICKLY THAT THE CLIENT AND FAMILY MAY NOT UNDERSTAND WHAT IS HAPPENING. THESE RAPID MOOD SWINGS ARE A RESULT OF DAMAGE TO THE BRAIN TISSUE AND ARE NOT AN INDICATION OF TRUE FEELINGS.

YOUR ROLE

Home care aides provide support to the client and family during the long road to recovery after a stroke.

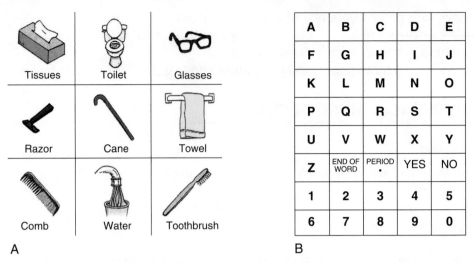

A	B	C	D	E
F	G	H	I	J
K	L	M	N	O
P	Q	R	S	T
U	V	W	X	Y
Z	END OF WORD	PERIOD ·	YES	NO
1	2	3	4	5
6	7	8	9	0

A   B

Fig 22-3 Communication charts. **A,** Picture communication chart. **B,** Alphabet communication chart.

Communicating

- Follow the guidelines in Chapter 3 for communicating with persons who are hearing impaired; clients may not be hard of hearing but usually have difficulty understanding and responding to speech.
- Ask questions that can be answered with a simple "yes" or "no."
- Use nonverbal communication: Gestures, pictures (Figure 22-3, *A* and *B*), chalkboards, flash cards, typewriters, and computers.
- Try to anticipate your client's need before he or she has to ask for something.
- Follow the instructions given by the speech-language therapist.

Maintaining a Safe Environment

- Assist with moving and walking.
- Follow the principles of safety in Chapter 8.
- Protect from infection.
- Discourage visitors with respiratory infections.

Performing ADL

- Follow the care plan; encourage the client to become as independent as possible.
- Use assistive devices (e.g., special toothbrushes, combs, soap-on-a-rope) as directed by occupational and physical therapists.
- Promote client mobility through range-of-motion exercises and ambulation, if possible.
- Change position every 2 hours, and check skin for injury; client should not lie on affected side any longer than 1 hour.
- Do not pull on or use the affected limb when lifting or moving the client.
- Apply a sling or elevate the paralyzed arm according to the care plan and directions from the physical therapist.
- Watch for swelling, discoloration, and pain in the affected limb.
- Schedule rest periods between activities; these clients tire easily.
- Take the client to the bathroom for elimination, if possible. A raised seat will make it easier for the client to use the toilet; a commode at the bedside may also be used. Clothing that is easy to get off will help to prevent accidents. See Chapter 15 for additional information on elimination.

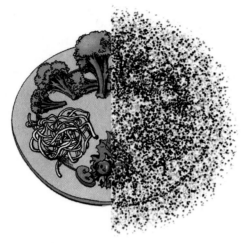

Fig 22-4 The client may only see half of the plate.

Maintaining Good Nutrition

- Remind the client to follow the speech-language therapist's instructions about proper swallowing techniques.
- Feed the client from the unaffected side; see Procedure 10-1, Feeding the Client, p. 159.
- Check the paralyzed side of the mouth to make sure no food is "pocketed" inside the cheek.
- Encourage the client to feed himself or herself when possible.
- Use assistive devices when needed.
- Rotate the plate so the client can see and eat all of the food; clients with perception problems may only see half the food on the plate (Figure 22-4).
- Feed slowly, and watch for choking and difficulty swallowing; know how to perform abdominal thrusts (Heimlich maneuver) (see Chapter 24).
- Follow the suggestions in Box 10-12 on p. 161 for clients with difficulty chewing and swallowing.

Handling Behaviors

- Be patient with your client; follow the suggestions found in Chapter 7, Working with Ill and Disabled Clients.

Assisting with Special Procedures

- Follow the care plan for special procedures to improve mobility, including turning, positioning, range-of-motion exercises, and ambulation with or without assistive devices.
- Assist the client to take medication according to schedule.
- Take the client's blood pressure on the unaffected side and pulse according to the care plan.

ORR   Observe, Record, and Report

- Coughing and choking when eating and swallowing
- Incontinence
- Constipation
- Skin changes
- Complaints of pain
- Depression
- Signs of infection

"I don't want to get out of bed today, and I don't want a shower, and I want you to go away," Father Kowalski told Rosina. She noticed that he had not eaten any breakfast. Father Kowalski began to cry. "Everything is so … so … what's the word? Oh, never mind … everything is so much. I can't, I can't, I can't …"

Rosina knows that frustration and depression are common reactions to a serious illness such as stroke. Rehabilitation (physical therapy, occupational therapy, and speech-language therapy) is long and hard work for the client. She understands how Father Kowalski must be feeling. Rosina fluffs his pillows and offers him a "nice hot cup" of tea. "Now you rest while I get the tea ready. I'll call my supervisor, too, just to let her know how you are feeling today."

CHRONIC OBSTRUCTIVE PULMONARY DISEASE (COPD)

DEFINITION

Chronic obstructive pulmonary disease (COPD) is a term used to describe a group of chronic diseases (adult asthma, chronic bronchitis, and emphysema) that causes the client to have difficulty inhaling and/or exhaling air from the lungs. Usually there are permanent physical changes in the lungs and alveoli. This condition is also known as *chronic lung disease.*

THE FACTS

More than 12 million Americans are living with chronic lung disease. Smoking, lengthy exposure to air pollutants, and chronic irritation from dust and fumes in the workplace are factors that contribute to COPD.

SYMPTOMS

Home care clients may show the following symptoms:
- Difficulty breathing when performing ADL and even when resting (in the later stages of the illness)
- Breathes through the mouth
- Inhaling is not as difficult as exhaling; may have pursed lips (Figure 22-5) in an effort to force out air that is trapped in the lungs
- Cyanosis of lips, nail beds, and skin
- Cough due to thick, hard plugs of mucus that are difficult to expel from the lungs
- "Barrel chest" because of enlarged rib cage
- Exhaustion; most of the energy is taken just to breathe
- Wheezing
- Decreased appetite

YOUR ROLE

Communication
- Use a calm, reassuring approach.
- Follow the guidelines listed in Chapter 3 if the client is hearing or visually impaired.
- Be patient; do not cut off the conversation if the client has difficulty talking. Practice your listening skills.

Fig 22-5 The client exhales through pursed lips.

Fig 22-6 The client sleeps best in an upright position.

Maintaining a Safe Environment

- Use safety precautions when clients receive oxygen; follow the safety guidelines listed in Chapter 18.
- Reduce the amount of dust in the air by damp dusting, especially in the client's bedroom; keep this room as dust-free as possible.
- Eliminate household odors from cleaning products by opening the window after use, when possible; environment should be free of aerosol sprays, perfume sprays, and so on.
- Teach the client the proper way to dispose of used tissues containing sputum.
- Use standard (universal) precautions when handling soiled tissues.
- Protect the client from visitors who have respiratory infections.

Performing ADL

- Assist the client with performing ADL according to instructions given by the occupational therapist or care plan.
- Help the client to maintain a comfortable sleeping or resting position (Figure 22-6).
- Follow the guidelines in Box 22-1 for assisting clients with low energy levels.

Maintaining Good Nutrition

- Encourage increased fluid intake to help in coughing up sputum, according to the care plan.
- Provide small, frequent meals; eating takes energy!
- Avoid gas-forming foods.
- Avoid milk and other dairy products: they tend to thicken mucous secretions and make coughing up sputum even more difficult.
- Follow the guidelines in Boxes 10-2 to 10-8 for ways to help your client maintain good nutrition.

Assisting with Special Procedures

- Help client to practice techniques to control the feeling of panic during coughing episodes; these techniques have been taught by the professional nurse or respiratory therapist and may be listed in the care plan.
- Support and encourage the client to use correct breathing and coughing techniques as taught by the respiratory therapist; if unsure of the technique, notify your supervisor for help.
- Assist client, as needed, to take medications orally or by means of metered-dose inhalers (see Procedure 18-6, p. 327).

Observe, Record, and Report

- Signs of infection
- Increase in panic attacks
- Severe difficulties in performing ADL
- Signs of depression

DIABETES MELLITUS

DEFINITION

Diabetes mellitus is a chronic illness in which the pancreas is unable to produce enough (or any) insulin to meet the body's needs for carbohydrate, fat, and protein metabolism. There are two types of diabetes.

- Diabetes mellitus, type 1: Clients take insulin daily.
- Diabetes mellitus, type 2: Clients usually do not take insulin but control the diabetes with a proper diet and oral medications; this type of diabetes usually occurs after 40 years of age.

THE FACTS

About 26 million children and adults in the United States have diabetes. Each year, almost 2 million people are diagnosed. Adult diabetics are two to six times more likely to have a heart attack or stroke than are those who are not diabetics. More than 50% have high blood pressure, and they are prone to many other problems, such as nerve damage (especially in hands and feet), blindness, leg and foot ulcers, kidney failure, impotence, infection, and poor healing. The disease is more common in Native Americans, African Americans, Hispanics, and Asian Americans than in whites. With the increase in obesity and sedentary lifestyles in children and adults, the number of diabetics will continue to rise.

SYMPTOMS

The symptoms vary according to the type of diabetes. Those who are already diagnosed and receiving treatment should have few disease symptoms. However, long-term effects of the disease may lead to serious problems, such as stroke, heart disease, leg ulcers, or amputation.

YOUR ROLE

Many times you will be caring for the client because of another condition, such as stroke, fracture, amputation. Remember that he or she is also a diabetic and requires special care.

Maintaining a Safe Environment

- Protect the client from injury; sense of touch may be missing in the hands and feet; burns or injuries may not be felt.
- Shoes or hard-soled slippers should be worn when walking; inspect ankles and feet (between and under toes) for changes in the appearance of the skin; report unusual findings; prompt treatment is essential to prevent infection and permanent damage to the tissues.
- Be alert for signs and symptoms of infection (see Box 11-2, p. 171).
- Dispose of used insulin syringes properly (see Chapter 11).

Performing ADL

- Assist the client with performing ADL according to the care plan.

Maintaining Good Nutrition

- The proper diabetic diet is prescribed for each client (see Chapter 10).
- Be sure the client eats the entire meal, no more and no less; if the client does not eat the entire meal, notify your supervisor.

Assisting with Special Procedures

- Assist the client to test the blood sugar level and record in a daily diary (see Chapter 18).
- Weigh the client according to the care plan.
- Assist the client to take medications according to the care plan.
- Be alert for signs of low blood sugar (Box 22-3): **THIS IS AN EMERGENCY.**
- If the client is able to swallow
  Give 4 ounces (120 mL) of orange juice.
  Notify your supervisor immediately, and follow the instructions given.
  Client should be better in a short amount of time. Have the client test blood sugar.
  If there is no improvement, call your supervisor again.

BOX 22-3 **Signs of Low Blood Sugar (Sometimes Called "Insulin Reaction")**

Early signs include
- Faintness
- Sudden weakness
- Excessive perspiration
- Irritability
- Hunger—"empty feeling" in stomach
- Palpitations
- Trembling
- Headache

Other signs
- Confusion
- Slurred speech
- Blurred vision
- Difficulty walking

If untreated, the client may lose consciousness and have seizures.

Treatment
- If the client can swallow, give 4 oz (120 mL) of orange juice; notify your supervisor.
- If the client is unable to swallow, call 9-1-1 or emergency medical services.

- If the client is unable to swallow
  Call 9-1-1 or emergency medical services immediately.
  Call your supervisor.

ORR Observe, Record, and Report
- Nausea and vomiting
- Excessive thirst
- Fruity odor to breath
- Rapid breathing
- Confusion
- Diarrhea
- Extreme fatigue
- Signs of low blood sugar (see Box 22-3)
- Not eating meals
- Sores on skin
- Any foot problems: Rash, sores, broken skin
- Signs of infection (see Box 11-2)

ALZHEIMER'S DISEASE

DEFINITION

Alzheimer's disease is a progressive, currently not treatable, and fatal disease that results from the gradual destruction of brain cells.

THE FACTS

Alzheimer's disease is the sixth leading cause of death in older adults. It usually occurs after 60 years of age but can be seen as early as 40 years of age. More than 5.1 million Americans are affected. It is *not* a normal result of aging.

CLIENT BEHAVIORS

There is no "typical" client with Alzheimer's disease. Symptoms and behaviors vary. As the disease progresses through various stages, the client loses more and more control over the ability to function mentally and physically. Families will often tell you how difficult it is to see their loved one change and be helpless to reverse these changes. Some health care professionals say that the family is the real victim of the disease. The client may not be aware of the devastating mental and physical changes.

The following are behaviors you may observe in your client:
- *Speech:* Slow, hesitant; difficulty completing a sentence; loses train of thought; struggles to use simple words; uses inappropriate words
- *Confusion:* May not know time of day and place
- *Changes in mood:* May have rapid mood swings; for example, may be calm, then have outbursts of anger, for no apparent reason
- *Personality changes:* May be anxious, agitated, aggressive, abusive, in a depressed state, or suspicious, or may show inappropriate or annoying behavior
- *Difficulty thinking:* Unable to think through a situation or reason; unable to make decisions
- *Difficulty in performing ADL:* Forgets how to dress, toilet, and groom self. Forgets what common objects are used for and how to use them, such as toothbrush
- *Difficulty remembering:* Forgets family members and location of key areas of the home (bathroom, kitchen, bedroom)

- *Wandering:* Particularly in late afternoon and evening
- *Eating:* Forgets how to feed self, chew, and swallow

YOUR ROLE

The needs of each client will vary according to how the disease is advancing and the types of behaviors the client shows. Follow the care plan carefully, and note any changes in the client's physical and mental condition. The following are some general rules to follow when caring for your client:

Communicating
- Speak slowly.
- Use simple words in short sentences.
- Repeat instructions as often as needed; reminders (e.g., "Brush your teeth.").
- Do not change topics suddenly.
- Follow the information in Chapter 3 on communicating with hearing-impaired clients (while the client may not be hearing impaired, the same principles apply).
- Place signs on doors to identify the bedroom, bathroom, and other rooms frequently used; a drawing on the signs may help (Figure 22-7).
- Wear a name tag with title to help the client remember; family members may also wish to wear name tags such as "Betty—Daughter" or "Bob—Husband."

Maintaining a Safe Environment
- Follow the guidelines on safety for confused clients in Chapter 21.
- Lock doors to unsafe areas (e.g., garage, basement).
- Keep doors to outside locked.
- Do not rearrange furniture; it may cause more anxiety and possible injury from tripping or falls.
- Place plastic bags out of reach; they may cause choking or suffocation.
- Remove artificial fruits, vegetables, or food-shaped kitchen magnets; client may try to eat them (Figure 22-8); also, remove items such as coins, safety pins, and other small objects—the client may confuse them with things to eat.

Fig 22-7 Labels help Alzheimer's clients to identify rooms.

Fig 22-8 Artificial "food magnets" may be confusing to the Alzheimer's client.

- Cover the thermostat so the client cannot reach the controls to raise or lower the temperature of the home.
- Remove control knobs from the stove.
- Unplug appliances when not in use.

Performing ADL
- Be alert for signs that the client needs help to perform ADL.
- Assist the client only when needed or when client shows signs of frustration.
- Do not rush; provide ample time for the activity.
- Divide an activity into steps that are easy to follow.
- Take one step at a time, and talk the client through each step as shown in the following examples of self-feeding.
  1. Pick up the spoon.
  2. Put pudding on the spoon.
  3. Bring the spoon up to your mouth.
  4. Open your mouth.
  5. Put food into your mouth.
  6. Put down the spoon.
  7. Chew the food.
  8. Swallow the food.
- Encourage and praise accomplishments.
- Do not force the client to perform the activity; if resistive, complete the task yourself, if possible; you may need to return later to perform the activity when the client is calmer.
- Be alert for signs that the client needs to use the bathroom (restlessness); the care plan may include a toileting routine.
- Lay out clothes in the order they are to be put on; clothing should be easy to put on and remove.

Maintaining Good Nutrition
- Provide extra time for eating.
- Encourage self-feeding; provide finger foods that the client can handle easily.
- Offer foods that are high in protein and complex carbohydrates for between-meal snacks, as indicated on the care plan.
- Give reminders on how to use utensils, if needed.
- Remind the client to chew food slowly.
- Remind the client to swallow food.
- Serve foods and liquids that are not too hot or too cold to avoid burns.
- Avoid possible confusion and frustration by doing the following:
  Reducing the number of food choices
  Placing one utensil and one food in front of the client at a time
  Using unbreakable plates and cups, if available
- Do not be concerned about poor table manners; give praise when the client attempts to feed self.

Handling Behaviors
- See Chapter 21 for ways of handling behaviors such as aggression, sexual acting out, anxiety, delusions, and hallucinations.

Wandering
- Approach the client calmly, walk with the client and gradually guide back, if client is found wandering outside the home.

Fig 22-9 Wandering clients should wear identification bracelets.

- Distract the client by offering a favorite snack or drink.
- Remain calm; do not use physical force or startle the client.
- Client should wear a bracelet engraved with the words *Memory Impaired* that includes client's name, address, and telephone number (Figure 22-9); this will help to identify the client who may wander from the home. Keep a recent photo of the client for easy identification.
- In some areas, clients may wear a "Project Lifesaver" bracelet. If they are lost, a tracking system can determine their location and a rescue team can be sent.

Hiding Objects/Suspiciousness
- Determine favorite hiding places (under bed, between chair cushions, under pillows); the care plan may provide this information.
- Ask the caregiver to remove valuables and lock them securely.
- Offer to help find the missing item (check favorite hiding places first).
- Do not argue with the client.
- Do not whisper; it just reinforces the client's suspicions.

ORR Observe, Record, and Report
- Changes in confusion or wandering
- Changes in ability to perform ADL and to communicate
- Signs of infection
- Refusal to take medications

Needs of the Informal Caregiver
The day-to-day responsibilities of caring for the person with Alzheimer's disease can affect the caregiver in a variety of ways. It is not unusual for him or her to experience feelings of helplessness, frustration, and anger. For many caregivers, the home care aide's visits may be the only contact with someone they can talk to and express these emotions. Take the time to listen to your client's caregiver and to express your understanding of the difficult situation they are handling each day. Recognize them as an important member of the home care team. Caregivers also appreciate words of praise for doing a good job!

MULTIPLE SCLEROSIS

DEFINITION
Multiple sclerosis is a chronic, slowly progressing disease of the central nervous system causing changes in the brain and spinal cord.

THE FACTS

Multiple sclerosis is a major cause of chronic disability in young adults.

SYMPTOMS

The symptoms of multiple sclerosis vary widely and may change almost daily. The disease is characterized by remissions and exacerbations of the symptoms, which include the following:
- Weakness, paralysis, poor coordination
- Stiffness or fatigue of a limb
- Walking problems: staggering, falling, inability to walk
- Visual disturbances: blurred vision, double vision, dark spots in front of the eyes
- Incontinence of bowel and bladder
- Mood swings, depression, irritability

YOUR ROLE

Activities of daily living present the most problems and challenges for the client. Some clients will be able to perform self-care within the limits of the disease, while others may be totally disabled and unable to perform any self-care.

Communicating
- Use large-print written materials for clients with visual problems.
- Follow the suggestions in Chapter 3 for communication with hearing-impaired clients when ringing in the ears may interfere with hearing.

Maintaining a Safe Environment
- Encourage the client to use assistive devices when walking.
- Remove any hazards in the home.
- Be alert for signs of infection; the risk of infection is always present.

Performing ADL
- Help the client as needed.
- Do not allow him or her to become tired.
- Schedule rest periods.
- Change positions every 2 hours; range-of-motion, ambulation, and other exercises will be used to ease stiff muscles.
- Observe output; record intake and output as ordered.
- Watch for constipation; watch for signs of a urinary tract infection: cloudy, foul-smelling urine, fever, pain when voiding.
- Keep skin clean and dry; watch for any sign of skin breakdown.

Maintaining Good Nutrition
- Buy food or prepare meals as indicated in the care plan.
- Offer foods from the entire MyPlate Food Guide; plenty of fluids (3000 mL) and high-fiber foods will help to prevent constipation.

Providing Emotional Support
- Help to maintain independence as much as possible. Mood swings are common and are often produced by fatigue, infection, or physical or emotional stress.
- Understand that clients and their families may grieve the losses caused by this disease. Many clients have a low self-image. They may be angry and depressed about

what is happening. Counseling services and support groups may be helpful. Some clients will find great comfort from spiritual support.

Assisting with Special Procedures
* Assist the client to take medications according to the care plan.
* Applications of heat or ice may be ordered to relieve muscle spasm before exercising.
* Use a wheelchair and other assistive devices as needed.

Observe, Record, and Report
* Signs of infection
* Increasing problems with the symptoms
* Severe behavioral and emotional changes
* Elimination problems: urinary retention, constipation, incontinence
* Skin breakdown

PARKINSON'S DISEASE

DEFINITION

Parkinson's disease is a chronic, slowly progressing degenerative disease of the central nervous system characterized by stiffness, slowed movements, and tremors.

THE FACTS

About 1 million Americans live with Parkinson's disease, and each year 60,000 are newly diagnosed. Men are 1½ times more likely to have the disease than women. Parkinson's disease usually occurs after 50 years of age. The total disability that occurs from this disease may take years to develop. Eventually, most clients will require care in a nursing home.

SYMPTOMS

* Fine tremors of hands
* Rigid muscles
* Slow movements
* Slow speech with a monotonous tone
* Slow, shuffling gait
* Expressionless face
* Drooling

YOUR ROLE

Self-care presents the biggest problem for client and family. As the disease progresses, the ability to perform ADL is lost, and the client needs more care. An effort is made to help the client maintain the abilities that are present for as long as possible.

Communicating
* Allow plenty of time for clients to answer your questions. Do not rely on their facial expressions to indicate understanding. While it may not appear that your client understands what you are saying, do not be fooled. They do understand but may

be very slow in responding. This is due to problems with muscle movement, not with intelligence or brain function.

- Encourage the client to perform exercises to strengthen speech and facial muscles as taught by the speech-language therapist.

Harold's caregiver is his wife, Helen. During your visit, she says, "You know, Harold is a very smart person; he may have trouble getting the words out of his mouth, but he's not dumb! It makes me mad when friends say to me, "Poor Harold, the disease has stolen his bright mind—now he seems so dull." Harold's friends could also learn from the communication tips listed above.

Maintaining a Safe Environment
- Remove clutter and hazards that may cause the client to fall.

Performing ADL
- Help the client as needed.
- Use assistive devices for grooming, bathing, and ambulation; clothing should be easy to put on and take off.
- Offer plenty of fluids and fiber in the diet, if possible; this is not always realistic because of chewing problems.
- Observe for constipation.

Maintaining Good Nutrition
- Remember that self-feeding, chewing, and swallowing are complex tasks involving the nerves and muscles (see Box 10-12 on p. 161).
- Offer foods from all groups of the MyPlate Food Guide.
- Use a spoon with a built up handle and a plate guard, if available; clients with tremors will have great difficulty using a fork or spoon.
- Serve foods that are easy to get to the mouth; avoid peas or other similar foods that are difficult to balance; spilling is common; protect the client's clothing from spills (Figure 22-10); clients are easily frustrated by spilling and the length of time it takes to eat, chew, and swallow.

Fig 22-10 Protect the client's clothing from spills.

- Provide small, frequent meals, instead of three large meals; they may be easier for the client to eat.
- Give lots of fluids, as much as 3000 mL per day.
- Encourage the client to practice exercises to strengthen muscles used in chewing and swallowing as taught by the speech-language therapist.
- Use adaptive equipment as ordered by the occupational therapist.

Providing Emotional Support
- Listen to the client, and allow him or her to express feelings. Clients express many feelings because of the enormous losses caused by this disease. Anger, frustration, low self-image, hopelessness, and worthlessness are common emotions associated with Parkinson's disease.
- Work with the family and agency staff to find ways to help the client cope with problems. Prayer and spiritual support can be uplifting for many of these clients. Regular visits from clergy or church members are welcomed by clients who have participated in religious activities. Support groups and counseling are also beneficial.

Assisting with Special Procedures
- Assist clients to take medications at the proper time; Parkinson's disease is treated with many medications; these do not stop the progress of the illness but do relieve the symptoms.
- Apply heat to reduce rigidity of the muscles, according to the care plan.
- Weigh the client according to the care plan.

ORR

Observe, Record, and Report
- Increasing problems with mobility
- Changes in behavior: severe anxiety, depression, withdrawal
- Signs of infection
- Problems with elimination
- Increasing difficulty with eating
- Weight loss

ARTHRITIS

DEFINITION

Arthritis is a group of conditions that damages the joints, cartilage, and connective tissue, causing pain and limitation in movement. About 100 different diseases are listed under the category of arthritis. The following are two common types:
- *Osteoarthritis (OA):* A localized, degenerative disease, involving the weight-bearing joints
- *Rheumatoid arthritis (RA):* A progressive, chronic inflammatory disease that causes joint changes; this is the more serious of the two diseases because other organs (heart, lungs, muscles, eyes) can also be affected.

THE FACTS

More than 50 million Americans have some type of arthritis; 4 million are completely dependent. They are unable to work, go to school, play, or carry out many activities of daily living. Arthritis is the leading cause of disability in the United States.

SYMPTOMS

Symptoms depend on the degree and the type of arthritis. Some common symptoms include the following:
- Swelling, redness, tenderness, and chronic pain in the affected area
- Stiffness, especially after being in the same position for a length of time, such as 30 minutes
- Inability to move the involved joints
- Weight loss
- Difficulty sleeping, moving, and performing ADL
- Chronic fatigue

YOUR ROLE

Maintaining a Safe Environment
- Prevent falls and injury.
- Use assistive devices, if needed, for safe ambulation.
- Protect the client from infection.

Performing ADL
- Allow the client to be as independent as possible. Grooming and hygiene activities may take a long time. Be patient; assist the client only when necessary. Stiffness occurs in the early morning and may take 1 or 2 hours to subside. A shower will ease the stiffness and helps to "get the client going."
- Encourage use of assistive devices. Clothing should be easy to put on and take off (Figure 22-11).
- Assist with range-of-motion exercises to prevent stiffening of joints. Some clients will have painful joints, so be careful when performing range-of-motion exercises. Do not hurt the client.

Maintaining Good Nutrition
- Use assistive devices for self-feeding.
- Use lightweight cups and glasses. Clients may not be able to lift cups and glasses that are full of liquid. Fill glasses halfway.
- Follow instructions from the occupational therapist regarding assistive feeding devices.

Fig 22-11 Clothing with Velcro or snaps makes dressing easier for the client.

- Offer foods from all groups of the MyPlate Food Guide; the client should remain at normal weight.

Providing Emotional Support
- Use listening skills to help client express feelings; clients can become discouraged and disgusted with their condition; it is hard to adjust to the lifestyle changes brought about by arthritis. NOTE: Clients will say they have "good days" and "bad days." On a good day, a person may do too much because he or she feels good—and pays for that overactivity for many days after. Learning to pace oneself is an important approach to coping with this disease.

Assisting with Special Procedures
- Assist the client to take medications as ordered; they are used to relieve inflammation and pain and can modify the progress of the disease.
- Apply heat and cold, according to the care plan, to relieve pain and stiffness.
- Use positioning devices, such as splints and slings according to the care plan.
- Lift, move, and position the client carefully to avoid pain in the joints; it is always best to have the client move himself or herself, even if it takes a long time.

Observe, Record, and Report
- Increasing pain and immobility
- Signs of infection
- Skin breakdown
- Swelling, redness, and tenderness in a joint
- Severe anxiety and depression

FRACTURES

DEFINITION
Fractures mean broken bones caused by injury, such as falls, or diseases that weaken bones.

THE FACTS
Each year, over 250,000 hip fractures occur in older adults, primarily due to falls in or nearby the home. Fractures are the leading cause of injury-related disability and death in older adults. See Chapter 19, Caring for Older Adults.

SYMPTOMS
The location of the fracture(s) and the method used to treat the fracture determine the type of symptoms your client may have. For example, the client with a fractured wrist will probably have a cast from the hand and extending to the upper arm. If the cast is on the dominant hand (right hand for a right-handed person), the client may have great difficulty feeding himself or herself with the other hand. But, the client who has had surgery to replace a fractured hip will not have difficulty eating because of the injury. However, learning to use a walker and exercising to strengthen the muscles of the injured leg are activities for this type of client.

Sometimes, you may care for a client who has both a fractured wrist and a fractured hip. The client may not return home until he or she is able to bear weight on the wrist and use a walker for support.

> **BOX 22-4** Check Limb with Cast for ... and Report to Your Supervisor
>
> - Skin color: White or bluish
> - Skin temperature: Cool or cold to the touch
> - Size: Swollen fingers, toes compared with the noncasted limb
> - Foul odor coming from cast
> - Movement: Difficulty or inability to move fingers, toes
> - Also report client complaints of
>   Pain under the cast
>   Pain when moving fingers, toes
>   Numbness or tingling in the area

YOUR ROLE

Caring for a Client with a Cast

Casts, made of fiberglass, are applied by the doctor to a part of the body to keep it immobile. The cast keeps the bones in proper position while healing takes place. The following are important points when caring for your client:

- Keep the cast clean and dry; wash with soap and water, if necessary; do not soak the cast.
- Be careful to avoid wetting the inside edges of the cast; they are difficult to dry and can cause irritation of surrounding skin.
- Cover the cast completely with plastic before assisting the client to take a shower, if permitted.
- Discourage the client from putting objects into the cast (coat hanger, "back scratcher") to relieve itching of the skin; notify your supervisor if the client complains of severe itching.
- Observe the limb for signs of problems affecting the circulation and nerves (see Box 22-4).
  Follow instructions in the care plan for
- Assisting with ADL
- Assisting with exercises or instructing the client about exercises to strengthen the limb or maintain range of motion, according to physical therapist's directions
- Observing the client's ability to use a walker correctly (see Chapter 12)
- Assisting with toileting, if needed
- Assisting at mealtime (cut food, butter bread, if wrist is casted)

Caring for a Client After Surgical Repair of a Fracture

Another way to repair the fracture is by placing pins in the bones to keep them in proper position for healing. Sometimes, the bone is so damaged that it must be replaced with an artificial part. Both procedures require surgery. After the initial postoperative period in the hospital, the client may be transferred to a rehabilitation center or other nursing facility to strengthen injured muscles and learn to perform various activities correctly, such as walking, transfer techniques, and ADL. Before returning home, the home care team may visit the primary caregiver and assess the home environment.

Follow the care plan, which may include the following:

- Assisting with mobility exercises as instructed by the physical therapist
- Assisting with ADL as instructed by the occupational therapist
- Encouraging the client toward independence; assist only when needed

ORR

- Observing that the client uses correct technique for
  Walker
  Crutches
  Transfers (see Chapter 12)
- Encouraging rest periods so the client does not become overtired, resulting in further injury

AIDS

DEFINITION

AIDS (acquired immunodeficiency syndrome) is an infectious, currently incurable, chronic disease caused by the HIV (human immunodeficiency virus). It breaks down the body's immune system and, therefore, destroys the body's ability to fight infection and illness. Not all persons with HIV will develop AIDS, but all AIDS victims have the HIV.

THE FACTS

Over 1.1 million people are living with HIV in the United States. One in five of them are not aware of their infection. About 56,300 become infected with HIV each year. Every 9½ minutes someone in the United States is infected with HIV, and each year more than 17,000 die from AIDS.

HIV is transmitted in several ways: having sex (homosexual or heterosexual) with someone who has HIV, sharing needles or syringes with an illicit drug user who has HIV, passing HIV from an infected mother to her infant during pregnancy and/or breast-feeding, and coming in contact with infected blood. There is no vaccine to prevent the HIV infection.

TRANSMISSION OF HIV

HIV **IS** transmitted from the client's body when the virus (contained in blood, vaginal secretions, breast milk, bloody urine, feces, or vomitus and other body substances, such as draining wounds) enters the caregiver's body through a break in the skin (e.g., open sore, cut).

HIV is **NOT** transmitted from client to caregiver during routine contact, such as touching, hugging, talking, transporting, bathing, or feeding. See Box 22-5 for myths and realities of AIDS.

When caring for the client with AIDS, it is very important that standard (universal) precautions and infection control procedures are followed. See Chapter 11 to review this information.

EFFECTS OF HIV ON THE IMMUNE SYSTEM

Clients infected with HIV may have no symptoms for a long time. However, the virus is multiplying and begins to affect the body's ability to fight infections and other diseases. The client may eventually show signs of infection, such as fever, fatigue, night sweats, diarrhea, and weight loss. These symptoms show that the body's natural defenses are no longer able to destroy the pathogenic organisms. Blood tests and a physical examination help the doctor to diagnose the client as having HIV. If diagnosed early in the course of the disease, the doctor prescribes a combination of powerful medications to increase the person's defense against the virus. THESE MEDICATIONS MUST BE TAKEN EACH DAY AT CERTAIN TIMES TO BE EFFECTIVE.

BOX 22-5   Myths and Realities of AIDS

The following are some myths and realities of the disease.

The Myth	The Reality
1. Only homosexuals and drug users get AIDS.	1. Anyone exposed to the HIV is at risk of contracting AIDS; HIV passes from the infected person into the other's bloodstream.
2. AIDS can be spread by touching, hugging, or being near a person with AIDS.	2. AIDS is not transmitted through casual contact.
3. Using public toilets and swimming pools are sources of the virus causing AIDS.	3. HIV is very fragile and does not survive for long outside the body.
4. Fewer people are becoming infected with HIV.	4. AIDS is increasing in adults who continue to practice high-risk behaviors such as unprotected sex and intravenous drug abuse.
5. HIV is primarily contracted by young adults 20 to 40 years of age.	5. The fastest growing group of those with HIV are older adults.

SKIPPING DOSES CAN BE DANGEROUS. While there is NO cure at the present time, early treatment of HIV has helped many people to live longer, more productive, and satisfying lives. This was not possible years ago. AIDS is the last stage of this chronic illness, but individuals with HIV often die of other illnesses.

Your client may have a variety of types of infections that affect many body systems. This is because the damaged immune system is no longer able to fight disease. As a result, both common and rare diseases may occur.

Caring for the client with AIDS means

• Using standard (universal) precautions to protect him or her from further infection

• Using standard (universal) precautions to protect yourself from the virus

THE CLIENT AS A PERSON

Sometimes, health care workers are so concerned with the proper procedures to take that they lose sight of the client as a person. Regardless of how HIV was acquired, the client is a human being who is living his or her life as fully as possible.

Because AIDS is a chronic illness, clients and their families may have times when they are discouraged and frustrated. Because AIDS is often a fatal illness, they may express many emotions, such as fear, anger, and sorrow. AIDS is an illness of many losses, and all concerned are deeply affected.

You can help both the client and family to cope with the effects of AIDS by showing, through action and communication, that you

• Accept the client as a person of worth

• Accept the family as they are—"family" may be the client's partner or friends

• Encourage both the client and family to express feelings and emotions

• Maintain a positive outlook

Families may be fearful of touching the loved one, afraid that AIDS is transmitted in this manner. Touching, caressing, and hugging are all ways of expressing tenderness and love. Encourage family members to have contact with the client through these means, if appropriate for their culture.

Sometimes, there may be conflicts between the client and other family members. Each may turn to you to express concerns. Your role includes listening and providing comfort and support. Use your listening skills. Share with your supervisor your own feelings and concerns about what they tell you.

Some clients will tell you how lonely it is to be homebound. Friends and family may not visit, fearing they will also become infected. Your visit may be the only contact the client has with another person.

SYMPTOMS

There are no "standard" symptoms for the client with AIDS. The types of symptoms vary according to the progress of the illness and the types of infection present. Some clients spend most of the day out of bed and may need some help with bathing and dressing. Others are so ill that they are in bed most of the time and require complete care.

YOUR ROLE

The client is at high risk for infection. Therefore, every action you take must be toward preventing possible infection. Listed below are some basic principles to follow. Your client's care plan will provide specific tasks to perform.

Communicating
- Follow the guidelines in Chapter 3 if your client is hearing- or visually-impaired.
- Use nonverbal communication to express your support; touch communicates just as well as words in many situations.
- Contact your supervisor if you believe that the client and/or family may need more assistance than you are able to give in handling the day-to-day problems of coping with AIDS.

Maintaining a Safe Environment
Safety includes using standard (universal) precautions when needed; disposing of client's waste according to policy and procedures of your agency; eliminating chances for infection; and maintaining home safety. Some tasks include the following:
- Keeping the living area well-ventilated, but avoiding drafts.
- Damp-dusting the client area, and keeping it as dust free as possible.
- Instructing the client about proper technique for coughing into tissues and disposing of them; many clients have pneumonia and cough up a lot of sputum.
- Discouraging persons who have colds or other infections from visiting the client.
- Following the directions in Chapters 8 and 9 for maintaining a safe, clean environment.
- Discouraging the client from cleaning birdcages, cat litter boxes, or fish tanks; organisms that live in these areas can easily travel to the client.
- Washing all fruits and vegetables thoroughly.
- Washing client's dishes with HOT, soapy water, using gloves; dishes do not have to be separated, unless indicated in the care plan.
- Following rules for standard (universal) precautions listed in Box 22-6 and Chapter 11.

Performing ADL
The amount of assistance required depends on the condition of the client. Fatigue is usually a common complaint. Follow the directions previously given in Box 22-1. Other tasks include the following:

> ### BOX 22-6   Basic Rules for Standard (Universal) Precautions
>
> - Wear gloves when there is a chance of being in contact with the client's blood, semen, vaginal secretions, mucous membranes, or other body fluids.
> - Wear gloves when the skin of your hands is broken or irritated.
> - Wash hands before applying gloves and immediately after removing gloves.
> - Wash hands immediately after being contaminated with blood or other body fluids.
> - Clean up blood or body fluid spills immediately with bleach and water solution (1:10); remember to prepare solution daily.
> - Do not handle used "sharps," such as needles or lancets.
> - Ask the client to place used "sharps," in puncture-resistant container or biohazard needle box container provided by your agency or community.
> - Wear personal protective equipment as required by your agency.
> - Avoid splashing when disposing of contents of bedpan, urinal, or commode; if splashing occurs, clean area immediately.
> - Wear gloves when disposing of soiled sanitary napkins or tampons.
> - Do not eat, drink, apply cosmetics, or handle contact lenses in areas where exposure to blood or other potentially infectious materials is possible.

- Using special care when performing oral hygiene, if the client has sores in the mouth, on the tongue or lips, or bleeding gums; be gentle, wear gloves, and follow directions given for cancer clients who have similar problems; the care plan may require the use of special medicated mouthwashes.
- Observing the skin for reddened areas or signs of skin breakdown: record and report.
- Encouraging good personal hygiene and grooming: assist as necessary.
- Following directions in the care plan for handling episodes of diarrhea, a common problem; wear gloves when washing anal area; when removing fecal material from clothing and bed linens; and when washing soiled materials.

Maintaining Proper Nutrition

One of the major symptoms of AIDS is loss of weight. As the illness progresses, clients lose a lot of weight. This is called *wasting*. Serving nutritious meals that the client will eat is a real challenge for the home care aide. Serving high-calorie supplements between meals may be ordered by the doctor. Listed below are some additional guidelines to follow.

- Avoid serving foods with high acid content (e.g., citrus, pineapple, tomatoes) for clients with sore mouths.
- Avoid serving foods containing raw eggs because of risk for infection.
- Encourage fluids, especially during episodes of diarrhea, to prevent dehydration.
- Boil tap water, according to directions in the care plan.
- Follow directions in Chapter 10 for clients who have nutrition problems caused by fatigue, difficulty swallowing, and so on.
- Prepare and store food properly: wash fresh fruits and vegetables thoroughly, and refrigerate leftovers immediately; see Chapter 10 for other directions to reduce the chance of infection from foods.
- Follow guidelines in Boxes 10-9, 10-11, 10-12, and 10-13 on pp. 156, 160, and 161.

Other Procedures

Your client may be receiving other treatments to handle a variety of problems, such as

- Oxygen, for difficulty breathing
- Intravenous fluids, for dehydration
- Intravenous medications, for infections
- Intravenous nutrition, for problems with nutrition

Follow the directions listed in Chapter 18 for caring for clients receiving these treatments.

Caring for clients with AIDS requires the home care aide to use all the knowledge learned in this program to give proper care. The care plan will give specific information to help you to give appropriate care to meet the client's needs. Unfortunately, the client will eventually develop an infection or disease that he or she can no longer fight. During this end stage of the illness, follow the information in Chapter 23 about caring for the client at the end of life.

ORR

Observe, Record, and Report
- Reddened areas on skin or skin breakdown
- Signs of infection
- Coughing, difficulty breathing
- Inability or failure to drink fluids or eat meals
- Unusual vaginal discharge
- Severe diarrhea
- Skin changes: Sores, draining wounds
- Decreased urinary output
- Confusion, changes in vision and hearing

THE POSTOPERATIVE CLIENT

DEFINITION

The term *postoperative* refers to the time after surgery.

THE FACTS

Some clients come home the day of surgery or the next day. Depending upon the type of operation, some people may be hospitalized for several days.

YOUR ROLE

Home care aides may care for postoperative clients. Your role depends on the following:
- Type of operation
- Condition of the client
- Type of care needed
  NOTE: Always follow the care plan.

Maintaining a Safe Environment
- Protect the client from falls.
- Support the client when ambulating.
- The surgical incision is an opening in the skin, the body's first line of defense against infection; nursing staff will change dressings and empty surgical drainage devices.
- Protect the client from **wound** infection.
- Report fever, pain in incision, and foul-smelling drainage on dressings.
- Practice standard (universal) precautions; do not handle anything stained with body drainage without wearing gloves.

- Wash hands according to the principles in Chapter 11.
- Teach the client to wash hands at appropriate times.
- Protect the client from infections of the respiratory tract by encouraging deep breathing, coughing (Procedure 22-1), moving, turning, and ambulation.
- Encourage the client to use an incentive spirometer (Figure 22-13) according to the care plan.
- Discourage visitors with respiratory infections.

PROCEDURE 22-1   Assisting Postoperative Clients to Deep Breathe and Cough

DEEP BREATHING

1. Explain what you are going to do.
2. Provide privacy (close door, shut drapes, pull shades).
3. Assist client into sitting position.
4. Have client place hands over lower end of rib cage with tips of middle fingers just touching each other.
5. Instruct client to deep breathe by
   a. Exhaling until the ribs move down as far as possible.
   b. Breathe in through the nose as deeply as possible. Client will be able to feel fingers separate during inhalation.
   c. Hold the breath for a count of three.
   d. Exhale slowly through pursed lips until the ribs move as far down as possible.
6. Repeat according to care plan, usually every 1 to 2 hours while awake.
7. Record what you have done. Report any unusual observations to your supervisor.

NOTE: An incentive spirometer is often used to assist clients with deep breathing. Follow instructions from your supervisor.

COUGHING

1. Explain what you are going to do.
2. Ask client to place interlaced fingers or a small pillow over the incision (chest or abdomen) (Figure 22-12, A and B).
3. Have client take two deep breaths (as above).
4. Tell client to take another deep breath, hold it for a count of 3, and then cough twice with the mouth open.
5. Repeat according to care plan, usually two or three coughs per hour.
6. Record what you have done. Report any unusual observations, such as bloody sputum or severe pain in operative area or chest.

CAUTION: Stand away from client. Do not let client cough on you. If client's hands are free, mouth should be covered with a tissue. Any sputum produced is coughed into tissue and discarded by client into waste container. If you are handling soiled tissues, wear gloves. If client is coughing on you, wear a mask.

Fig 22-12 **A,** The client places interlaced fingers over the incision. **B,** The client places a small pillow over the incision.

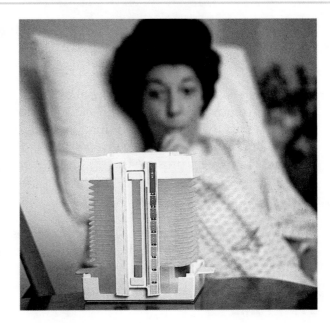

Fig 22-13 An incentive spirometer. (From Potter PA, Perry AG: *Fundamentals of nursing*, ed 7, St. Louis, 2009, Mosby.)

Performing ADL

- Assist as necessary; encourage movement and independence as permitted; most clients will be permitted to ambulate.
- Change position every 2 hours, and carry out range-of-motion exercises, if bed rest is ordered; leg exercises help to prevent formation of blood clots.
- Check output; be alert for constipation.

Maintaining Good Nutrition

- Offer fluids regularly.
- Follow special diet according to care plan.
- Use suggestions in Box 10-11 on p. 160 for loss of appetite, which is a common post-operative problem.

Providing Emotional Support

- Encourage the client to try to move and become more independent.
- Follow suggestions in Chapter 7, Working with Ill and Disabled Clients.

Special Procedures

- Assist with medications at the correct time.
- Reinforce dressings as necessary.
- Apply elastic stockings or bandages as directed.
- Encourage the client to perform exercises taught by the physical therapist.

Observe, Record, and Report

- Signs of infection
  Fever
  Foul-smelling drainage
  Coughing up sputum
  Redness and swelling at site of incision
- Fresh blood on dressings
- Nausea and vomiting
- Constipation
- Pain in chest and/or difficulty breathing
- Leg pain, especially in calf muscles

CARING FOR A CLIENT WITH A PROSTHESIS

DEFINITION

A prosthesis is a mechanical device used to replace a part of the body that has been surgically removed (amputated) because of disease or injury. Sometimes a prosthesis replaces a part that is deformed due to a birth defect. Prostheses are specially made to fit the client by a specialist, called a *prosthetist*. Plastic, metal, and wood are some materials used to make a prosthesis.

THE FACTS

Prostheses are very expensive. One that replaces an upper or lower leg may cost more than $35,000. Circulatory problems and diabetes are two of the most frequent causes of amputation.

SYMPTOMS

After recovering from surgery, the client often goes to a rehabilitation center. Learning to adjust physically and emotionally to the loss of a limb can be a long, difficult process. Clients may mourn their loss in silence or express their feelings verbally or nonverbally. It is not unusual for them to be sad during this period of adjustment.

Some clients will tell you about pain, tingling, or numbness in the missing limb. This is called *phantom limb pain,* and it is due to changes in the region of the brain that once controlled the function of the now-missing limb. These feelings are real and should not be viewed by others as "silly" or "crazy." Medical researchers are experimenting with ways to eliminate these symptoms.

YOUR ROLE

While at the rehabilitation center, the client learns to apply and remove the prosthesis. If a part of the arm or leg is amputated, the prosthesis fits over the stump. A stockinette covers the stump to protect the skin. Learning the proper care and maintenance of the prosthesis is very important for both client and caregiver. The physical therapist instructs the client about exercises to perform so that the remaining muscles of the limb remain strong. The occupational therapist teaches the client to perform ADL using the prosthesis.

Your role in assisting the client may include the following:
- Placing the prosthesis near the client so that it can be reached
- Assisting the client to put on or remove the prosthesis, if necessary
- Storing the prosthesis properly after the client has removed it
- Washing and drying the stockinette, if the client is unable to perform this activity. Wash with mild soap and water. Rinse well before drying. Store stockinette in proper location.

ORR Observe, Record, and Report
- The condition of the stump; note any signs of pressure, such as redness, bluish color, bruising, or skin breakdown
- Signs of pressure in areas where the prosthesis touches the skin, other than the stump (redness, bluish color, bruising, pressure ulcer)
- Signs of infection
- Complaints of pain or discomfort in the stump or other area

SUPPORT GROUPS

Many communities sponsor support groups to assist clients and caregivers to cope with the day-to-day aspects of living with the illnesses described in this chapter. These groups, usually led by a health professional and/or counselor, provide the chance for members to share their experiences, discuss ways to handle typical problems, and express feelings and concerns. Through participating in support groups, clients and caregivers say that they receive encouragement and renewed strength to cope with the limitations of the illness.

Sponsors of support groups include local hospitals and medical and rehabilitation centers. Local chapters of national organizations, such as the Alzheimer's Association, American Lung Association, American Heart Association, and the American Cancer Society, also sponsor support groups. Information about where and when the groups meet can be obtained by telephoning the sponsoring agency/association, or by checking their Internet website that contains valuable information about services available to clients and caregivers.

CHAPTER SUMMARY

The home care aide cares for clients with many conditions.
- Frequently seen conditions are
  - Cardiovascular diseases
  - Cancer
  - Stroke (CVA)
  - Chronic obstructive pulmonary disease (COPD)
  - Diabetes mellitus
  - Alzheimer's disease
  - Multiple sclerosis
  - Parkinson's disease
  - Arthritis
  - Fractures
  - AIDS
  - Amputation with prosthesis
- Your role includes
  - Communicating with client and family
  - Maintaining a safe environment
  - Performing ADL
  - Maintaining good nutrition
  - Assisting with special procedures
- Clients returning after surgery require special care. The home care aide watches for and reports abnormal signs and symptoms.
- Support groups provide caregivers and clients with the opportunity to
  - Share experiences
  - Express feelings and concerns
  - Discuss ways to cope with the day-to-day aspects of living with the illness
- Home care aides provide emotional support to clients and family members coping with illness.
- Standard (universal) precautions and infection control practices are essential in the care of all clients.

STUDY QUESTIONS

1. Select six conditions described in this chapter, and give two ways in which you will do the following:
   a. Communicate with the client
   b. Maintain a safe environment
   c. Perform ADL
   d. Maintain good nutrition

   Also, list three observations to report to your supervisor (Observe, Record, and Report).
2. Describe the care of a postoperative client. What will you watch for and report to your supervisor?

Continued

STUDY QUESTIONS—cont'd

3. Identify a support group in your community. Where does it meet? How often? What are its purposes?

4. List two ways the home care aide can provide emotional support for the client (or family) with the following:
   a. AIDS
   b. Alzheimer's disease
   c. Stroke
   d. Cancer
   e. Multiple sclerosis
   f. Amputation
   e. Cardiovascular disease

5. Discuss how you will use the principles of standard (universal) precautions and infection control when caring for clients with the following:
   a. COPD
   b. AIDS
   c. Diabetes
   d. Cancer
   e. Parkinson's disease
   f. Arthritis
   g. Surgical wounds

23

Caring for the Client at the End of Life

OBJECTIVES

After you read this chapter, you will be able to:

1. Recognize your own feelings about death and dying.
2. Discuss the emotional reactions of clients and their families to a terminal illness.
3. Define the terms *living will, durable power of attorney,* and *DNR (do not resuscitate)*.
4. Understand the hospice approach to caring for clients who have a terminal illness.
5. Explain how the home care aide meets the physical, emotional, social, and spiritual needs of the dying client.
6. Identify the signs of approaching death and the signs of death.
7. Give postmortem care.

KEY TERMS

AND Abbreviation for "allow natural death"
Bereaved Those who mourn the death of a loved one
DNR Abbreviation for "do not resuscitate," meaning do not artificially restart the heartbeat
Durable power of attorney Advance directive that names another to make health care decisions if a person becomes unable to do so
Empathy Understanding the feelings of another

End-stage disease Terminal or final illness
Expire Die
Living will Advance directive that specifies treatment to be given or withheld if a person becomes terminally ill or incapable of making decisions himself or herself
Postmortem After death
Rite(s) Formal ritual(s) used in religious or solemn practices
Terminal illness Illness that causes the end of life

Louis Roupp has been having much difficulty breathing and is using his portable oxygen all the time. When Russ Larson visited yesterday, he noticed that Louis' lips and nails were bluish. His pulse was weak and rapid. "I'm so tired and my chest hurts. I can't take care of myself much longer. I'm so afraid." Russ put his arm around Louis' shoulder and comforted him. "Mr. Roupp, I'm going to call my supervisor to tell her how you are feeling," said Russ. After discussing his observations with Mrs. Randolph, Russ called 9-1-1 as she had directed and waited with Mr. Roupp for the ambulance to arrive. Mr. Roupp was admitted to the hospital. His condition was very serious. Russ thought, "This will probably be the last time I see Mr. Roupp alive." His eyes started to tear.

> **BOX 23-1   Attitudes About Death**
>
> - When did you first learn about death?
> - Who died?
> - Who told you about death?
> - What feelings do you remember?
> - What did you do about those feelings?
> - Did you attend the funeral/memorial service/burial?

At some time during your career as a home care aide, you may be assigned the care of a client who will not recover from his or her illness. This client is said to have a terminal illness or end-stage disease. No matter which term is used, the client is expected to die.

You may feel uncomfortable being around a person who is dying. You may not know what to say or do for this client. Because of your own feelings about death and dying, you may want to avoid spending time with your client. This behavior, of course, causes the client to feel abandoned, rejected, and isolated. It is important for you to examine and understand your own feelings about death (Box 23-1). We learned these from family members, and they may change as we grow older. Religious and cultural influences affect our attitudes about death. Some people believe that death is the end of everything; others believe in an eternal afterlife, where the good are rewarded and the evil are punished. Others may believe in reincarnation into a new life or life form. Whatever your attitudes or beliefs, the fact remains that we all will die. Humans do not live forever.

Most clients are told that they are dying. This is done by the physician or a family member. Sometimes, the family does not want the client to know that the illness is terminal. In this case, you must follow their wishes. This can be very difficult for you because you may feel as if you are lying to your client. Discuss these feelings and your concerns with your supervisor. Other times, clients learn their diagnosis without being told. They make this discovery by

- Reading their medical records when no one is looking
- Overhearing conversations about their condition
- Realizing that they are becoming sicker, not better
- Recognizing that the treatment is no longer effective and may be stopped

EMOTIONAL REACTIONS TO DEATH AND DYING

We all know that we are going to die some day. No one gets out of this world alive. Someone has said that "we are all dying of a terminal illness, it is called life." However, the news that one has a fatal illness can be overwhelming, and there are many emotional reactions in response to this information. Some feelings will come and go; there will be peaks and valleys—like riding on a roller coaster (Figure 23-1). Clients' families, too, will have these reactions. In some cases, feelings will be verbally expressed. In other cases, nothing will be discussed—it will all be held inside, within a wall of silence. Reactions may include but are limited to those that follow.

DENIAL

Denial is a defense mechanism that protects the client from unpleasant reality. "Oh, no, it can't be true." "Not me, the lab must have made a mistake." These quotes are expressions of denial. (See Reactions of the Client to Illness in Chapter 7.)

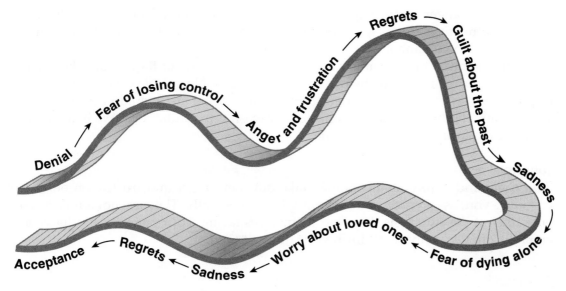

Fig 23-1 Roller coaster of emotions.

The family, too, may express denial. "How could this happen?" "He never smoked—and now they say that he has lung cancer. It just can't be true."

Your Role
Adjusting to the diagnosis of an end-stage illness is overwhelming and devastating. It takes some time to get used to the idea that there may not be a cure for this illness. Try to understand everyone's need to deny what is happening. Partial acceptance may follow, but sometimes denial will continue. In this case, do not argue with your client and/or the family. Do not try to change their thinking. Accept the client's behavior, and understand the reasons for it. Discuss your feelings with your supervisor.

FEAR AND WORRY

Clients are afraid of many things: pain, loss of control, dying alone, rejection by family and friends, not knowing what is going to happen, and when and how the disease will affect them. They worry about finances, family responsibilities, and being a burden to loved ones. Families, too, have similar emotions and concerns about being caregivers of a dying person, caring for their own health, and carrying out their responsibilities of daily life.

Your Role
Listen to the client and the family as they express their concerns. This is a very difficult time for everyone. Provide reassurances, if appropriate. Your supervisor can arrange assistance from the agency, perhaps from the social worker.

ANGER AND FRUSTRATION

These emotions may be expressed verbally. "If I had only followed my doctor's instructions." Or, they may be focused on others. "I lived a good life—why am I being punished by God, now?" "Agnes, you're my wife, you should have insisted that I quit smoking. Now, I have terminal lung cancer and it's all your fault." Anger and frustration may also be directed at you, the home care aide. "You do everything wrong; why can't you do something right!"

Sometimes, anger is not expressed verbally, but by the client's actions (e.g., not speaking to relatives, friends, or even the home care aide) or by facial expression and other types of body language.

Family members may be angry and frustrated for many of the reasons the client is angry. "She never followed the doctor's instructions. Now, I have to assume all this responsibility. It's not fair!" "I tried to help him, but he just wouldn't listen. What a selfish man." "Why am I being punished? It wasn't my fault." Or, "We had so many plans for the future. Now, it's too late."

Your Role

Both client and family members may take out their anger and frustration on others including you, as caregiver. But, do not take it personally. They are not angry at you, but rather at the situations they find themselves facing. Your patience, kindness, and empathy are very important during this difficult time.

SADNESS

Anger can also turn to sadness when the client realizes that what caused the anger cannot be changed. The illness is progressing, and past events cannot be changed, either. Some reasons for sadness include: (1) Regrets about the past—what could have been or should have been. (2) Loss of physical strength and normal daily activities (e.g., shopping with friends, bowling) and loss of normal body functioning (e.g., incontinence). (3) The "unfinished business of life" that will never happen—taking that long-planned-for trip. (4) Loss of the future—not being able to attend the high school graduation of a grandchild or not celebrating another wedding anniversary. (5) Helplessness—unable to control the advancing illness or unable to provide financial help for family and loved ones.

Family members also experience sadness as they see the physical changes in their loved one. They are coping with their own day-to-day roller-coaster emotions. They, too, may have regrets about their relationship with the dying person. Coping with the physical and emotional aspects of caregiving may be a new experience for them. Handling one's emotions while caring for a loved one can be exhausting. Remember that the family is also in the process of losing the future—a future without the loved one. So, sadness is an emotion felt by both client and family.

Your Role

There are many reasons for both the client and family's feelings of sadness. Do not attempt to "cheer them up" or try to comfort them by saying "Everything will be okay" or "Don't cry." Sadness is a normal reaction, and crying is "okay." In fact, crying can help to relieve stress, even though it is temporary. When appropriate, a touch on the hand, a hug, or placing your arm around the shoulder may provide the comfort needed by your client or family member. If the client or family wants to talk, use your listening skills. Be careful not to give advice. Sadness is part of the preparation for death and final separation for both client and family.

GUILT

Both the client and family members may express the feeling, "I should have gone to the doctor earlier." "I could have _____." "If only I/we had _____." These are common statements signifying guilt. Some clients may see the terminal illness as punishment from God for something they did (or did not do) earlier in life.

Your Role

Reassure client and family that they did the best they could at the time. Now they view things differently because they have new and different information. For those who feel that they are being punished, comfort and reassurance may be offered by a member of the clergy. Discuss this with your supervisor. He or she may be able to assist the client and family to work out some of the feelings of guilt.

ACCEPTANCE

The client is neither depressed nor angry. The client is just there and seems to have almost no feelings. At this time, the family needs support because the client begins to withdraw from them. Many times family members cannot understand why the client is "giving up" and will not fight the disease any longer. However, there comes a time when the body is no longer able to fight, no matter what the family wants. Of course, not all clients quietly accept death, close their eyes, and die. Some will fight the illness and continue treatment for as long as possible.

Your Role

This may be a difficult time for the family—the reality of death is near. Or, they may feel a sense of relief that their loved one is at peace. Provide the kinds of support discussed earlier in the chapter. Your calm, quiet presence may be most appreciated at this time.

ADVANCE DIRECTIVES

Advance directives are documents in which a person states choices for medical treatment (or appoints others to make treatment choices) if he or she should lose decision-making ability.

Advance directives include the living will and durable power of attorney.

LIVING WILL

- Written instructions
- Called a living will because it takes effect while the person is still alive
- Specifies treatment to be provided or withheld if a person becomes terminally ill and/or incapable of making decisions himself or herself; for example, the document may specify
  Organ donation after death (which organs)
  DNR (do not resuscitate)
  AND (allow natural death) is a newer advance directive term. It means not interfering with the natural dying process.

DURABLE POWER OF ATTORNEY

- Written instructions
- Names another person (called a "proxy") to make health care decisions if the person is unable to do so
  An advance directive can be changed or canceled at any time. It does not go into effect until the time when the client can no longer make or communicate decisions for himself or herself. Loved ones should be included in advance directives discussion and decision making.

The home care agency provides all adult clients with information about their rights under state and federal laws to make health care decisions. This includes the right to refuse or accept treatment and the right to carry out advance directives. This is clearly explained in the Client's Bill of Rights. **IF YOU OR YOUR CLIENT (AND FAMILY) HAVE ANY QUESTIONS CONCERNING ADVANCE DIRECTIVES, NOTIFY YOUR SUPERVISOR.**

HOSPICE

Some people who are at home with end-stage disease will be in a hospice program sponsored by the community home care agency. Hospice care is also available in special units of hospitals or in residential homes in the community. Hospice is a special concept of care designed to provide comfort and support to clients and their families when a life-limiting illness no longer responds to cure-oriented treatments. These programs provide physical, social, emotional, and spiritual care given by a medically supervised team of professionals and volunteers. One of the main goals of hospice care is to help clients live comfortably until they die and to help the family live with them as they are dying. The focus is on *caring* rather than on curing. All services are provided through the hospice program. As death approaches, there are no calls to 9-1-1 for emergency medical services. All calls are directed to the hospice. You will direct calls and questions to your supervisor.

The principles of hospice care include
- Providing comfort when cure is no longer possible with special emphasis on controlling client's pain and discomfort
- Giving care to the whole person and whole family
- Placing the client and family at the CENTER of the hospice team (Figure 23-2)
- Offering education, preparation, and support about the natural process of dying
- Having a system of care that supports the client and family 24 hours a day, 7 days a week
- Supporting the bereaved for 1 year or longer after the client's death

To work in a hospice program is a commitment to be there for the client and family—for the "long haul." They rely on the hospice team, especially the home care aide, to provide personal care and hygiene for the client.

It is almost as if you become a family member; you are "in it" with them. Clients have a great fear of being deserted; do not abandon them. If you will be late for work

Fig 23-2 The client and caregiver are at the heart of the hospice program.

or absent, notify your supervisor so the family will not worry about you and a substitute can be sent.

Mrs. Stevens has been treated for cancer for many months. She has had chemotherapy and radiation, but now she's weaker, has lost more weight, and has a lot of pain. Mrs. Stevens asks her daughter to come with her for her checkup at the oncologist's office. During the visit, the doctor explained to both of them that the cancer was spreading. "There are some experimental drugs that may help. Are you interested in trying more treatments?" asked the doctor. "No, I've had enough. I just want to have less pain and be as comfortable as I can for the time I have left," said Mrs. Stevens. Then the doctor recommends the services of hospice and explains how hospice can help both Mrs. Stevens and her family. After discussing the situation with her daughter and other family members, Mrs. Stevens agrees to have the local hospice coordinator visit the next day to make the necessary arrangements.

CARING FOR THE DYING CLIENT

The following principles are important to remember when caring for clients with end-stage disease.

HELP CLIENTS LIVE UNTIL THEY DIE

- Encourage socialization (Figure 23-3).
- Use listening skills. **ALWAYS BE HONEST; YOU WILL BE ASKED MANY QUESTIONS THAT YOU WILL BE UNABLE TO ANSWER. SAY, "I DON'T KNOW, BUT I'LL ASK MY SUPERVISOR"** (Box 23-2).
- Help the client to finish any unfinished business. For example, Mr. Schmidt wanted to make a quilt for each one of his children. His home care aide gathered all the materials and placed them within Mr. Schmidt's reach so he could complete his work. The aide arranged Mr. Schmidt's schedule so that he would have the energy to do what was important to him.
- Offer your clients some control over their lives. Give them choices regarding routines, foods, activities, and so on.

Fig 23-3 Encourage socialization for dying clients.

> ### BOX 23-2 Communicating with the Dying Client
>
> - Sit at eye level with the client.
> - Gently touch the client; place your hand on the client's hand or forearm.
> - Let the client talk or not, as he or she wishes.
> - Do not worry if the client is silent; he or she knows that you are there. Just be quiet and "be there."
> - Listen, without judging. Clients may feel anger, guilt, and sadness.
> - Be truthful; if the client says he or she is going to die, do not contradict him or her. Use your listening skills (see Chapter 3).

- Promote independence; encourage your client to do as much as possible within his or her ability and energy level.
- Offer comfort and support.

ENCOURAGE HOPE

- Hope is present throughout the process of dying.
- Hope keeps the client going through the time of suffering; it maintains the spirit and helps people to go on.
- Hope changes. Clients hope for a better day tomorrow, a good sleep tonight, less pain, expecting the best and preparing for the worst.
- Hope for a "miracle" of a complete cure is always present. We all hope for this along with the client and family. While this is not realistic, it is always in the "back of one's mind." Do not discourage the client's hope and demand that he or she be realistic. Research has revealed that people with hope live longer and have a better quality of life than do those who are hopeless. If and when acceptance comes, and hope seems to be gone, just listen to your clients and care for their needs. Hope for recovery may not be appropriate at this time.

RELIEVE PAIN

Review the information on observing pain in Chapter 6, pp. 78–82.

- Assist the client to take medications as ordered. These are usually taken every 4 hours (q4h) around the clock, instead of when needed.
- When pain medication is to be taken as needed (PRN), clients should take it when the pain begins and not wait until the pain becomes unbearable.
- Keep the client's environment as quiet and calm as possible to promote rest and sleep. Music may be soothing and comforting.
- Good hygiene, a back rub, and clean bed linens also promote comfort and will enhance the effect of the pain-relieving medications (Figure 23-4).
- If activity causes pain, provide personal care about 1 hour after the client takes his or her medication.

Notify your supervisor, if the following occur:

- Medication is not effective in relieving pain
- Client wants to take more medication than what was prescribed
- Client wants to take the medication more frequently
- Client refuses to take the pain medication
- Client has difficulty having bowel movements; observe the stool, and report problems (many pain medications cause constipation)

Fig 23-4 A back rub can help clients to rest and relax.

Fig 23-5 The chaplain attends to the client's spiritual needs.

ASSIST WITH RELIGIOUS CONSOLATION

- Some clients will find their own relationship with God a strong source of strength at this time. Clients may want you to read scriptures or other religious books to them. Do so.
- Allow time for visits from clergy, the chaplain, or others from the client's religious community or the hospice program (Figure 23-5). Have the client ready for the visit. Whenever possible, schedule personal care and hygiene activities before the visit so the client feels and looks as good as possible.
- Catholic clients who wish to receive the Sacrament of Reconciliation will need private time alone with the priest. For Sacrament of the Sick, the priest anoints the client with blessed oils and prays for healing. Family members may be present and pray with the priest. For those clients who are receiving Holy Communion (Eucharist), have a glass of water nearby.
- When a client's religious belief is unfamiliar to you, ask the family or your supervisor to explain the belief and its rites to you.
- If your client does not belong to any specific faith tradition and wants to see a clergyperson, the hospice team will be able to help. Notify your supervisor about your client's need.
- Some clients will not find religion to be a source of help. Recognize that each person has his or her own needs and beliefs that are to be respected.
- Do not perform religious activities unless the client asks you to do so.

PROVIDE GOOD PHYSICAL CARE

- Meet client's needs for grooming, hygiene, and toileting.
- Keep skin clean and dry; change positions and perform range-of-motion exercises; skin breaks down very quickly.
- Report any skin changes to your supervisor immediately.
- Give mouth care before meals.

- Offer foods and liquids that the client likes and is able to consume.
- Do not force the client to eat.
- Follow the care plan regarding protein supplements and special preparation of food.
- Feed the client as necessary. (See Chapter 10 to review information on feeding clients.)
- As body systems fail, increasing physical care is needed. Always practice standard (universal) precautions to prevent infection.
- Try to anticipate your client's needs.

NEEDS OF CAREGIVERS

This is a difficult and stressful time for caregivers. Accept their feelings, listen to them, and demonstrate your concerns for them. Acknowledge their problems. Caregivers will express many emotions: anger, fear, guilt. Other problems may be expressed, including watching a loved one die, worry about income, worry about their own physical problems, exhaustion, and so on. You cannot solve all of the caregiver's problems. Let your supervisor know what is happening. The hospice program can provide assistance, such as a social worker or volunteer to visit the caregiver. Perhaps some time off can be arranged to relieve (briefly) the stress of caregiving.

NEEDS OF THE HOME CARE AIDE

Caring for dying people is hard work, both physically and emotionally. You will have many feelings about working with hospice clients. Do not withdraw from your client and caregiver. Discuss your feelings with your supervisor. You may participate in hospice team meetings. Do not be afraid to discuss your feelings and observations with team members. Perhaps you just need to express what you are feeling and know that it is "okay" to feel this way. Perhaps you need some time off or a different assignment. The most important thing is to remember that you have needs, too, so take care of yourself, as well as your client.

SIGNS OF APPROACHING DEATH

As death approaches, physical changes can be seen as each system shuts down. Many clients slip into death very much like the way they have fallen asleep during life. Seizures, hemorrhages, and a "death agony" are quite uncommon, although these may happen. If family members are present, let them stay with the client and assist with personal care, if they are able.

THE LAST SENSE TO LEAVE THE DYING PERSON IS HEARING. REMEMBER, THE CLIENT MAY BE ABLE TO HEAR WHAT IS GOING ON, EVEN IF HE OR SHE IS UNABLE TO RESPOND. Everyone should speak with the client knowing he or she understands and needs to know who is there and what is happening. Holding the loved one's hand, saying "I'm here" is very comforting. This, too, may be the time to say any last words and good-byes to the dying person.

On her last visit to Mrs. Stevens, Rosina realized that her client was much weaker and much sicker than before. It was hard for Mrs. Stevens to breathe. Her respirations were very fast, and it was hard for her to talk. She could just about whisper, and it took almost all of her strength. Rosina bathed Mrs. Stevens, gave her a back rub, and changed the linens on her hospital bed. Mrs. Stevens looked so clean and comfortable that Rosina smiled, knowing that she had helped her client feel a little better.

When Rosina was ready to leave, Mrs. Stevens held her hand and whispered, "Rosina, I might not be here the next time you come. So, I just want to thank you for taking such good care of me. You are like a part of my family—I love you." Rosina and Mrs. Stevens both began to cry as they held each other's hands. "I'll never forget you and all the things you told me about your life and living on this farm," Rosina told her client. "I will miss you, Mrs. Stevens. Good-bye."

As Rosina walked down the path to her car, she thought about the first time she cared for a client with a terminal illness. "I was so scared, but I am not scared anymore. I am privileged to meet people like Mrs. Stevens and to help them in the last stage of their lives. I am blessed to be able to help their families, too, when they are having such a hard time. I know Mrs. Stevens is going to die very soon. I will really miss her, her husband, and coming out to this farm. I did my best to give her comfort and rest. I think I did a good job."

Common physical changes in the near-to-death client include the following:

- Circulation is slowed. The pulse becomes rapid and weak, almost impossible to count. The skin becomes cold, especially the arms, legs, hands, feet, and nose. Cover the client with a light blanket, and elevate the limbs to return the flow of blood to the heart. A heavy blanket will make the client too warm and restless from trying to remove the covers. Lips and nail beds may be cyanotic. Oxygen may be given.
- Respirations are slow, irregular, and shallow until breathing stops. Clients breathe through the mouth. Give oral hygiene frequently. Be careful the client does not aspirate liquids. Moisten and lubricate lips and tissues of the mouth frequently. Breathing may become noisy from mucus in the throat, the "death rattle."
- Incontinence may occur. Keep the client clean and dry. Provide good skin care to prevent additional discomfort from skin breakdown.
- The client becomes very still. Movement is almost absent. Sensations gradually disappear.
- Appetite and thirst are lost, although some clients awaken from an unconscious state and take tiny sips of fluids or small pieces of ice.
- The client is usually unconscious.

Death may come quickly, over a period of hours, but, for some persons, the process of active dying may take several days. This is emotionally and physically draining for family and caregivers. You will know that death has occurred when your client has stopped breathing for a few minutes and you cannot feel a pulse. Note the time, and call your supervisor.

You may feel very sad that your client has died. You may even cry along with the family and loved ones (Figure 23-6). This is normal. Home care agencies and hospices hold "support sessions" for staff members whose clients have died. It helps, and it is important to discuss your feelings and experiences when your client expires.

CARE AFTER DEATH

Care of the body after death is called postmortem care. Once you have notified your supervisor of the client's death, the doctor and funeral director are notified. Before the funeral director can remove the body, the client must be legally/officially pronounced dead. The procedure for this pronouncement varies from state to state. Your agency will know what to do.

Fig 23-6 Sharing your sorrow with the client's family is a normal and natural reaction.

The body is prepared for removal from the home. The family may need some time alone with the client to say the final good-byes. Some specific religious or cultural practices may be followed at this time. Special preparation of the body may be done by the caregiver or others according to religious rites. These should be done only after the legal pronouncement of death. Check with your supervisor concerning religious and cultural practices. Some families may wish to have their clergyperson notified.

When appropriate, and according to agency policy, prepare the body in the following manner:

- Place one pillow under the head.
- Bathe the body, if necessary; clean the genital area if there has been any incontinence. Use standard (universal) precautions.
- Reinforce dressings if needed (don't forget to wear gloves).
- Close eyes; put dentures in mouth, if possible.
- Keep the body flat on back, legs straight, arms folded over the abdomen.
- Follow agency policy regarding jewelry; if taken by family members, be sure to record who took what off the body.
- Do not try to straighten limbs if there are contractures.

After the body is removed from the room, strip the bed and wash the linens, if there is sufficient time. Equipment is removed; rented equipment is returned to the providers. The hospice program arranges to have equipment returned.

You may wish to attend the viewing and funeral of your client. This will give you a chance to say good-bye and to let the family know that you really did care for the client. This is your decision; there is no right or wrong. You must do what is best for you.

CHAPTER SUMMARY

- The home care aide's feelings about death and dying will influence his or her ability to care for dying clients. You may feel uncomfortable caring for dying persons; this is normal.

- Both client and family react to the diagnosis of a terminal illness. Typical emotions include the following:
  Denial
  Anger and Frustration

CHAPTER SUMMARY—cont'd

Fear and Worry
Sadness
Guilt
Acceptance

- Advance directives are documents in which a person states choices for medical treatment if he or she should lose decision-making ability.
- Hospice is a program that provides total care for dying clients, which includes the physical, social, emotional, and spiritual needs of the client.
- Guidelines for caring for dying persons include the following:
   Help client live until he or she dies
   Encourage hope
   Relieve pain
   Assist with religious consolation
   Provide good physical care
- Caring for dying persons is hard work, both emotionally and physically. If you have concerns, questions, and uncomfortable feelings, you are not unusual. Discuss these feelings with your supervisor.
- The home care aide recognizes the signs of approaching death and offers comfort to both client and family.
- Follow agency policy and procedures when the client has died.

STUDY QUESTIONS

1. What are two factors that influence our attitudes about death?
2. How do people find out they have a terminal illness? What are the "typical" emotional reactions?
3. Define the following terms:
   Advance directives
   Living will
   Durable power of attorney
   DNR
   AND
   Hospice
4. List five principles to remember when caring for clients with end-stage disease. Explain three ways the home care aide can implement each.
5. List five signs of approaching death.
6. What are the home care aide's responsibilities when the client has died?
7. Discuss appropriate behavior for the home care aide whose client has expired.

24

Emergencies

OBJECTIVES

After you read this chapter, you will be able to:

1. Define the term *emergency*.
2. Describe three ways to prepare for medical emergencies.
3. Discuss five rules to follow when there is an emergency.
4. List the information needed to report an emergency by telephone.
5. Describe first aid procedures to follow for four common medical emergencies.
6. Discuss the importance of recording and reporting your actions in an emergency to your employer.
7. Describe the use of standard (universal) precautions when giving first aid.

KEY TERMS

First aid Immediate care given before treatment by trained medical personnel
Medical crisis Event requiring immediate attention

Shock Condition in which the circulatory system is not able to transport adequate amounts of blood to all parts of the body

Russ Larson has just entered the front door of his client's (Marjorie) apartment house when her daughter runs from the elevator screaming and crying. She pulls his arm and leads him into the kitchen of the apartment. Russ finds Marjorie sitting at the table, unable to speak or breathe, with her hands around her neck. Her face is turning blue, but she is conscious. The daughter says that her mother started to choke while eating a piece of meat and then stopped breathing. Russ tells the daughter to call 9-1-1 for help. He immediately performs abdominal thrusts (Heimlich maneuver) to help Marjorie cough up the meat from the windpipe and begin to breathe again. The piece of meat comes out after the second thrust. "You are a miracle worker," says Marjorie. "I thought I would die—you came just in time."

Recognizing an emergency, calling for help, and giving first aid calmly and skillfully are responsibilities of the home care aide.

WHAT IS AN EMERGENCY?

The term *emergency* is used when the following are present:
- Serious situation
- Arises suddenly
- Threatens the life or welfare of a person or group of persons

Emergencies may be due to accidents (injury to leg due to falling from a ladder), a medical crisis (chest pain), or natural disasters (injuries due to a hurricane or tornado).

Each emergency situation needs immediate action. This is called first aid. It is the immediate care given to the person before treatment by trained medical personnel.

PREPARING FOR EMERGENCIES

Because emergencies arise suddenly, using time wisely is critical. For example, taking time to search for emergency telephone numbers so help can be called is not wise. SO, PLANNING FOR EMERGENCIES IN ADVANCE IS VERY IMPORTANT.

EMERGENCY TELEPHONE NUMBERS

In Chapter 8, Box 8-8 on p. 118 is a sample of information needed in case of a household emergency. This information can also be used in medical emergencies. Most communities have a 9-1-1 number to contact emergency medical services (EMS). The person answering the telephone is called an "emergency dispatcher" who has special training in handling crisis situations over the telephone. The dispatcher will ask questions to find out what type of help is needed (police, fire, or medical services). **Answer the questions as completely and clearly as possible.** The dispatcher will also give directions about what to do while waiting for emergency medical personnel to arrive. **Do not hang up the telephone unless told to do so.** See Box 24-1 for the types of questions you should be prepared to answer.

KNOWING WHAT TO DO

This chapter gives some common medical emergencies that may occur in the home and other places. However, it does not include all possible emergency situations. You are encouraged to take a first aid course and be certified to perform cardiopulmonary resuscitation (CPR). This is a procedure used to maintain critical oxygen and blood flow to the heart and brain until EMS personnel arrive. Another procedure, hands-only CPR, involves no mouth-to-mouth contact. Agencies in your community offer such courses, including the local evening adult school or community college, local chapter of the American Red Cross, or your own home care agency. Being trained in first aid and using these skills in an emergency can mean the difference between life and death for the victim. Being prepared helps to reduce fears and panic that many feel when an emergency occurs. Panic can make a person immobile. THE WORST THING TO DO IN AN EMERGENCY IS NOTHING.

BOX 24-1   Reporting an Emergency

Answer the questions that the dispatcher asks. Typical questions are
1. What is the exact location or address of the emergency?
   - Give name of town, city, or area, and address
   - Give landmarks, nearest cross streets
   - Give building name, floor, room, or apartment number
   - Give other information that will help in finding the location
2. Where are you calling from?
   - Provide telephone number
3. Who are you?
   - Give your name and title
4. What happened? How many people are involved?
   - Give as much information as possible, as briefly as possible
5. What is the condition of the victim(s)?
   - Provide information as requested
6. What first aid is being given?
   - Tell what you are doing

Stay on the telephone until you are told to hang up or the dispatcher hangs up.

Fig 24-1 Four signs of a life-threatening emergency.

CALLING FOR HELP

When in doubt, call for help. The following situations require an immediate call for help:

The victim
- Is unconscious
- Has no pulse
- Is not breathing or has difficulty breathing
- Is bleeding severely (Figure 24-1)

Sometimes, the victim may not want you to call for help, but you must use your judgment. **When in doubt about calling for help, CALL.** In many situations, minutes, even seconds, count in getting the proper care for the person.

When a telephone is not available, you should know where the nearest telephone is located. If another person is in the home, ask him or her to make the call for help. Prepare the person to answer questions about the victim. In this case, your role is to stay with the victim until help arrives. If you are alone and there are neighbors nearby, shout for help.

THE FIRST AID KIT

Having a first aid kit available is another way to prepare for an emergency. A kit should be available to use in the home, automobile, workplace, and other locations (e.g., boats,

BOX 24-2   Important Parts of the First Aid Kit

- Adhesive tape
- Cotton balls
- Gauze pads and roller gauze
- Scissors and tweezer
- Adhesive bandages (assorted sizes)

- Antiseptic solution
- Antibiotic ointment
- Hand cleaner
- Disposable gloves and face mask

BOX 24-3   The Four Cs of Emergency Care

Caution is always taken; never put yourself in danger.
Check the victim's condition and area where found.
Call 9-1-1 or your local emergency number.
Check the victim until help arrives, using the first aid skills you have learned.

BOX 24-4   Preventing Infection

FIRST AID SITUATIONS THAT INCREASE THE HOME CARE AIDE'S RISK FOR INFECTION

Victim Is

- Bleeding
- Vomiting
- Coughing up sputum
- Incontinent

The Wound Is

- Bleeding
- Weeping fluid
- Caused by a bite (animal or insect)
- Caused by chemicals

Take Precautions

- Create a barrier between yourself and any body fluids and/or mucous membranes.
  Use disposable or utility gloves, if available.
  or
  Use a plastic bag or plastic wrap to cover your hands, if available.
  or
  Use a sterile dressing; clean, dry pad; or clean, dry clothing to cover a wound.
- Wash your hands thoroughly after giving first aid.

restaurants). First aid kits may be purchased or assembled. Box 24-2 gives the essential supplies needed.

GUIDELINES FOR HANDLING EMERGENCIES

Although each emergency situation is different, listed below are general guidelines to follow (Box 24-3).

- Do not put yourself in danger; check the scene for hazards (e.g., live electrical wires, broken stairs).
- Protect yourself from the victim's body fluids (Box 24-4).

ORR

- Remain calm and in control; it helps you, and it helps the victim to feel more secure.
- Observe the victim. Is he or she conscious? Is there a pulse? Is there severe bleeding?
- Observe the area. Try to find out what happened, what caused the emergency, and how the victim was injured.
- Talk to the victim; reassure him or her, and try to find out what happened; bystanders may be able to provide additional information; try to get as much information as possible from the victim and others.
- Explain to the victim what you are doing and that help is being called.
- Call 9-1-1 or your local emergency number.
- Give first aid as needed.
- Cover the victim with a blanket, coat, or sweater to maintain body temperature.
- Do not move a seriously injured victim unless there is an immediate danger (e.g., strong odor of gas, fire, flooding); then, move carefully according to the procedures you learned while taking the first aid course; ask the victim not to move because moving can cause additional injury and pain.
- Do not give any food or fluids.

Bystanders may provide some help to you (according to the situation), such as comforting the victim or other persons involved.

WHEN EMS PERSONNEL ARRIVE

Your role in caring for the victim ends when EMS personnel arrive. They may ask more questions about the victim or about the first aid you have been giving. Answer the questions accurately and quickly. Time is very important. If they need your assistance, they will ask for help. Otherwise, do not interfere. Remain with other family members to provide comfort and support.

Some home care aides have said that EMS personnel ignored them and did not give them credit for giving first aid. In many cases, this is true. EMS personnel are highly trained to handle all types of emergencies. Their focus is on the victim, giving the necessary emergency care, and transporting him or her to the hospital as quickly as possible. There is usually not much time for them to recognize your contributions to helping the victim.

ORR

REPORTING TO YOUR AGENCY

As soon as possible following the emergency, contact your agency and report the following:

- Your name
- Your client's name or name of victim
- The emergency
- Where and when it happened
- What you did (first aid given; called 9-1-1 or EMS)
- What happened when EMS arrived
- Results (client or victim to hospital?)

Record this information right away, before you forget what you did during the emergency situation in your client's home. Your agency needs to know exactly what happened because they are legally responsible for the client's care while you are in the home. This information will become a part of the client's record and may be used to plan his or her care when returning home.

Your agency will give you further directions to follow. Remember to record the information listed above in the client's record. Most agencies will ask you to complete and sign an Incident Report. Your agency will provide you with the form and give you special directions for its completion (see Chapter 6).

COMMON EMERGENCIES

The following is a discussion of a few of the more common emergencies home care aides may see.

CHOKING

The airway is blocked by a piece of food or other object (e.g., candy, marbles, small pieces of plastic). While common in infants and children, more adults die from choking than children. Choking can result from such activities as trying to swallow large pieces of poorly chewed food; eating too fast; eating while laughing; or running with food or other objects in the mouth.

Partially Blocked Airway

The victim is getting enough air in and out of the lungs to cough, make wheezing noises, and may even be able to talk. Encourage the person to continue coughing. If the object is not expelled, call 9-1-1 or EMS for help.

Totally Blocked Airway

No air can get in or out of the lungs. The victim cannot speak, cough, or breathe, and may turn blue (cyanosis). Sometimes, the person may make high-pitched sounds or cough weakly. He or she usually puts his hand around the throat—a universal sign of choking (Figure 24-2). This is a very frightening experience for the victim and a life-threatening emergency. ACT AT ONCE.

Action

Have someone call 9-1-1 or EMS while you begin to give abdominal thrusts (Heimlich maneuver). This is a series of thrusts to the upper abdomen above the navel and below the ribcage. These thrusts force air out of the lungs and the object is pushed out, like a cork from a champagne bottle. Follow these directions for giving abdominal thrusts.

Fig 24-2 The universal sign of choking.

Fig 24-3 Stand behind the victim, and wrap your arms around the victim's waist.

Fig 24-4 Make a fist with one hand, and place the thumb side against the middle of the victim's abdomen, just above the navel and below the ribcage.

Fig 24-5 Grab your fist with your other hand, and give quick inward and upward thrusts into the abdomen.

Fig 24-6 To give yourself abdominal thrusts, press your abdomen into a firm object, such as a kitchen countertop.

Directions for Abdominal Thrusts

Victim Is Standing or Sitting

1. Stand behind victim and wrap your arms around the victim's waist (Figure 24-3).
2. Make a fist with one hand and place the thumb side against the middle of the victim's abdomen, just above the navel and below the ribcage (Figure 24-4).
3. Grab your fist with your other hand and give quick inward and upward thrusts into the abdomen (Figure 24-5).
4. Repeat these thrusts until the object is forced out.

   NOTE: If victim is noticeably pregnant or extremely overweight, give chest thrusts. Place your fist against the center of the breastbone. Grab it with your other hand and give quick thrusts into the chest.

When You Are Alone and Choking

1. Lean over and press abdomen against a firm object, such as the back of a chair or kitchen sink. Avoid using an object with sharp edges or corners that can cause further injury (Figure 24-6).
2. Use your hands to give abdominal thrusts as listed above.

NO BREATHING

When breathing stops, the person will lose consciousness very shortly. If breathing is not restored, the heart stops beating, and blood does not circulate throughout the body. Lack of oxygen to the tissues causes other body systems to fail, leading to death. Breathing must be restored for the person to stay alive.

Action

If the victim is not breathing and there is no pulse, CPR must be started. It is highly recommended that all home care aides take a course in CPR to learn the proper techniques for maintaining the oxygen and blood flow throughout the body until EMS personnel arrive. If you are certified to give CPR, it is important to keep your skills current through annual continuing education.

BLEEDING

Bleeding occurs when capillaries and blood vessels are injured. Severe bleeding (hemorrhage) is caused when one or more large blood vessels are involved. If untreated, the victim may die within a short period of time.

There are two types of bleeding.

- *External:* Bleeding is visible and comes from an open wound.
- *Internal:* Bleeding occurs inside the body. The location of the bleeding cannot be seen, but the victim's symptoms show that the injury is internal. For example, the victim vomits bright red blood. Sometimes, the vomitus appears like coffee grounds. This means that the gastric juices of the stomach have acted on the blood.

When severe bleeding occurs, the person may also show the following signs:

- Rapid, weak pulse
- Moist, cool skin
- Pale or bluish skin
- Very thirsty
- Swollen, tender, hard areas of the body, such as the abdomen
- Confusion, drowsiness, or unconsciousness

Action

Severe bleeding is a medical emergency. Assist the victim to a comfortable position, usually lying down, and keep him or her from getting chilled or overheated.

For External Bleeding from an Open Wound

- Put on disposable gloves, if available. If not available, place a barrier (dressing, cloth, plastic bag, plastic wrap) between you and the blood.
- Place a clean dressing over the wound, and apply direct pressure. If a sterile dressing is not available, use anything that is clean and dry (clean towel, face cloth, shirt, blouse, sock). If dressing becomes soaked with blood, apply another dressing over it and continue to apply pressure. Do not remove the original dressing or peek under the dressing(s) to see if the bleeding has stopped. This could cause blood clots to be dislodged and cause more bleeding.
- If the victim can help, ask him or her to apply pressure to the wound.
- Raise the injured area above the level of the heart, if possible. If you suspect that the wound involves a fracture, *do not* move the person.
- Apply a bandage snuggly over the dressing to keep it in place.
- Wash your hands immediately after giving care.
- Call 9-1-1 or EMS for help.
- Do not give food or fluids.

For Signs of Internal Bleeding
- Save specimen containing blood (vomitus, feces, urine, sanitary pad, or other specimen containing blood).
- Wear gloves, if possible, when handling blood. If not available, place a barrier between you and the blood (see above).
- Wash hands immediately after care.
- Call 9-1-1 or EMS for help.
- Do not give food or fluids.

SHOCK

Shock is a condition in which the circulatory system is not able to transport adequate amounts of blood to all parts of the body. Some causes of shock include: severe bleeding, electrical shock (victim is in contact with live electrical wires), serious bodily injury, severe burn, allergic reaction, and emotional reaction to sudden illness. Shock can also be caused by an insulin reaction (see Chapter 22).

Signs of shock include the following:
- Weak, rapid pulse
- Shallow, irregular, labored breathing
- Cold, clammy skin
- Paleness in light-skinned persons; grayish in dark-skinned persons
- Restlessness
- Dazed look: Eyes dull and pupils wide
- May be confused

Action
- Do not touch the victim until the source of electrical current is turned off, if electrical shock is suspected.
- Assist the victim into position with head lower than legs: this helps to keep the blood flowing to the brain (Figure 24-7). If you suspect head, neck, or back injuries, keep the victim flat.
- Loosen any tight clothing to make breathing easier.
- Cover the victim's body to keep warm.

Fig 24-7 Elevate the victim's legs approximately 12 inches.

- Remain with the victim until help arrives; have someone call 9-1-1 or EMS.
- Reassure the victim that help is coming.

STROKE

Care of the client with a stroke was discussed in Chapter 22. However, first aid for the victim who has signs of a stroke is very different. Signs appear suddenly and may include the following:
- Weakness or paralysis on one side of the body
- Drooping of eyelid, mouth, facial muscles
- Loss of movement of arms, fingers, legs, toes
- Tingling sensations in weakened areas
- Lack of ability to grasp objects, poor grip in hand
- Trouble seeing in one or both eyes
- Severe headache, with no known cause
- Slurred speech or aphasia
- Staggering gait
- Conscious, but may be confused
- Unconscious
  RECEIVING TREATMENT QUICKLY CAN GREATLY REDUCE THE RISK OF PERMANENT BRAIN DAMAGE.

Action
- Place the victim in a comfortable position; if lying down, keep head and shoulders raised; if unconscious, turn the victim to the affected side to allow saliva to drain from the mouth.
- Keep the victim calm; reassure him or her.
- Cover the victim's body to keep warm.
- Have someone call 9-1-1 or EMS.
- Remain with the victim until help arrives.

FALLS AND FRACTURES

Throughout this textbook, safety for both client and home care aide have been discussed. However, many people are not safety conscious. Falls are a common medical emergency for all ages. Most falls happen in or around the home because of carelessness or physical conditions of the victim. The risk of fractures is always present when falls occur. The following are some general signs of fractures:
- Pain or tenderness in the area of the fracture
- Deformity of the affected limb
- Loss of function; the victim cannot move or has difficulty moving
- Swelling in the area; bruising of the skin
- Victim may say that he or she felt or heard the bone snap or pop

Action
- DO NOT move the victim unless he or she is in danger. If the victim *must* be moved, try to get help. If no help is available, gently move the victim to a safe area. Protect the injured area from further damage. A first aid course will give instruction on the proper ways to keep the part immobile.
- Do not attempt to straighten the limb or have the victim try to move it.
- Maintain body temperature, and keep the victim as comfortable as possible.
- Have someone call 9-1-1 or EMS for help.
- Remain with the victim; provide reassurance.

BURNS

Burns are injuries to tissues of the body caused by heat, electricity, chemicals, radiation, or gasses. Burns are classified according to the amount of damage caused to the skin: epidermis, dermis, and structures beneath the skin (i.e., muscles, nerves, bones). They are described by degree, as follows:

- *First degree:* Involves only the outer layer of skin, the epidermis. The skin appears red and dry. Swelling may be present. The area is painful.
- *Second degree:* Involves the epidermis and the upper part of the dermis. The skin is red with blisters. Blisters may open and weep clear fluid making the skin appear wet. Swelling may be present. The area is painful.
- *Third degree:* Involves the epidermis, dermis, and any or all structures beneath the skin such as nerves, blood vessels, and fat. The skin appears to be charred. Structures underneath may appear to be white. There may be an odor of burned flesh. The area may be painful or not, depending on the amount of injury to the nerve endings.

A first-degree burn of the finger can be painful, but it is not life threatening. Third-degree burns are very serious and can be life threatening when they cover large amounts of skin surface.

Action

When the victim is burned, take the following action:

- Remove the victim from the source of the burn, such as putting out flames (smother with blanket, roll victim on floor to put out flames) (Figure 24-8).
- For first-degree burns that involve small areas

    Apply ice packs. Wrap ice in clean cover (e.g., dish towel, washcloth), and hold pack on area for 20 minutes. Remove for 10 minutes and reapply.

    Do not leave ice pack on any longer than 20 minutes to prevent further skin damage (see Chapter 18, Procedure 18-12, p. 334).

    If the burned area is large, call 9-1-1 or EMS.

- For second- and third-degree burns

    Remove any clothing surrounding the burn that has not stuck to the burn area.

    Cover the burn using a dry, sterile dressing (if available) or dry, clean cloths to prevent infection; loosely bandage to keep them in place.

    Do not apply ice, cold water, or ointments to the burned area.

    Call 9-1-1 or EMS for help.

    See Box 24-5 for burn care cautions.

Fig 24-8 Stop, drop, and roll to smother flames and stop the burning process.

BOX 24-5	Burn Care Cautions

- Do not try to clean up the burned area by
    Removing pieces of clothing or jewelry that stick to the burn
    Washing the area with soap and water
- Do not apply ointments, butter, cooking oil, burn creams, or other substances to burned areas.
- Do not break blisters; they protect the injured skin below.
- Do not apply ice to second- or third-degree burns or when large surfaces have been burned.

SEIZURES

A seizure (convulsion) occurs when the normal functioning of the brain is interrupted by injury, infection, or disease. Seizures may occur because the victim has epilepsy, a chronic condition usually controlled by medication. Seizures may be mild blackouts or a sudden, uncontrolled series of muscle contractions. They may last for several minutes.

Action
- Protect the victim by
    Loosening clothing around the neck
    Placing him or her on the floor, if possible
    Removing furniture or other objects that the victim might strike against during uncontrolled body movements
    Placing a folded towel or clothing under the head
    Remaining with the victim during the entire seizure
- If there is saliva, blood, or vomitus in the victim's mouth, roll the victim onto his or her side to allow fluid to drain from the mouth. This is done with two people: one turns the head and neck, the other turns the legs and torso. Both do the turning at the same time to prevent injury to the victim's neck.
- **Do not place anything in the victim's mouth.**
- Do not restrict the victim's movements during the seizure; this could cause more injury.
- Have a family member call 9-1-1 or EMS for help.

POISONING

A poison is a substance that, when taken into the body, can cause injury, illness, or death. There are four ways poisons enter the body.
1. *Respiratory System*
    Examples: Breathing in carbon monoxide gas (Box 24-6) or fumes from paints or from drugs (crack cocaine)
2. *Digestive System*
    Examples: Eating foods containing poisons; drinking household cleaning products; abusing or misusing drugs
3. *The Skin*
    Examples: Handling fertilizers or pesticides improperly; contact with certain poisonous plants
4. *Circulatory System*
    Examples: Injecting poisons into the body through bites or stings of insects, animals; drugs injected by needle and syringe

---

BOX 24-6 Carbon Monoxide Poisoning

Carbon monoxide is an odorless gas, most commonly found in exhaust fumes from cars and from fumes of wood-burning stoves. Carbon monoxide poisoning is a condition that leads to death if not treated immediately. It results from inhaling fumes that cause a decrease in the ability of the blood cells to carry oxygen. The person does not know that he or she is breathing in the deadly gas. He or she may complain of headache or drowsiness. Mental confusion is also a symptom.

   If you suspect that there may be carbon monoxide in the home or the carbon monoxide detector alarm sounds, ACT IMMEDIATELY—THIS IS AN EMERGENCY.
- Get yourself and your client out of the home immediately.
- Call 9-1-1 or EMS.
- Open all windows and doors to the outside if you cannot get the client out, and call 9-1-1 or EMS.
- Breathe in fresh air; it is the best treatment until emergency medical personnel arrive.

BOX 24-7 Do's and Don'ts When Caring for a Suspected Poisoning Victim

DO

- Call 9-1-1, or EMS.
- Try to find out what caused the poisoning (e.g., an empty bottle of pills) and when it happened; give this information to the 9-1-1 dispatcher, or local EMS personnel.
- Listen for directions about caring for the victim until help arrives.
- If fumes were inhaled, get the victim to fresh air, if possible (open windows).

DON'T

- Cause the victim to vomit if poison has been swallowed.
- Follow directions on the container's label; they may not be correct.

Action

Signs of poisoning vary according to the type of poison and how it entered the body. If you suspect that poisoning has occurred, take the following action:
- Call 9-1-1 or the local emergency number.
- Follow the directions given.
- See Box 24-7 for additional guidelines.

CHEST PAIN

Chest pain is the major symptom of a heart attack. A heart attack is a condition in which the heart muscle is not receiving enough blood due to damage of the blood vessels in the area. The only way to know if the victim is having a heart attack is by medical examination and tests. Therefore, getting medical help as quickly as possible is very important. While chest pain can be a symptom of other problems, the person who is having chest pain should be treated as if he or she is having a heart attack. Signs of heart attack include the following:
- Squeezing, uncomfortable pressure, fullness or dull pain in the center of the chest that lasts for more than 2 minutes
- Pain that radiates to shoulders, arm, neck, or jaw (Figure 24-9)
- Signs of shock (see p. 466)

Fig 24-9 Signs of a heart attack. **A,** The feeling of pressure in the chest. **B,** Pain that spreads from the chest, up the neck, and down the left arm. **C,** Dizziness and sudden sweating.

NOTE: Women may have symptoms different from men, such as: mid-back pain, unexplained tiredness, nausea and/or vomiting, shortness of breath, and symptoms that seem like indigestion.

Action
- Help the victim into a comfortable position, usually sitting.
- Loosen tight clothing.
- Encourage victim to remain quiet.
- Take pulse and respirations.
- Have someone call 9-1-1 or EMS for help.
- Remain with the victim until help arrives.
- Comfort and reassure the victim; chest pain is very frightening.

CHAPTER SUMMARY

- *Emergency* is a term used to describe a serious situation that arises suddenly and threatens the life or welfare of a person or group of persons. The immediate action taken is called *first aid.*
- Preparing in advance for an emergency is very important. This includes knowing the correct emergency telephone number to call, the types of questions the dispatcher may ask, and how to care for common medical emergencies until help arrives.
- Taking a first aid course is highly recommended.
- There are several general guidelines to follow when emergencies occur.
- Reporting to your agency following the emergency is very important. Do not forget to record in the client's care record what happened and what first aid care you gave.
- Medical emergencies, such as choking, difficult or no breathing, severe bleeding, lack of a pulse, and unconsciousness, require immediate action and an immediate call to 9-1-1 or EMS for help.
- If you suspect that the victim has been poisoned, call 9-1-1 immediately.
- Shock is a condition that can result from severe bleeding, serious bodily injuries, severe burns, allergic reactions, and emotional reaction to sudden illness. Prompt treatment is important.
- Always practice standard (universal) precautions when giving first aid.

STUDY QUESTIONS

1. What does the term *emergency* mean? Give four examples of medical emergencies.
2. Give three ways you will prepare for medical emergencies.
3. List five rules to follow when an emergency happens.
4. The emergency dispatcher will ask you several questions. Identify six questions that the dispatcher usually asks.
5. Select four medical emergencies from the following list, and describe the first aid you will give for each emergency.
   a. Choking
   b. Shock
   c. Chest pain
   d. Poisoning
   e. Fracture
   f. Severe external bleeding
   g. Third-degree burns
   h. Seizure
   i. Stroke
6. Why is it important to record your actions on the care record (if the victim is your client) and prepare an incident report for your agency?
7. When you are waiting in line to check out at the supermarket, an elderly man falls to the floor and lies there bleeding. You and the manager go to the victim's assistance. How can you avoid contact with the victim's blood?

25

Getting a Job and Keeping It

KEY TERMS

Employment agencies Private or government agencies that match job seekers and potential employers

Evaluation Process of judging employee performance to determine suitability to remain in the job

Job application form Form to be filled out when applying for a job

Job placement counselors Persons in public or private agencies who provide services to those seeking employment

Mandatory Required

Networking Informal method of exchanging information about job openings

Personnel policies Set of rules and regulations to be followed by employees, usually pertaining to employer and employee rights and responsibilities

Reference Person who will speak in another's behalf

Resume Listing of educational and work experience to be used in getting a job

Supervision Process of observing employees doing their jobs

Janet and Jorges sing in the same choir. They both have successfully finished a training program for home care aides. Janet was hired and trained by her agency, so she already has a job. Jorges took the home care aide course at a local technical school, and he needs to find a job.

Anna Petrova's husband, Sergei, has accepted a better job in an area that is 300 miles from where they now live. Both Anna and Sergei are excited about moving to another part of the country and having the chance to improve financially. However, this decision means that Anna must leave her job at the home care agency. "I love my job and everyone at the agency; I've made a lot of friends. I sure will miss them. I know that the agency has an office where we'll be living. Maybe there's a job opening for me."

Just as training to become a home care aide takes time and energy, so does finding the right job. There is preparation and thought involved.

- Locating job openings
- Writing a **resume** and sending it electronically
- Completing the **job application form** in person or online
- Preparing for an interview
- Participating in the interview
- Deciding whether to take the job

This chapter presents the guidelines to follow in your job search. Remember that looking for the right job should be done in an organized and orderly manner. Job-seeking, job-getting, and job-keeping skills are important to develop.

LOCATING JOB OPENINGS

Sources of information that can help you identify job openings in your area are as follows.

1. Networking

   This is an informal way to find out about job openings. **Networking** takes place when you let other people (those who work in home care and those who do not) know that you are looking for a job. For example, Janet may be able to tell Jorges if her employer is looking for more home care aides. If Anna works for an agency with offices in other states, her employer may have some job leads. Also, other persons in your community, church, PTA, or other groups might know of job openings. If you have a computer, do not forget to check the online Websites.

2. Reverse Search

   You look for jobs by calling local Home Care Agencies to see if they are accepting applications. Locate them on Internet search engines such as Google or Yahoo. You may also visit their websites to see if they are hiring.

3. Internet job sites

   These are locations on the World Wide Web that are devoted to listing job openings. Some feature all kinds of jobs, while others are specifically for certain occupations. Examples include the following:

   a. CareerBuilder, Monster

   b. State, county, and municipal sites

   c. Federal jobs: www.opm.gov/job_seekers/

   d. Health-related jobs: www.heathcarejobsite.com

4. Newspaper

   Newspaper advertisements give a general listing of the jobs open in your community. Look in the special section that lists medical/health care jobs. Also, check for

TABLE 25-1   Want Ad Abbreviations and Meanings

ABBREVIATION	MEANING	ABBREVIATION	MEANING
Cert.	Certification	HHA	Home health aide
CHHA	Certified Home Health Aide	Lic.	License
		M-F	Monday through Friday
Comp.	Companion		
Eve.	Evenings	Reim.	Reimbursed
Excel.	Excellent	Req.	Required
Exp. Pref'd	Experience Preferred	Wknd	Weekend
F/T	Full time	EOE	Equal Opportunity Employer
HCA	Home care aide		

the listing, HOME CARE AIDES in the general Help Wanted ads. There is an art to reading want ads: a basic understanding of abbreviations used and reading "between the lines" will help you to understand the ads (Table 25-1). These ads are usually linked to Internet job sites or e-mail addresses.

5. **Employment agencies**

There are two types of employment agencies: private and public. Both match job seekers with potential employers.

a. Public employment agencies are sponsored by State Government Departments of Labor. You can locate the "career one stop" location in your area by visiting the U.S. Department of Labor's website, America's Job Bank, at www.ajb.dni.us, where you will be directed to your own State Department of Labor. Here you will be able to create a job seeker account, post your resume, locate job openings, and find the location of your "One Stop Job Center." These centers are staffed with on-site professionals who can assist you in obtaining employment.

b. Private employment agencies are staffing services. They hire and provide employees for employers. These jobs are usually temporary or part-time. There is no fee for the applicant; however, the employer does pay the agency for your services. YOU SHOULD NEVER BE REQUIRED TO PAY A FEE TO GET A JOB.

6. **Job placement counselors**

Employed by public or private employment agencies, these counselors match the client's abilities to jobs available in the community.

7. Your instructors

Your teachers are excellent sources of contacts in the home care field. They have had experience working with you in your program. They can often supply leads to your first job or to a new and more challenging one. Do not be afraid to ask for their help. Ask them, too, if you can use their name as a reference.

PREPARING A RESUME AND COVER LETTER

A resume gives the employer information about you before the job interview takes place. In fact, the main purpose of a resume is to help you GET the job interview. It should give the person enough information about your education, work experience, and other important points so that he or she will want to interview you for the job (Figure 25-1). A cover letter is sent with the resume. This letter explains briefly what job you are seeking and why you believe you have the necessary skills and abilities to do the job. "First impressions are lasting ones"—this old saying is very true, especially when it comes to the cover letter and resume. It is your chance to "sell" yourself. It

Jorges Ortiz
456 Bridge Street
Any Town, NJ 012345
Phone 555-687-9012
ortizj@noaddress.com

OBJECTIVE: To obtain an entry-level position as a home care aide.

EDUCATION

Any Town Technical School, Home Care Aide Program, Any Town, NJ; received
"Most Caring Student" Award

Riverview High School, Riverview, NJ

SPECIAL SKILLS

Fluent in Spanish and English
Certified in CPR
Special ability to communicate easily with clients.

SKILLS AND EXPERIENCE
Acquired at Any Town Technical School

Performed client's personal care: bathing, grooming, dressing, feeding, transfers and walking
Practiced infection prevention, medical asepsis and bloodborne pathogen training
Observed, documented and reported information, including vital signs.
Maintained client's home environment: light cleaning and laundry
Performed special procedures and specimen collection
Completed clinical experience
Career oriented, dedicated to superior client care. Enjoy working with clients of all ages.
Punctual, reliable, and hard working

WORK HISTORY

Waiter	Seafood Buffet Restaurant	Atlantic Beach, NJ

Selected "Best Waiter in Summer" in competition
2xxx and 2xxx

Retail Sales Associates	Ralph's Tall Men's Shop	Nearby, PA

OTHER ACTIVITIES

Member, Any Town Rescue Squad, beginning volunteer. Certified in CPR

References available on request.

Fig 25-1 Sample resume.

546 Bridge Street
Any Town, NJ 01234
ortizj@noaddress.com
October 28, 2xxx

Ms. Arlene Weller
Personnel Manager
ABC Community Home Care Services
99 Elm Drive
Any Town, NJ 01235

Dear Ms. Weller:

The home care aide position with ABC Community Home Care Services, listed in the classified ads section of the October 27, 2xxx edition of *The Gazette*, interests me very much. Please consider me an applicant for the position.

I have completed the Home Care Aide course at Any Town Technical School and am a Certified Home Care Aide. Also, I have had extensive experience working with people of all ages. I understand the importance of good communication and working as a team member. My client care skills, along with my work experience, have given me the abilities needed to be successful as a home care aide.

I would like to discuss the possibility of employment with you at your convenience. You may contact me at the above address or by e-mail to arrange for an interview. I look forward to hearing from you.

Sincerely,

Jorges Ortiz

Jorges Ortiz

Enclosure

Fig 25-2 Cover letter.

shows off your special abilities and skills even before you appear in person for the interview. Therefore, use a computer to prepare both the resume and cover letter. Neatness counts. Also, be careful to use correct grammar and punctuation.

Resumes may be written several different ways. Your State Department of Labor has many resources available that can help you select the best way to write your resume. Job websites will have a standard resume form for you to use. Listed below are tips to use when preparing a resume and cover letter.

THE COVER LETTER

- Use business letter style (Figure 25-2) and unlined white bond paper.
- Address the letter to the correct person. Telephone the agency to get the correct spelling of the person's name and title, if unsure.

- Clearly state the job you are interested in getting.
- Give the reason you are interested in working for the agency.
- Briefly discuss your education and any related experiences you have had.
- Request an interview, and give information on where you can be reached.
- Sign the letter.

THE RESUME

- Prepare one page of information (or two, if necessary). Use unlined white bond paper.
- Make sure the resume contains the following important elements:

  Personal information: Your name, address (with ZIP code), telephone number (with area code), and e-mail.

  Objective: The title of the job you are seeking

  Summary of qualifications: A statement about your education and the experiences you have had that make you suitable for the job

  Education: Name and address of the school, type of program, date completed, any special courses or training (e.g., Red Cross First Aid)

  Work history: Most recent employment (list first), dates employed, employer's name and address, job title and duties; include volunteer activities, if appropriate to the job you are seeking

  References: You may use the statement "References available on request." Bring a printed list of references to the interview. List the full name, title, address, and telephone number of each reference. Prior approval is *required before* listing the person's name. Give the list to the interviewer if he or she requests references, or list them on the application form.

- Be sure that information in your resume (and cover letter) is accurate.
- Enclose your resume with the cover letter.

NOTE: Ask a relative or friend to look for any errors, misspelled words, or incorrect grammar in the letter or resume. Correct and reprint, if necessary.

SUBMITTING A COVER LETTER AND RESUME

There are three ways to send your cover letter and resume to the future employer:
1. Regular mail: Do not fold. Place the documents in a 9- by 12-inch envelope; add proper postage and mail.
2. Internet: Send the letter of interest and your resume by e-mail via computer. Remember that you must have an e-mail address of your own so the future employer can contact you.
3. Hand carry: Place the documents in a large 9- by 12-inch envelope. Be sure to have your address on the envelope. Deliver the documents "in person" to the agency. Ask the receptionist for a receipt.

ELECTRONIC JOB SEEKING

Electronic resumes are submitted over the Internet (Figure 25-3). They must be written on the specific form provided. Resumes are sorted by specific key words, so use them whenever possible (e.g., *performed, practiced, observed, good memory,* and *sense of responsibility*).

It is a good idea to have two versions of the resume—one electronic copy for a computer to read online and one hard copy for people to read.

ELECTRONIC JOB SEEKING

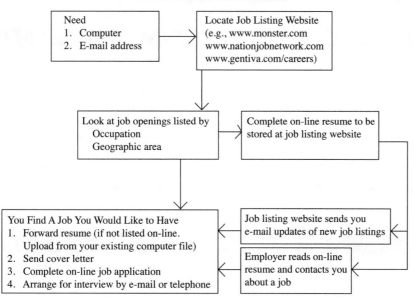

Fig 25-3 Electronic job-seeking chart.

COMPLETING THE JOB APPLICATION

When you have located a possible job opening, call, e-mail, or visit the agency in person to find out if this is true.

Some employers will send a job application online; others will require you to complete a paper application at the agency office. This is usually done just before the interview. IF YOU COMPLETE AN ONLINE JOB APPLICATION, BE CAREFUL... DO NOT GIVE ANY CONFIDENTIAL INFORMATION SUCH AS SOCIAL SECURITY NUMBER, CERTIFICATION NUMBER, DRIVER'S LICENSE OR BANK ACCOUNT NUMBERS. ALL THESE CAN BE PROVIDED ONCE YOU ARE HIRED. INTERNET SCAMS ARE A CONSTANT PROBLEM, SO ALWAYS PROTECT YOUR PERSONAL CONFIDENTIAL INFORMATION.

You will need the following in order to complete the paper application as a part of the hiring process:

- Social Security card
- Proof of citizenship or legal residency
- Names and addresses of personal references and former employers (if applicable)
- Certification
- Driver's license (if applicable)
- A pen and paper or pad for writing notes
- Resume

Always completely fill out the application in ink and print all information so it is easy to read (Figure 25-4). Be truthful. Do not give any false information.

PREPARING FOR THE INTERVIEW

MAKE AN APPOINTMENT

Most employers will set up an interview when you call or after you submit a resume and/or completed application form. Once the appointment time has been set, be sure to get there before the time arranged. If it is not possible to keep the appointment, notify the person *immediately* to explain why you cannot come and to set up another

APPLICATION FOR EMPLOYMENT
(Please print clearly)

Date:_____

PERSONAL INFORMATION

Name_____
                 Last   First   Middle Initial

Address_____
            Street   City   State   Zip Code

Telephone_____ Social Security No._____
         Area Code   Number

If under 18 years of age, do you have a work permit? ❑ Yes ❑ No

If not a U.S. citizen, do you have the right to remain permanently and work in the U.S.A.? ❑ Yes ❑ No

    Alien Reg. No._____

EMPLOYMENT DESIRED

Position applied for: _____

Shift you can work: ❑ Day ❑ Evening ❑ Either   Hours desired: ❑ Full time ❑ Part time ❑ Temporary

How did you learn of this opening? _____

Date you can start: _____
                 Month   Day   Year

Have you ever applied to this company before? ❑ Yes ❑ No When _____

Have you ever worked for this company before? ❑ Yes ❑ No

When _____ Supervisor_____

Reason for Leaving _____

_____

EDUCATION

Highest grade completed (circle):   9 10 11 12   1 2 3 4
                                High School   College

Name and location of last school attended _____

Vocational or trade training _____

Extracurricular
activities while in school _____

Area of specialization
or major interest _____

Professional organization memberships, honors received, volunteer or community service or other qualifications you have
which you feel are related to the position for which you are applying:

_____

_____

_____

_____

Fig 25-4 An application form. (Courtesy Briggs Corporation, Des Moines, Iowa.)

REFERENCES

List three persons who know you well. Do not include relatives or former employers.

Name	Address	Phone	Years Acquainted With You

FORMER EMPLOYERS

List below your work experience, starting with your present or last place of employment.

Date Employed	Name and Address of Employer	Name of Supervisor	Position(s) Held
from_____ to _____			start _____ finish_____
from_____ to _____			start _____ finish_____
from_____ to _____			start _____ finish_____
from_____ to _____			start _____ finish_____
from_____ to _____			start _____ finish_____

May we contact your present employer at this time? ❑ Yes ❑ No

EMPLOYMENT UNDERSTANDING (Please Read and Sign)

This institution does not discriminate in hiring or any other decision on the basis of race, color, sex, citizenship, national origin, ancestry, Vietnam era veteran status, or on the basis of age or physical or mental disability unrelated to the ability to perform the work required. No question on this application is intended to secure information to be used for such discrimination.

I voluntarily give this institution the right to make a thorough investigation of my past employment and activities, agree to cooperate in such investigation and release from all liability or responsibility all persons, companies or corporations supplying such information. I consent to take the physical examination, and such future physical examinations as may be required by this institution at such times and places as the institution shall designate. I understand that an offer of employment may be contingent on passing the physical examination which relates to the essential duties I would be required to perform.

I understand that my employment is at will, and that either party is free to terminate the employment relationship at any time without cause. I also understand that my employment may be terminated for any misstatement or omission of fact appearing on this application form.

If employed, I will be required to complete an Employment Verification Form (I-9), and within three days show satisfactory evidence of identity and eligibility for employment.

Applicant's Signature_____ Date_____

APPLICATION FOR EMPLOYMENT

Fig 25-4, cont'd

appointment. Otherwise, the employer may decide that you are unreliable. If you do not know the exact location of the office where you will be interviewed, a practice trip may be helpful. It will give you an idea of how much time you need to get there. Remember, YOU need the job. If you miss the interview without notifying the potential employer, you may not get another chance.

GATHER INFORMATION

Get to know some facts about the employer and the agency. Get the agency's brochure from the office. Is it a branch of a national agency? Is it Medicare approved? What kind of services does it offer? What do others in your community and the health care field have to say about it?

PREPARE QUESTIONS

Make a list of questions to ask during the interview about job responsibilities and the agency.
- How long has the agency been open?
- What types of clients do you serve? How many clients do you serve?
- How many home care aides do you employ? What other staff do you employ?
- Are there other responsibilities not listed in the ad?
- Will I wear a uniform?
- What geographic area(s) does your agency cover? What area(s) will I work in?
- Will I use public transportation? Drive my own car?
- Tell me about your infection control plan.
- What is your job orientation procedure?
- Are there opportunities for further education?
- Are there any other questions I can answer for you?
- When can I expect to hear from you?

Asking questions shows that you are interested in the agency and the job. Avoid asking questions about sick time, vacations, or pay raises unless the interviewer gives no information about them. Questions that focus almost entirely on pay, vacations, and holidays give the impression that you are more interested in "off-time" benefits rather than the responsibilities of the job.

PREPARE ANSWERS

Most interviewers have a basic set of questions they ask all applicants. It is impossible to guess all the questions that might be asked, but the following are often included.
- Tell me about yourself.
- Why are you interested in working here? What do you know about us?
- What experience have you had in home care?
- Have you worked in any other health field?
- What makes you a good home care aide?
- Why did you select this field of health care?
- What personal qualities are necessary for success as a home care aide?
- What are your strengths? Weaknesses? Why should we hire you?
- If already employed, why do you want to change jobs?
- What do you see yourself doing in one year? Five years?
- Are you willing to work overtime, nights, and weekends?

Preparing answers to these questions (before the interview) may be helpful so you can be ready to answer if any of the topics are discussed.

There are some questions that interviewers cannot ask because they violate a person's civil rights. According to federal law, the following questions may not be asked by the employer before employment.

- When were you born?
- How old are you?
- How many children do you have?
- Do you have any children?
- Do you have a boyfriend/girlfriend?
- How much do you weigh?
- What type of military discharge do you have?

If any of these questions is asked during the interview, you have the right to refuse to answer the question.

DRESS APPROPRIATELY

It is said that interviewers make their decisions about hiring an applicant within a few minutes after the initial contact. Therefore, first impressions are extremely important. Preparing for the interview means being well groomed and dressing professionally (Figure 25-5). Do not wear shorts, cut-off jeans, yoga pants, sweats, and so on, for an interview (Figure 25-6). Your appearance is a preview of your grooming while "on the job." Box 25-1 lists some tips on dressing and grooming for a job interview.

Fig 25-5 Correct dress and grooming for a job interview.

Fig 25-6 Incorrect dress and grooming for a job interview.

BOX 25-1	**Dressing and Grooming for a Job Interview**

- Dress as you would for the first day on the job (unless the agency requires a uniform).
- Wear neat, casual clothes and comfortable shoes (e.g., skirt and blouse, slacks and shirt).
- Hair should be neatly combed; shoes and clothes clean.
- Males should be cleanly shaven. If facial hair is worn, be sure it is neatly trimmed.
- Do not wear excessive jewelry, makeup, or cologne.

PARTICIPATING IN THE INTERVIEW

PURPOSE

The interview is the most important step in obtaining the job. The actual interview lets the employer
- Get to know you
- Consider you as a future employee
- Explain the details of the job
- Tell you about the agency and the clients served
  You will have the opportunity to
- Explain why you are suitable for the job
- Ask specific questions about job responsibilities, working conditions, benefits, and so on
- Ask other questions
  The interview helps to answer two basic questions.
1. "Is this the person for the job?" (employer)
2. "Is this the job for me?" (applicant)

   If you have prepared ahead of time, you should feel confident and ready for the interview. Arrive about 10 minutes before the appointment. This shows your interest and reliability. It also gives you a chance to calm down and concentrate on the upcoming interview. Remember, you are prepared. You have the skills the employer needs. You are a winner. Go for it!

GUIDELINES

The following "do's and don'ts" will help you through the interview:

Do
- Turn off your cell phone or other electronic device.
- Greet the receptionist politely.
- Give your name and reason for being there.
- Remove your coat (and hat) before the interview.
- Complete the job application form; read it completely before starting.
  Use your resume.
  Complete the entire form; print "None" or "N/A" for parts that do not apply to you.
- Take several deep breaths to relax before you enter the interview area.
- Firmly shake hands with the interviewer, and greet by name when introduced; smile.
- Maintain eye contact during the interview.
- Speak clearly; use proper grammar.
- Be polite.
- Maintain good posture; sit up straight.
- Answer all questions honestly.
- Emphasize your strong points.
- Think about the question asked and how to answer it before you begin to speak.
- Give clear, short answers.
- Be honest.
- Ask questions you have prepared in advance (use notes you have made).

Don't
- Text or answer your cell phone.
- Bring children or friends to the interview.
- Write in spaces labeled "office use only" on the application form.
- Fidget, squirm, wiggle, or move nervously.

- Chew gum, smoke, eat, or drink (coffee, bottled water) during the interview.
- Use slang expressions or obscene words or gestures.
- Interrupt the interviewer when he or she is speaking.
- Brag about yourself.
- Rush when giving answers.
- Talk too much or too long.

At the end of the interview, thank the person for the opportunity to be interviewed. Firmly shake his or her hand, and leave the room.

A positive interview may result in a job offer. Sometimes you may be offered the position immediately. If not, the interviewer will tell you when you will hear about the job.

After the interview, send a follow-up letter to the interviewer thanking the person for the chance to be interviewed. State again, briefly, your interest in the job and why you are the best applicant for the job. Many times the "thank you" letter will give you an edge over the other applicants. It is definitely worth the time and energy that it takes (Figure 25-7).

While you are waiting to hear about the job, keep looking for another one. After all, an interview does not guarantee a job offer. Even if you are not the successful candidate

---

546 Bridge Street
Any Town, NJ 01234
ortizj@noaddress.com
November 18, 2xxx

Ms. Arlene Weller
Personnel Manager
ABC Community Home Care Services
99 Elm Drive
Any Town, NJ 01235

Dear Ms. Weller:

Thank you for the opportunity to interview for the home care aide position on November 15, 2xxx. I appreciate the time spent with me during the interview and the tour of the agency's offices.

I believe that I have gained the skills and knowledge needed by graduating from the Home Care Aide program at Any Town Technical School. My present and past work experience and home care aide certification make me an excellent and qualified applicant for the position.

I look forward to hearing from you soon and am grateful for your consideration.

Sincerely,

Jorges Ortiz

Jorges Ortiz

Fig 25-7 A "thank you" letter.

for the job, you have been through the job-seeking process and have learned what to do and what not to do. Keep trying; do not give up. There IS a job for you.

DECIDING WHETHER TO TAKE THE JOB

Now that you have completed the application and interview, the next step is deciding if the job is for you. Some factors to consider in the decision are

1. *Starting wages or pay (salary):* Weekly, every other week, monthly? Can I budget myself to live on the amount offered?
2. *Pay raises:* How often? How much? Based on length of employment and/or performance?
3. *Benefits:* Medical insurance (type of plan, insurer, cost to employee)? Dental insurance? Disability insurance? Life insurance? Pension plan? Plan for prescription drugs? Eyeglass plan?
4. *Paid sick leave:* How much? Can it be carried over from 1 year to another?
5. *Vacation:* How much? Based on length of employment?
6. *Holidays:* How many?
7. *Location of areas where you will work:* Close to public transportation? Fares paid or reimbursed? Personal automobile needed? Amount reimbursed per mile? Type and amount of automobile insurance required? Safety of areas served?
8. *Uniform worn?* Paid for by agency? Self? Any allowance for uniform maintenance?
9. *Education:* Continuing education or in-service education available?
10. *Conference/office time:* How often? How long? Paid?
11. *Hours:* Work schedule?

MAKING YOUR DECISION

Put all of the information about the job(s) offered to you in writing, and compare the positive and negative aspects. Also, consider the following questions:
- Will the job meet my career goals?
- Will I find job satisfaction?
- Can I work comfortably and safely for this employer in this agency?
- Will I be able to give good care to clients as an employee of this agency?
- Will I be able to safely use my skills and abilities?

Once you have answered all of these questions, you are ready to make your decision. It's your choice!

PRE-EMPLOYMENT SCREENING

The last part of the employer's hiring process is the pre-employment screening. This happens when the agency intends to offer the job to the applicant when he or she successfully passes the following screening:
- Background check and fingerprinting to determine criminal record, outstanding claims, damages, and so on.
- Credit check to review credit history and reports, outstanding debts, and so on.
- Substance abuse screening to rule out presence of illegal substances or other controlled substances.
- Physical examination including medical history to determine physical health to perform the duties of a home care aide.

Upon employment, you will be asked to complete an Employment Verification Form (I-9) and to provide evidence of your identity and eligibility for employment.

CERTIFICATION

Certification is recognition by a government or nongoverment agency that a person has met certain qualifications. The home care aide must attend a training program that is approved by the certifying group. Sometimes, an examination is given to test the aide's knowledge and competence. You must apply and pay a fee to take this test. Your instructor can tell you how and what to do. In some states, certification is obtained when a student successfully finishes a training program. He or she applies to the appropriate state regulating agency and pays a fee for certification. In some states, certification is mandatory.

Each state has its own requirements for certification. If you move from one state to another, you may be required to contact the appropriate regulating agency in that state to apply for certification. Remember, in order for your agency to receive Medicare reimbursement for your services, you must be a certified home care aide.

To keep your certification active, you must meet the requirements set up by your state. This may involve participating in educational programs and/or working a specific number of days within a certain time period. For example, you must work a minimum of 14 days within 2 years. In addition, you will have to follow the rules and regulations for certified home care aides in your state. These usually govern what tasks you can legally perform. Honesty, safety of clients, and substance abuse are also concerns of the regulating agency. Some states require that certification be renewed every year or every 2 years. A fee is charged for renewal.

Certification is very valuable to you. It demonstrates that you have met a required level of knowledge and competence. And, it gives you the opportunity to work in many agencies.

Certification is also a valuable resource. Protect it—do not let it expire. Keep it current by participating in your agency's in-service education program. Failure to keep your certification up-to-date may result in losing your job. And remember to keep drug free and always follow the agency's code of behavior as discussed in Chapter 3.

For additional information about certification
1. Consult your instructor or agency.
2. Consult the state regulatory agency (state health department, state board of nursing).
3. Write to: National Association for Home Care & Hospice
        228 Seventh Street, SE
        Washington, DC 20003
        www.nahc.org

EMPLOYMENT: A PARTNERSHIP

Employment is a partnership. If the partnership is a good one, both employer and employee benefit. The employer has agreed to pay you for the services that you will provide. You have agreed to perform these services to the best of your ability. In this way, both you and the employer will benefit. The home care agency receives monies from the client based on the services given by its employees. Because the employees perform these services accurately and skillfully, the employer is able to pay the employees from monies received from the client (Figure 25-8).

Fig 25-8 Employment is a partnership between employer and employee.

It is this mutual agreement—employer to employee and employee to employer—that makes the real difference. Unfortunately, there are many employees, in all types of businesses, who do not understand that the employer *cannot* pay the employee unless the product or service being produced is *sold* or *used*. In the automobile industry, the product is the car. In the home care industry, the product is not as easy to see or touch. The product is the delivery of a variety of home care services to many different clients (i.e., mothers and their newborn infants, children, younger and older adults). Your ability to produce the desired services will affect your employer's ability to have enough monies to pay you. Therefore, performing your duties and responsibilities accurately and skillfully is very important.

EMPLOYER AND EMPLOYEE RIGHTS

In this partnership, both parties have rights. Some of the rights of your employer and some of your rights are listed in the sections that follow:

EMPLOYER RIGHTS

- Right to expect that the home care aide will perform the duties properly
  That you will
    Practice your skills correctly
    Perform your duties and responsibilities accurately
    Know what you are **not** permitted to do
    Give care according to the care plan
    Refuse to perform skills that you are not trained to perform or not permitted to do
- Right to expect that the home care aide will keep accurate records of client care given and billable time
  That you will
    Use the correct forms, provided by your agency, to record client care and billable time
    Use other forms, such as Incident Report forms, when necessary
    Be honest in recording the time spent caring for your client and the care given to your client

- Right to expect that the home care aide will use correct safety practices to protect himself or herself and the client
  That you will
  - Practice safety awareness at all times
  - Use standard (universal) precautions and infection control procedures when needed
  - Report to your supervisor situations in the client's home that you believe to be unsafe
- Right to expect the home care aide to follow the agency's personnel policies and procedures
  That you will
  - Follow all personnel policies and procedures; look and act professionally (see Chapter 2)
  - Ask your employer to explain any policies or procedures you do not understand
- Right to supervise and evaluate the home care aide's job performance and to discipline him or her, if necessary
  That you will
  - Accept constructive criticism offered by your supervisor
  - Follow suggestions for improving your job performance
- Right to expect that the home care aide will protect and respect the client's privacy and property
  That you will
  - Keep all information confidential about the client and family (see Chapter 3)
  - Treat the client's property with respect and consideration
- Right to expect that the home care aide will treat all agency personnel with respect
  That you will
  - Follow the agency's code of behavior (see Chapter 3)
- Right to expect that the home care aide will remain free from substance abuse and free from disqualifying crimes
  That you will
  - Keep your certification current

EMPLOYEE RIGHTS

- Right to be paid for the work you perform
  That your employer will
  - Provide payment according to an agreed-upon rate and according to the agency's pay schedule
  - Provide the correct amount of money for the time worked
  - Provide a direct bank deposit if available
  - Provide additional monies for extra time worked (e.g., overtime, holidays)
  - Keep accurate records of work time, income taxes, and Social Security paid
- Right to a safe working environment
  That your employer will
  - Provide the necessary equipment and supplies to protect you from possible infection (e.g., mask, gloves)
  - Remove you from situations in the home where there is danger to your well-being
  - Follow federal regulations regarding exposure to bloodborne pathogens (see Chapter 11)

- Right to be supervised properly
  That your employer will
  - Supervise you on the job regularly
  - Inform you of the results of the supervision, verbally or in writing
  - Explain how you can improve your performance, if needed
  - Respond promptly when you contact the agency to report abnormal or unusual conditions in your client
  - Let you know when a job is well done
- Right to be evaluated and to be informed if your performance is not satisfactory
  That your employer will
  - Evaluate your performance on a regular basis
  - Inform you of the results of the evaluations—verbally and in writing
  - Inform you about ways to improve your performance
  - Inform you about what will happen if your performance does not improve
- Right to receive copies of the agency's personnel policies, including code of behavior, and job description
  That your employer will
  - Give you copies of the personnel policies and job description
  - Answer any questions, if you do not understand the meaning of any policy or procedure
  - Honor the personnel policies as printed
- Right to attend in-service education programs provided by the employer to maintain your skills and develop new ones
  That your employer will
  - Provide in-service education programs regularly
  - Keep records of your attendance
- Right to be treated with respect by all agency staff
  That your employer will
  - Treat you with respect and dignity at all times
  - Recognize that you are an important part of the home care team

SUPERVISION AND EVALUATION

Supervision is a process used by employers to observe employees doing their jobs. The purpose is to assist them to improve client care skills and to perform their duties and responsibilities more effectively.

Evaluation is the process employers use to find out how well the employee performs on the job and how well he or she relates to the client/family and members of the home care team.

From time to time, you will be supervised and evaluated by your employer. You will be told how often supervisory visits will be made during the year. You may or may not be given advance notice. Remember that these visits are made to help you to improve your client care skills, organization, and home management abilities. Supervisory visits give you the chance to ask questions and receive helpful hints from your employer. After each visit, your supervisor records the observations and discussions with you about your performance, including directions given for improvement.

Employee evaluations are given according to a time schedule (every 6 months or yearly), which your employer will explain. As a new employee, you may be evaluated more frequently. One of your rights as an employee is to know in advance what areas will be covered in the evaluation. Figure 25-9 shows a sample evaluation form.

ABC Home Care Agency
Employee Observation/Evaluation

☐   Observation   ☐   Evaluation

Employee _____   Position _____   Date of Hire _____

Employee:	Yes	No	N/A
Plans and/or follows the care plan.			
Uses equipment properly.			
Follows rules and regulations of agency.			
Records accurately and completely.			
Reports pertinent information to supervisor in timely manner.			
Attends required in-service education programs.			
Carries out assignment tasks correctly and safely.			
Relates well to clients.			
Relates well to client's family members.			
Cooperates with other team members.			
Is properly dressed and well groomed.			

Rate Employee	Superior	Average	Below Average
Work Attitude and Courtesy			
Adaptability			
Initiative			
Punctuality/Attendance			
Cooperation/Communication Skills			

Comments:

Fig 25-9 A sample evaluation form.

Quality of Work and Job Skills:

Other Comments:

Evaluator's Recommendations:

Employee Comments:

Signature of Employee	**Title**	**Date**

Signature of Observer/Evaluator	**Title**	**Date**

Fig 25-9, cont'd

After evaluating your performance, your employer will meet with you privately to discuss the findings. He or she should discuss your strengths and those areas that need improvement. The purpose of the evaluation is to help you to progress on the job. It is to your employer's advantage to assist you to improve; it is to your advantage to follow your employer's recommendations.

There is space on the evaluation form for the employer and employee to give written comments. You may agree or disagree with the evaluation. Give your reasons in writing, sign, and date the form. Each evaluation is kept as a permanent, confidential part of your employee record. The employee gets a copy. If you do not receive it, ask for it. Keep it in a safe place at home.

CONTINUING YOUR EDUCATION

We are living in a time when approaches to health care change rapidly. New techniques and procedures are being developed to improve the care given to clients at home. Sometimes procedures we have been taught are changed; sometimes new procedures need to be learned to replace outdated ones. It is very important to keep up with these changes so that your skills remain sharp and current. One way to do this is by participating in continuing education programs offered by your employer. Ask your supervisor about the types of programs given.

Some states consider continuing education to be so important that certification renewal depends on proof of the person's participation in these activities. Your employer can give you more information about your state's requirements.

DECIDING TO LEAVE YOUR JOB

Leaving a job can be a most frustrating, difficult, and stress-producing experience. It need not be, however, if approached properly. There are many reasons for deciding to leave a job. Perhaps you, like Anna Petrova, are moving to another area of the state or country. Or, you are planning to continue your education full-time. Maybe there are people you work with whose behavior is causing you difficulty in performing your job effectively.

The final decision to leave should be based on careful thought. It should not be a decision made in haste, on the spur of the moment. Some employees storm the employer's door with the statement, "I quit!" This behavior shows that the person's decision is probably based on the immediate problem rather than on a review of the factors leading to the actual event. At any rate, should you decide that the only thing to do is to leave the job, it is important that you have a new job **before** leaving your old one. It is much more difficult to find a job after you have already left your employer, no matter what the reason.

Before deciding to leave, you need to think about the reasons for leaving. If a problem situation exists, have you taken the steps necessary to solve the problem? Can it be solved? Have you talked to your supervisor about it? The best approach to handling the situation may not be to leave your employer. Talking to your supervisor about the problems and possible solutions may help you to decide whether to leave or to stay.

LEAVING THE JOB GRACEFULLY

According to the latest statistics, the average worker in the United States will change jobs at least ten times during one's work life. Therefore, it is important to develop skills needed to leave the job gracefully. Once you have decided to leave, the following steps need to be taken.

1. Follow your agency's policy about notifying superiors about your decision. For example, your agency may require 2 weeks' notice of resignation. Make sure that you honor this policy. Let your employer know as soon as possible so that there will be time to hire a replacement.
2. Speak to your supervisor and explain why you are leaving.
3. Avoid discussing your intentions to leave with coworkers before speaking with your supervisor. It is poor practice to inform everyone but those who really need to know. Information spreads rapidly through the "grapevine," and you do not want your employer to hear about your leaving from this source.
4. Share the news with your client(s) after you have told your employer. Your client will appreciate your telling him or her yourself.

Some agencies conduct an exit interview with each employee who is leaving. This gives the employer the chance to ask you for information about the job you are leaving. Your honest answers help the employer to improve working conditions in the future. Do not take this opportunity to gripe about your supervisor or other staff members. You may, at some future time, want to return to the agency. Do not "burn your bridges"—always leave the interview on a positive note.

Take the opportunity during this exit interview to ask the employer if

- You can use their name as a reference
- There are other offices located in the new area (if you are moving to a new location)

Anna Petrova and Mrs. Quick met at the agency office for an exit interview. "I have been dreading this meeting," Anna said. "It means that I am really leaving. Part of me is very sad. I don't want to leave my clients, my coworkers, and my friends. I will miss them very much—but another part of me is so excited. I am happy that Sergei has a better job, with regular hours and more pay. Still, starting all over again, many miles away…"

Mrs. Quick smiled and said, "Well, Anna, you started all over when you came to the United States. Look at how well you and Sergei and the children have done. You are young, healthy, talented, and smart; you can do it again. But, I, too, have mixed feelings. I hate to lose such a fine home care aide. Your work has been outstanding. Your clients love you; where will I find another like you?"

"You are embarrassing me," Anna said. "I have enjoyed my work here very much, and now I must find a new job."

Mrs. Quick said, "Well, Anna, as you know this office is a branch of a large home care agency. I believe we have an office near to your new home. I'll give you the address and telephone number, and you can contact them when you're ready."

"Oh, Mrs. Quick," Anna replied, "thanks so much, and would it be okay if I used you as a reference?"

"Anna, you may use me as a reference at any time. As I said, you are an excellent home care aide; thank you for working with us and giving excellent care to your clients." Mrs. Quick stood up and shook Anna's hand. "Good luck," she said. "Please let us hear from you once in a while."

"Oh, I will," said Anna. She smiled and left the office.

As Anna closed Mrs. Quick's office door, she saw Russ Larsen. "Anna," he said, "come into the conference room so I can copy down your new address."

The conference room was right next door to Mrs. Quick's office. When Russ and Anna went in, all of the home care aides from the agency were there with a cake, balloons, cards, gifts, and good luck, good-bye wishes.

Anna began to cry. "New beginnings always come after endings; they are bittersweet," she said. And she thought, "How lucky I am to have good friends, wonderful clients, and a great career."

CHAPTER SUMMARY

- Seeking, finding, and keeping a job are important skills to develop.
- There are several resources for obtaining information about job openings, including
  Networking
  Reverse search
  Newspaper advertisements
  Employment agencies
  Computer websites
  Job placement counselors
  Your instructors
- Prepare for the job interview by
  Writing a resume
  Making an appointment
  Gathering information
  Preparing questions and answers
  Dressing appropriately
- Certification is recognition by a government or nongovernment agency that you have met specific qualifications as a home care aide.
- Both employers and employees have rights.
- Evaluation and supervision are important to the employer, employee, and client.
- Continuing education helps you learn new information and skills that will help you give better care to your clients.
- Follow agency personnel policies regarding resignation when possible.

STUDY QUESTIONS

1. Locate a job opening using any two of the following sources:
   a. Local newspaper
   b. Your instructor
   c. Home care agency within your community
   d. Computer website
2. Write a list of four questions to ask during a job interview.
3. Select four questions (from this chapter) that an interviewer might ask you. Write answers for each question.
4. Prepare a resume that lists the information you will need during an interview.
5. How is certification obtained in your state? Is certification mandatory? Gather the same information about another state that is the closest to your home state.
6. List two reasons for employee evaluation. How can you use the results of evaluation and supervision by your employer?
7. List six rights of employers and six rights of employees.
8. Your coworker complains about attending the agency's continuing education programs. How would you respond?
9. Give two reasons for leaving a job, and explain how you would do this.

Glossary

Abuse Mistreating or causing harm.

Acute illness Illness with a rapid onset and severe symptoms and of short length.

Advance directive Document that indicates a client's wishes about health care.

Aerobic Able to live in the presence of oxygen.

AIDS Abbreviation for *acquired immunodeficiency syndrome*, an infectious disease caused by a virus and spread through contact with blood, body fluids, and/or unprotected sexual intercourse.

Ambulate To move the body with or without assistance; to walk.

Anaerobic Able to live without air or oxygen.

Analysis Determining the substances present in a specimen.

AND Abbreviation for "allow natural death."

Anorexia Loss of appetite.

Antiembolism stockings Elastic stockings worn to prevent the formation of blood clots in the legs.

Anxiety A state of intense worry and/or fear.

Aphasia Absence of speech.

Areola Colored, circular area surrounding the nipple.

Aspiration Breathing in or inhaling a substance into the bronchial tubes and lungs.

Assess To determine the client's needs for home care services.

Assistive devices Equipment or other items to help clients perform activities of daily living more easily.

Atrophy Decrease in size or a wasting away of tissue.

Baby boomers Those born between 1946 and 1964.

Bacteria Microorganisms that cause disease.

Basic need Requirement for survival.

Bed cradle A device to keep the top bedding from resting on the client's legs and feet.

Behavior Actions and interactions with clients.

Bereaved Those who mourn the death of a loved one.

Bias(es) To like or dislike someone or something without a good reason; prejudice.

Biohazard A biologic agent, such as harmful bacteria or viruses, or condition, such as chemical fumes, that threatens human life or health; potential danger, risk, or harm from exposure to such organisms or agents.

Blood pressure Pressure of blood in the large arteries.

Bloodborne pathogens Pathogenic microorganisms that are present in human blood and can cause disease in humans.

Body mechanics Proper use of muscles to move and lift objects and to maintain correct posture.

Body structure(s) Construction and arrangement of cells, tissues, organs, and organ systems.

Bond Emotional attachment between infant and parents, especially the mother.

Bony prominence Part of the bone that is near the skin's surface.

Calculi Stones formed in the body due to the accumulation of mineral salt.

Carbon dioxide Gas that is eliminated from the lungs during exhalation.

Care record Permanent written record of a client's progress during illness and rehabilitation; also contains information about client care.

Carrier A person or animal that spreads disease to others but does not become ill.

Catheters Hollow, flexible tubes made of soft plastic or rubber that can be inserted into the body to withdraw or to insert fluids.

Certification Recognition by a government or nongovernment agency that a person has met certain requirements.

Cesarean birth Surgical procedure in which the baby is delivered through an incision in the abdomen.

Chart To record in writing information on the client's record.

Chronic illness Disease with little change and slow progress and of long duration; not an acute illness.

Client Person receiving care at home.

Clinical experience Practicing the skills learned in the classroom in a client care setting.

Combustible Capable of catching on fire and burning.

Communication Sharing of thoughts, information, and opinions with others.

Compress (compresses) Gauze, washcloths, or small towels applied to a body area; may be moistened with hot or cold solution.

Confidential Private information that is not to be discussed.

Confidentiality Something written or spoken in confidence; in secret (in private).

Congenital Present at birth.

Constrict To narrow.

Contaminated Dirty and/or exposed to harmful organisms, making the object unsafe for use as intended.

Contamination Introduction of harmful organisms.

Contract To become smaller and tighter.

Contracture Shortening of a muscle whereby a joint becomes permanently immovable.

Crisis A critical time.

Defense mechanisms Unconscious reactions that protect a person from real or perceived threats.

Deficiency A lack of one or more essential nutrients in the diet.

Dehydrated/Dehydration Excessive water loss from body tissues resulting from insufficient fluid intake.

Denial A refusal to admit the truth.

Depression/Depressed A prolonged feeling of intense sadness.

Diabetes Disease resulting from lack of insulin secreted by special cells of the pancreas; causes blood sugar level to be elevated.

Diagnose(d) To determine the type and cause of an illness or a condition based on a variety of information.

Diastole Relaxation of the heart muscle that causes its chambers to fill with blood.

Diastolic (blood) pressure Force of blood pushing against walls of the large arteries when the heart is relaxing.

Digestion Complete physical and chemical breakdown of food.

Dilate Expand or open wider.

Disability Physical, mental, or emotional condition that interferes with abilities to carry out activities of daily living.

Discipline System of rules that governs the way we act.

Disinfect To destroy germs.

Disinfectant Chemical that can be applied to objects to destroy germs.

Disoriented Unable to give correct information about time, place, or identity of persons or objects, or to perform activities correctly.

Diuretic(s) Drug or other substance that causes an increase in the production and excretion of urine.

DNR Abbreviation for "do not resuscitate," meaning do not artificially restart the heartbeat.

Document To describe in writing observations or action taken; also called *recording* or *charting*.

DRG (diagnosis-related group) Listing of diagnoses used to establish reimbursement by Medicare and Medicaid for hospitalization and medical care.

Durable power of attorney Advance directive that names another to make health care decisions if a person becomes unable to do so.

Dysuria Difficult or painful urination.

Ecologically Relating to the environment.

Edema Abnormal amount of fluid in the tissues (swelling).

Elimination Process of removing waste products from the body.

Embolus Blood clot that travels through the circulatory system until it lodges in a distant blood vessel.

Embryo Stage of human development during the first 2 months of pregnancy.

Emergency (emergencies) A serious situation that comes on suddenly and threatens life or well-being.

Emesis basin A kidney-shaped basin that fits against the neck to collect vomitus.

Empathy Understanding the feelings of another.

Employment agencies Private or government agencies that match job seekers and potential employers.

Endocrine Glands that secrete hormones directly into the bloodstream.

End-stage disease Terminal or final illness.

Entry-level Beginning, just starting.

Ethics Code of behavior or conduct.

Ethnic A group of people with the same origins or common traits.

Evaluation Process of judging employee performance to determine suitability to remain in the job.

Exacerbation(s) Return of symptoms of illness or disease following a remission.

Exocrine Glands that secrete substances into a duct.

Expire Die.

Exposure incident A specific eye, mouth, other mucous membrane, nonintact skin, or parenteral contact with blood or other potentially infectious material that results from the performance of an employee's duties.

Fatigue Loss of strength and endurance.

Feces Formed body waste that is discharged from the bowels.

Fetus Stage of human development from the third month of pregnancy to birth.

Fever Abnormal elevation of body temperature.

First aid Immediate care given before treatment by trained medical personnel.

Flammable Burns easily.

Flatus Air or gas in the intestine that is released through the anus.

Fontanel(s) Space covered by tough membranes between bones of the infant's skull (soft spot[s]).

Footboard A positioning device used to keep the client's feet in an upright position.

Footdrop Inability to keep the foot in a normal walking position.

Fracture Broken bone.

Full term Completion of 37 to 40 weeks of pregnancy.

Function(s) Action(s) performed by any structure.

Genetic Inherited through the genes from mother and father.

Genitalia (genitals) Organs of reproduction, usually external organs.

Gerontologists Specialists in the study of aging.

Gestation Period of time between conception and birth.

Grief Physical and emotional responses associated with extreme sorrow or loss.

Grievance A wrong, considered as grounds for a formal complaint.

Habit A repeated pattern of involuntary behavior or thought.

Health State of physical, mental, and social well-being.

Hemianopsia Blindness or defective vision in one half of the field of vision.

Hemiplegia Paralysis of one side of the body.

Hemorrhoids Enlarged veins in the rectum or anus.

Hepatitis B, hepatitis C Infectious diseases of the liver caused by a virus and spread through contact with blood, body fluids, and/or unprotected sexual intercourse.

HIV Abbreviation for *human immunodeficiency virus*; the virus that causes AIDS.

Hormones Chemicals produced by endocrine glands.

Hospice Program of care that assists the dying client to maintain a satisfactory lifestyle during the end stage of an illness.

Hospital discharge planner Person who arranges for the care of a patient on release from the hospital; may be a professional nurse or social worker.

Humidifier Equipment used to increase the amount of moisture in an oxygen delivery system.

Hypertension High blood pressure.

Hypotension Low blood pressure.

Illness State of being sick.

Impaction The presence of a large, hard mass of feces in the rectum or colon.

Impulse(s) Sudden, uncontrollable urge(s).

Incentive spirometer Instrument that is used to encourage the client to breathe deeply and correctly.

Incident Unexpected event.

Incontinent The inability to control urination or bowel elimination.

Infection Occurs when harmful organisms enter the body and grow, causing illness or disease.

Informal caregivers Unpaid persons, usually family members, who care for clients on a voluntary basis.

Intravenous (IV) infusions Administration of nutrients or medications through a vein or veins.

Invasive Entering the body.

Job application form Form to be filled out when applying for a job.

Job placement counselors Persons in public or private agencies who provide services to those seeking employment.

Lancets Short pointed blades used to obtain blood from capillaries.

Lifting or turning sheet Folded sheet placed under the client from shoulders to thighs.

Living will Advance directive that specifies treatment to be given or withheld if a person becomes terminally ill or incapable of making decisions himself or herself.

Lochia Discharge from the vagina after childbirth.

Lubricant A fluid, an ointment, or another substance for reducing friction between parts that rub together and for making a surface slippery; it protects skin and prevents drying.

Malignant Becomes progressively worse and causes death; for example, cancer.

Malnutrition Any disorder of nutrition.

Mandatory Required.

Medicaid State and federal insurance program that pays for hospitalization and health care for low-income persons of all ages.

Medical asepsis Use of techniques and practices to prevent the spread of pathogenic organisms.

Medical crisis Event requiring immediate attention.

Medicare Federal program of hospitalization, prescription drugs, and health care insurance for persons older than 65 years and/or those with permanent disabilities; participation is voluntary.

Medications Substances used in the treatment of disease or illness; drugs.

Menarche First menstrual period.

Menopause Permanent end of menstruation.

Mental illness Brain disorder that affects thoughts, emotions, and behavior.

Metabolism Burning of food to produce heat and energy in the body.

Microorganisms Living plants or animals that can be seen only through a microscope.

Microscope Instrument for viewing objects that cannot be seen with the naked eye.

Mourn Process of grieving caused by great personal loss.

Mourning Reaction to a great personal loss.

Muscle atrophy Wasting of muscle.

Muscle tone Readiness of the muscle to work.

Nasal cannula Two-pronged device that delivers oxygen; short prongs are inserted into client's nostrils.

Neglect Inability or failure to provide needed care.

Networking Informal method of exchanging information about job openings.

Nonpathogenic Usually not capable of causing or producing a disease.

Nonverbal communication Communication without the use of words.

Normal Conforming to a standard or following the rule.

Normal saline solution A solution of table salt and water in the same concentration as in the body.

Nutrition The process by which food is taken in and used by the body.

Observe (observation) Act of watching carefully and attentively.

Output All fluids lost from the body that can be measured.

Oxygen Gas that is essential for life.

Parasites Organisms that live in or on another organism.

Parenteral Piercing mucous membranes or skin through needlesticks, human bites, cuts, and/or scrapes.

Pathogenic Capable of causing or producing a disease.

Peers People who are one's equals.

Perception Ability to recognize sensations through the senses.

Perineal (perineum) Pertaining to the perineum, the area between the legs; in women, the area between the vagina and the anus; in men, the area between the scrotum and the anus.

Peristalsis Rhythmic involuntary movement that occurs in hollow tubes of the body.

Personal protective equipment (PPE) Specialized clothing or equipment worn by an employee for protection against a biohazard.

Personnel policies Set of rules and regulations to be followed by employees, usually pertaining to employer and employee rights and responsibilities.

Physiological Pertaining to the normal functioning of the body.

Pigment Coloring matter in the body.

Pneumonia Inflammation of the lung.

Policy (policies) Set of rules and regulations.

Postmortem After death.

Postpartum period First 6 weeks after the birth of the baby.

Prefix Word part that is attached to the beginning of the word root to modify its meaning.

Prejudice Having or forming a preconceived judgment or opinion without fair reasons.

Pressure ulcer Sore on the skin caused by prolonged pressure on the part; also called *bed sore* or *decubitus ulcer*.

Primary caregiver Person who provides most of the care early in one's life.

Prognosis Educated guess about the probable outcome of an illness.

Prostheses Devices used by disabled people to replace a missing body part.

Psychotherapy Method of treating mental disorders, primarily by "talk therapy."

Pulse Throbbing felt over the arteries with each beat of the heart.

Pursed lips Lips positioned for whistling.

Reference Person who will speak in another's behalf.

Reimbursement To make payment for an expense incurred.

Remission(s) Partial or complete disappearance of symptoms of illness or disease.

Reservoir A place where a pathogen is stored and can live and grow.

Respiration(s) Act or process of breathing.

Respite care Short-term care provided so that main caregivers in the family can have a break from their responsibilities.

Resume Listing of educational and work experience to be used in getting a job.

Rite(s) Formal ritual(s) used in religious or solemn practices.

Role The usual function of a person.

Rooting reflex Normal reaction infants have that makes them begin to suck when their cheeks are stroked.

Scope of practice A term used by licensing agencies that describes what procedures and actions are permitted by law for a home care aide to perform.

Secrete (secretion) Release of a substance that serves a special function in the body.

Sedative(s) Substance, procedure, or measure that has a calming effect.

Self-actualization State of reaching one's full potential and being able to cope with problems.

Self-esteem Thinking and feeling good about yourself.

Semen Fluid containing sperm.

Shearing Pressure against the surface of the skin and skin layers as the client is being moved; one surface rubs against another surface.

Shock Condition in which the circulatory system is not able to transport adequate amounts of blood to all parts of the body.

Sibling Brother or sister.

Sphincters Rings of voluntary and involuntary muscles that surround external and internal body openings.

Sputum Material coughed up from the lungs and spit out through the mouth.

Standard Gauge that is used as a basis for judgment.

Standard (universal) precautions An approach to infection control, designed to prevent the spread of bloodborne and other pathogens.

Stereotype Generalization about a form of behavior in an individual or a group.

Sterile Free of living organisms.

Suffix Word part that is attached to the end of the word root to modify its meaning.

Supervision Process of observing employees doing their jobs.

Surgical incision A cut produced surgically by a sharp instrument creating an opening into an organ or space.

Surrogate One who is appointed to act for another.

Systole Contraction of the heart muscle that causes blood to leave the heart.

Systolic (blood) pressure Force of blood pushing against walls of the large arteries when the heart is contracting.

Temperature Amount of heat produced by the body as it uses food for energy.

Terminal illness Illness that causes the end of life.

Thermometer Instrument for measuring temperature.

Thrombus Blood clot.

Toxic Poisonous.

Traction To put under tension, by means of weights and pulleys, to straighten or immobilize a body part or to relieve pressure on it.

Transfer Moving the client from one place to another.

Transmitted Passed from one person or place to another.

Trauma Injury caused by external force or violence.

Tremors Purposeless, continuous, quick movements of skeletal muscles, especially in the hands.

Unit prices Method of pricing food.

Universal precautions See standard precautions.

Urinate Process of eliminating urine.

Verbal communication Communication using the spoken or written word.

Vital signs Essential signs of life: temperature, pulse, respirations, and blood pressure.

Vomitus Material expelled from the stomach when vomiting.

Word root Word part that is the core of the term; contains the basic meaning of the word.

Wound Physical injury causing a break in the skin during surgery or an accident.

Index

A

Abandonment, 363
Abbreviations, 91–92, 92t, 475t
Abdominal cavity, 56
Abdominal position, 199, 200b
Abdominal thrusts, 464, 464f
Absorbent undergarments, 268
Abuse, 363–364. *See also* specific types of
  of child/children, 391b
  of elderly, 363–364
  signs of, 364
Acceptance, of dying client, 449
Accidents, elderly risk of, 106, 360b
ACE bandages, 341–343, 341b, 343b
Acquired Immune Deficiency Syndrome (AIDS), 88, 169,
    175–176, 435–439
  defining, 435
  facts about, 435
  HIV, effects on immune system, 435–436
  home care aide, role of, 437–439
  myths about, 436b
  realities of, 436b
  symptoms of, 437
  transmission of, 435
A.C.T., 107
Activities of daily living (ADL)
  for AIDS, 437–438
  for Alzheimer's disease, 424, 426
  for arthritis, 432
  for cancer, 415
  for cardiovascular diseases, 412
  for cerebrovascular accident, 417–418
  for chronic obstructive pulmonary disease, 421
  for diabetes mellitus, 423
  for low energy level clients, 412b, 412f
  mental illness affecting, 397
  for multiple sclerosis, 428
  occupational therapists role in, 16
  during old age, 346f–347f
  for Parkinson's disease, 430
  for postoperative client, 441
  suspicion and performing, 405
Acute illness, 14, 95
Acute pain, 78
Adaptive eating utensils, 158f
Adolescence/adolescents, 50–51, 50f
  characteristics of, 50
  dress code for, 395f
  needs of, 50–51
Adrenal glands, 64
Adulthood/adults, 51–52, 51f. *See also* Older adult/adulthood
  characteristics of, 51
  needs of, 51–52
Advance medical directives, 449–450
Aerobic organisms, 167

Age/aging
  adjusting to, 349b
  as bias, 29
  myths about, 348t
  physical signs of, 353–359, 353f
  process of, 345–346
  pulse, factor effecting, 305
  realities about, 348t
Ageism, 349
Agency, 16, 31, 462–463
Aggression, 404–405
Aids for dressing/undressing, 256–257
Airborne transmission, 170
Alcohol/alcoholism, 21–22, 365, 407
Alphabet communication charts, 418f
Alternate exit, 113
Alternating pressure mattress, 222, 222f
Alveoli, 69
Alzheimer's Association, 443
Alzheimer's disease, 88, 346, 424–427
  artificial food magnets for, 425f
  behaviors associated with, 424–425
  defining, 424
  facts about, 424
  home care aide, role of, 425–427
  labels to help, 425f
Ambulation, 211–212, 212t
American Cancer Society, 413, 443
American Heart Association, 443
American Lung Association, 443
American Red Cross, 459
American's Job Bank, 475
Amino acids, 142
Anaerobic organisms, 167
AND (allow natural death), 449
Anger, 100–101, 447–448
Animals, transmission of infection through, 170
Anorexia, 160
Answers, preparing for interview, 482–483
Antiembolism stockings, 341, 341b–342b
Anxiety, 101–102, 402–403
Aphasia, 417
Appetite, loss of. *See* Poor appetite
Arm pain, 417
Arteries, 66
Arthritis, 88, 431–433
  defining, 431
  facts about, 431
  home care aide, role of, 432–433
  symptoms of, 432
Arthroscope, 90
Artificial food magnets, 425f
Aspiration of fluid, 234
Assignment sheet, 83
Assistive devices, 103, 207–211, 209f
  mechanical lift, 209–211
  sliding board, 207–208
  transfer belt, 207
  trapeze, 208–209
Automatic blood pressure monitor, 314, 315b

Page numbers followed by "b" indicate boxes, "f" indicate figures, and "t" indicate tables.